Epigenetics Protocols

METHODS IN MOLECULAR BIOLOGY™

John M. Walker, SERIES EDITOR

300. **Protein Nanotechnology:** *Protocols, Instrumentation, and Applications,* edited by *Tuan Vo-Dinh, 2005*

299. **Amyloid Proteins:** *Methods and Protocols,* edited by *Einar M. Sigurdsson, 2005*

298. **Peptide Synthesis and Application,** edited by *John Howl, 2005*

297. **Forensic DNA Typing Protocols,** edited by *Angel Carracedo, 2005*

296. **Cell Cycle Protocols,** edited by *Tim Humphrey and Gavin Brooks, 2005*

295. **Immunochemical Protocols, Third Edition,** edited by **Robert Burns, 2005**

294. **Cell Migration:** *Developmental Methods and Protocols,* edited by *Jun-Lin Guan, 2005*

293. **Laser Capture Microdissection:** *Methods and Protocols,* edited by *Graeme I. Murray and Stephanie Curran, 2005*

292. **DNA Viruses:** *Methods and Protocols,* edited by *Paul M. Lieberman, 2005*

291. **Molecular Toxicology Protocols,** edited by *Phouthone Keohavong and Stephen G. Grant, 2005*

290. **Basic Cell Culture,** *Third Edition,* edited by *Cheryl D. Helgason and Cindy Miller, 2005*

289. **Epidermal Cells,** *Methods and Applications,* edited by *Kursad Turksen, 2004*

288. **Oligonucleotide Synthesis,** *Methods and Applications,* edited by *Piet Herdewijn, 2004*

287. **Epigenetics Protocols,** edited by *Trygve O. Tollefsbol, 2004*

286. **Transgenic Plants:** *Methods and Protocols,* edited by *Leandro Peña, 2004*

285. **Cell Cycle Control and Dysregulation Protocols:** *Cyclins, Cyclin-Dependent Kinases, and Other Factors,* edited by *Antonio Giordano and Gaetano Romano, 2004*

284. **Signal Transduction Protocols,** *Second Edition,* edited by *Robert C. Dickson and Michael D. Mendenhall, 2004*

283. **Bioconjugation Protocols,** edited by *Christof M. Niemeyer, 2004*

282. **Apoptosis Methods and Protocols,** edited by *Hugh J. M. Brady, 2004*

281. **Checkpoint Controls and Cancer, Volume 2:** *Activation and Regulation Protocols,* edited by *Axel H. Schönthal, 2004*

280. **Checkpoint Controls and Cancer, Volume 1:** *Reviews and Model Systems,* edited by *Axel H. Schönthal, 2004*

279. **Nitric Oxide Protocols,** *Second Edition,* edited by *Aviv Hassid, 2004*

278. **Protein NMR Techniques,** *Second Edition,* edited by *A. Kristina Downing, 2004*

277. **Trinucleotide Repeat Protocols,** edited by *Yoshinori Kohwi, 2004*

276. **Capillary Electrophoresis of Proteins and Peptides,** edited by *Mark A. Strege and Avinash L. Lagu, 2004*

275. **Chemoinformatics,** edited by *Jürgen Bajorath, 2004*

274. **Photosynthesis Research Protocols,** edited by *Robert Carpentier, 2004*

273. **Platelets and Megakaryocytes, Volume 2:** *Perspectives and Techniques,* edited by *Jonathan M. Gibbins and Martyn P. Mahaut-Smith, 2004*

272. **Platelets and Megakaryocytes, Volume 1:** *Functional Assays,* edited by *Jonathan M. Gibbins and Martyn P. Mahaut-Smith, 2004*

271. **B Cell Protocols,** edited by *Hua Gu and Klaus Rajewsky, 2004*

270. **Parasite Genomics Protocols,** edited by *Sara E. Melville, 2004*

269. **Vaccina Virus and Poxvirology:** *Methods and Protocols,* edited by *Stuart N. Isaacs, 2004*

268. **Public Health Microbiology:** *Methods and Protocols,* edited by *John F. T. Spencer and Alicia L. Ragout de Spencer, 2004*

267. **Recombinant Gene Expression:** *Reviews and Protocols, Second Edition,* edited by *Paulina Balbas and Argelia Johnson, 2004*

266. **Genomics, Proteomics, and Clinical Bacteriology:** *Methods and Reviews,* edited by *Neil Woodford and Alan Johnson, 2004*

265. **RNA Interference, Editing, and Modification:** *Methods and Protocols,* edited by *Jonatha M. Gott, 2004*

264. **Protein Arrays:** *Methods and Protocols,* edited by *Eric Fung, 2004*

263. **Flow Cytometry,** *Second Edition,* edited by *Teresa S. Hawley and Robert G. Hawley, 2004*

262. **Genetic Recombination Protocols,** edited by *Alan S. Waldman, 2004*

261. **Protein–Protein Interactions:** *Methods and Applications,* edited by *Haian Fu, 2004*

260. **Mobile Genetic Elements:** *Protocols and Genomic Applications,* edited by *Wolfgang J. Miller and Pierre Capy, 2004*

259. **Receptor Signal Transduction Protocols,** *Second Edition,* edited by *Gary B. Willars and R. A. John Challiss, 2004*

258. **Gene Expression Profiling:** *Methods and Protocols,* edited by *Richard A. Shimkets, 2004*

257. **mRNA Processing and Metabolism:** *Methods and Protocols,* edited by *Daniel R. Schoenberg, 2004*

256. **Bacterial Artifical Chromosomes, Volume 2:** *Functional Studies,* edited by *Shaying Zhao and Marvin Stodolsky, 2004*

Books are to be returned on or before

METHODS IN MOLECULAR BIOLOGY™

Epigenetics Protocols

Edited by

Trygve O. Tollefsbol

Department of Biology
University of Alabama
Birmingham, AL

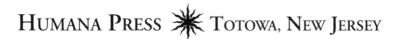

HUMANA PRESS ✳ TOTOWA, NEW JERSEY

© 2004 Humana Press Inc.
999 Riverview Drive, Suite 208
Totowa, New Jersey 07512

www.humanapress.com

All papers, comments, opinions, conclusions, or recommendations are those of the author(s), and do not necessarily reflect the views of the publisher.

This publication is printed on acid-free paper. ∞
ANSI Z39.48-1984 (American Standards Institute)

Permanence of Paper for Printed Library Materials.

Cover design by Patricia F. Cleary.

Cover illustrations: Disrupting Hsp90 function induces heritable epialleles that cause homeotic transformation in a sensitized *Drosophila melanogaster* strain (foreground; Chapter 12, Fig. 1; *see* complete legend and discussion on p. 154). (Background) An area negative for p16 hypermethylated DNA (Chapter 20, Fig. 1B; *see* complete legend on p. 265 and discussion on p. 264).

For additional copies, pricing for bulk purchases, and/or information about other Humana titles, contact Humana at the above address or at any of the following numbers: Tel.: 973-256-1699; Fax: 973-256-8341; E-mail: humana@humanapr.com; or visit our Website: www.humanapress.com

Photocopy Authorization Policy:

Printed in the United States of America. 10 9 8 7 6 5 4 3 2 1

eISBN 1-59259-828-5
ISSN 1064-3745

Library of Congress Cataloging-in-Publication Data

Epigenetics protocols / edited by Trygve O. Tollefsbol.
    p. ; cm. -- (Methods in molecular biology ; 287)
   Includes bibliographical references and index.
   ISBN 1-58829-336-X (alk. paper)
   1. Chromatin--Laboratory manuals. 2. Telomere--Laboratory manuals. 3. ADP-ribosylation--Laboratory manuals. 4. Epigenesis--Laboratory manuals. [DNLM: 1. Chromatin Assembly and Disassembly--genetics-Laboratory Manuals. 2. Chromosome Structures--metabolism--Laboratory Manuals. 3. DNA Methylation--Laboratory Manuals. 4. Epigenesis, Genetic--Laboratory Manuals. 5. Histone Code--genetics--Laboratory Manuals. 6. Histones--metabolism--Laboratory Manuals. QU 25 E64 2004] I. Tollefsbol, Trygve O. II. Series: Methods in molecular biology (Clifton, N.J.) ; v. 287.
QH599.E65 2004
572.8'7--dc22

                  2004002870

Preface

The field of epigenetics has grown exponentially in the past decade, and a steady flow of exciting discoveries in this area has served to move it to the forefront of molecular biology. Although epigenetics may previously have been considered a peripheral science, recent advances have shown considerable progress in unraveling the many mysteries of nontraditional genetic processes. Given the fast pace of epigenetic discoveries and the groundbreaking nature of these developments, a thorough treatment of the methods in the area seems timely and appropriate and is the goal of *Epigenetics Protocols*.

The scope of epigenetics is vast, and an exhaustive analysis of all of the techniques employed by investigators would be unrealistic. However, this volume of *Methods in Molecular Biology*™ covers three main areas that should be of greatest interest to epigenetics investigators: (1) techniques related to analysis of chromatin remodeling, such as histone acetylation and methylation; (2) methods in newly developed and especially promising areas of epigenetics such as telomere position effects, quantitative epigenetics, and ADP ribosylation; and (3) an updated analysis of techniques involving DNA methylation and its role in the modification, as well as the maintenance, of chromatin structure.

The protocols presented in *Epigenetics Protocols* are intended to provide investigators with a contemporary set of tools that can be applied to research in the field. These tools include recent breakthroughs in epigenetic analysis such as techniques for determining changes in native chromatin, methods of microarray analysis as applied to epigenetics, and methylation-sensitive single-strand conformation techniques. These methods, as well as many others provided in *Epigenetics Protocols,* have strong potential for further facilitating developments in this promising and rapidly developing field.

Trygve O. Tollefsbol

Contents

Preface v

Contributors ix

1 Methods of Epigenetic Analysis
   Trygve O. Tollefsbol 1

2 Chromatin Immunoprecipitation Assays
   Yan Yan, Haobin Chen, and Max Costa 9

3 Native Chromatin Immunoprecipitation
   Alan W. Thorne, Fiona A. Myers, and Tim R. Hebbes 21

4 Q-PCR in Combination With ChIP Assays to Detect Changes
   in Chromatin Acetylation
   Ryan A. Irvine and Chih-Lin Hsieh 45

5 Restriction Endonuclease Accessibility as a Determinant
   of Altered Chromatin Structure
   William M. Hempel and Pierre Ferrier 53

6 Measuring Changes in Chromatin Using Micrococcal Nuclease
   Nicolas Steward and Hiroshi Sano 65

7 DNaseI Hypersensitivity Analysis of Chromatin Structure
   Qianjin Lu and Bruce Richardson 77

8 Inhibition of Histone Deacetylases
   Cheng Liu and Dawei Xu 87

9 Site-Specific Analysis of Histone Methylation and Acetylation
   David Umlauf, Yuji Goto, and Robert Feil 99

10 Analysis of Mammalian Telomere Position Effect
   Joseph A. Baur, Woodring E. Wright, and Jerry W. Shay 121

11 Activity Assays for Poly-ADP Ribose Polymerase 1
   **Eva Kirsten, Ernest Kun, Jerome Mendeleyev,
   and Charles P. Ordahl** 137

12 Multigenerational Selection and Detection of Altered Histone
   Acetylation and Methylation Patterns:
   Toward a Quantitative Epigenetics in Drosophila
   **Mark D. Garfinkel, Vincent E. Sollars, Xiangyi Lu,
   and Douglas M. Ruden** 151

13 Profiling DNA Methylation by Bisulfite Genomic Sequencing:
     Problems and Solutions
     Liang Liu, Rebecca C. Wylie, Nathaniel J. Hansen,
     Lucy G. Andrews, and Trygve O. Tollefsbol 169

14 Methylation-Sensitive Single-Strand Conformation Analysis:
     A Rapid Method to Screen for
     and Analyze DNA Methylation
     Jean Benhattar and Geneviève Clément 181

15 SIRPH Analysis: *SNuPE With IP-RP-HPLC*
     for Quantitative Measurements of DNA Methylation
     at Specific CpG Sites
     Osman El-Maarri 195

16 Real-Time PCR-Based Assay for Quantitative Determination
     of Methylation Status
     Ulrich Lehmann and Hans Kreipe 207

17 Denaturing Gradient Gel Electrophoresis
     to Detect Methylation Changes in DNA
     Masahiko Shiraishi 219

18 Photocrosslinking Oligonucleotide Hybridization Assay for
     Concurrent Gene Dosage and CpG Methylation Analysis
     Risa Peoples, Michael Wood, and Reuel Van Atta 233

19 Methylation-Specific Oligonucleotide Microarray
     Pearlly S. Yan, Susan H. Wei, and Tim Hui-Ming Huang 251

20 Methylation-Specific PCR *In Situ* Hybridization
     Gerard J. Nuovo 261

21 Relative Quantitation of DNA Methyltransferase mRNA
     by Real-Time RT-PCR Assay
     John Attwood and Bruce Richardson 273

22 DMB (DNMT-Magnetic Beads) Assay: *Measuring DNA*
     Methyltransferase Activity In Vitro
     Tomoki Yokochi and Keith D. Robertson 285

Index 297

Contributors

LUCY G. ANDREWS • *Department of Biology, University of Alabama at Birmingham, Birmingham, AL*

JOHN ATTWOOD • *Cancer Center and Geriatrics Center, University of Michigan, Ann Arbor, MI*

JOSEPH A. BAUR • *Department of Cell Biology, The University of Texas Southwestern Medical Center, Dallas, TX*

JEAN BENHATTAR • *Institute of Pathology, Centre Hospitalier Universitaire Vaudois, Lausanne, Switzerland*

HAOBIN CHEN • *Department of Environmental Medicine, New York University School of Medicine, Tuxedo, NY*

GENEVIÈVE CLÉMENT • *Institute of Pathology, Centre Hospitalier Universitaire Vaudois, Lausanne, Switzerland*

MAX COSTA • *Department of Environmental Medicine, New York University School of Medicine, Tuxedo, NY*

OSMAN EL-MAARRI • *Institute of Experimental Haematology and Transfusion Medicine, Bonn, Germany*

ROBERT FEIL • *Institute for Molecular Genetics, CNRS UMR-5535 and University of Montpellier II, Montpellier, France*

PIERRE FERRIER • *Centre de Immunologie, INSERM-CNRS-Université de la Méditerranée, Marseille Cedex, France*

MARK D. GARFINKEL • *Department of Environmental Health Sciences, University of Alabama, Birmingham, AL*

YUJI GOTO • *Institute for Molecular Genetics, CNRS UMR-5535, and University of Montpellier II, Montpellier, France*

NATHANIEL J. HANSEN • *Department of Biology, University of Alabama at Birmingham, Birmingham, AL*

TIM R. HEBBES • *Institute of Biomedical and Biomolecular Sciences, School of Biological Sciences, University of Portsmouth, Portsmouth, UK*

WILLIAM M. HEMPEL • *Department of Research Technologies, Pfizer Global Research and Development, Fresnes Cedex, France*

CHIH-LIN HSIEH • *Department of Urology and Department of Biochemistry and Molecular Biology, University of Southern California, Los Angeles, CA*

TIM HUI-MING HUANG • *Division of Human Cancer Genetics, Department of Molecular Virology, Immunology and Molecular Genetics, The Ohio State University, Columbus, OH*

RYAN A. IRVINE • *Department of Urology and Department of Biochemistry and Molecular Biology, University of Southern California, Los Angeles, CA*

ix

EVA KIRSTEN • *Department of Anatomy, Cardiovascular Research Institute, School of Medicine, University of California, San Francisco, CA*

HANS KREIPE • *Institute of Pathology, Medizinische Hochschule Hannover, Hannover, Germany*

ERNEST KUN • *Department of Cellular and Molecular Pharmacology, Cardiovascular Research Institute, School of Medicine, University of California, San Francisco, CA*

ULRICH LEHMANN • *Institute of Pathology, Medizinische Hochschule Hannover, Hannover, Germany*

CHENG LIU • *Department of Medicine, Division of Hematology, Karolinska Hospital, Stockholm, Sweden*

LIANG LIU • *Department of Biology, University of Alabama at Birmingham, Birmingham, AL*

QIANJIN LU • *Cancer Center and Geriatrics Center, University of Michigan, Ann Arbor, MI*

XIANGYI LU • *Department of Environmental Health Sciences, University of Alabama, Birmingham, AL*

JEROME MENDELEYEV • *Department of Anatomy, Cardiovascular Research Institute, School of Medicine, University of California, San Francisco, CA*

FIONA A. MYERS • *Institute of Biomedical and Biomolecular Sciences, School of Biological Sciences, University of Portsmouth, Portsmouth, UK*

GERARD J. NUOVO • *Department of Pathology, Ohio State University Medical Center, Columbus, OH*

CHARLES P. ORDAHL • *Department of Anatomy, Cardiovascular Research Institute, School of Medicine, University of California, San Francisco, CA*

RISA PEOPLES • *Naxcor, Mountain View, CA*

BRUCE RICHARDSON • *Cancer Center and Geriatrics Center, University of Michigan, Ann Arbor, MI*

KEITH D. ROBERTSON • *Epigenetic Gene Regulation and Cancer Section, National Cancer Institute, National Institutes of Health, Bethesda, MD*

DOUGLAS M. RUDEN • *Department of Environmental Health Sciences, University of Alabama, Birmingham, AL*

HIROSHI SANO • *Research and Education Center for Genetic Information, Nara Institute of Science and Technology, Nara, Japan*

JERRY W. SHAY • *Department of Cell Biology, The University of Texas Southwestern Medical Center, Dallas, TX*

MASAHIKO SHIRAISHI • *DNA Methylation and Genome Function Project, National Cancer Center Research Institute, Tokyo, Japan*

VINCENT E. SOLLARS • *Kimmel Cancer Institute, Thomas Jefferson University, Philadelphia, PA*

NICOLAS STEWARD • *Institut Jacques Monod, Paris Cedex, France*

ALAN W. THORNE • *Institute of Biomedical and Biomolecular Sciences, School of Biological Sciences, University of Portsmouth, Portsmouth, UK*

TRYGVE O. TOLLEFSBOL • *Department of Biology, University of Alabama at Birmingham, Birmingham, AL*

DAVID UMLAUF • *Institute for Molecular Genetics CNRS UMR-5535 and University of Montpellier II, Montpellier, France*

REUEL VAN ATTA • *Naxcor, Mountain View, CA*

SUSAN H. WEI • *Division of Human Cancer Genetics, Department of Molecular Virology, Immunology and Molecular Genetics, The Ohio State University, Columbus, OH*

WOODRING E. WRIGHT • *Department of Cell Biology, The University of Texas Southwestern Medical Center, Dallas, TX*

MICHAEL WOOD • *Naxcor, Mountain View, CA*

REBECCA C. WYLIE • *Department of Biology, University of Alabama at Birmingham, Birmingham, AL*

DAWEI XU • *Department of Medicine, Division of Hematology, Karolinska Hospital, Stockholm, Sweden*

PEARLLY S. YAN • *Division of Human Cancer Genetics, Department of Molecular Virology, Immunology and Molecular Genetics, The Ohio State University, Columbus, OH*

YAN YAN • *Department of Environmental Medicine, New York University School of Medicine, Tuxedo, NY*

TOMOKI YOKOCHI • *Epigenetic Gene Regulation and Cancer Section, National Cancer Institute, National Institutes of Health, Bethesda, MD*

1

Methods of Epigenetic Analysis

Trygve O. Tollefsbol

Summary

Epigenetics encompasses heritable changes in DNA or its associated proteins except mutations in gene sequence. Many investigators in the field of epigenetics focus on histone modifications and DNA methylation, two molecular mechanisms that are often linked and interdependent. A variety of methods are applied to the study of epigenetic processes, and the past decade has witnessed an exponential increase in novel approaches to elucidate the molecular mysteries of epigenetic inheritance. This chapter summarizes some of the most contemporary methods used to study epigenetics presented throughout the book.

Key Words: Epigenetics; DNA methylation; chromatin; methods; histone; technique.

1. Introduction

Epigenetic processes are stable changes in DNA and its chromatin environment that are important in processes as diverse as gene expression, X-chromosome inactivation, and telomere position effects. These heritable changes do not involve mutations, but rather modifications of DNA or its associated proteins such as the histones. Major epigenetic mechanisms include (but are not limited to) DNA or histone methylation and histone acetylation. Interest in these processes has increased exponentially over the past decade as the potential for novel therapeutic approaches involving the targeting of histone modifications and DNA methylation has emerged. For example, enzymes such as the histone acetyltransferases (HATs) and deacetylases (HDACs) as well as the DNA methyltransferases (DNMTs), which mediate many of the epigenetic processes, have been the recent focus of novel drug-development strategies and potential targets of anticancer agents (1,2). A greater understanding of epigenetics and the therapeutic potential of intervention into these processes can best be achieved through improved methods for analysis of epigenetic modifications.

From: *Methods in Molecular Biology, vol. 287: Epigenetics Protocols*
Edited by: T. O. Tollefsbol © Humana Press Inc., Totowa, NJ

Studies of chromatin remodeling have been greatly improved in the last decade with the development of modifications of the chromatin immunoprecipitation (ChIP) assay. For instance, it is now possible to analyze native chromatin using the native ChIP (nChIP) technique and to monitor quantitative changes in processes such as histone acetylation. Other modes of chromatin analysis such as those using restriction endonuclease accessibility, micrococcal nuclease analysis of chromatin changes, and DNaseI hypersensitivity analysis have continued to yield important information about the epigenome. Methods for inhibiting the HDACs and analysis of site-specific histone methylation are also showing great promise in identifying the specific genes affected by epigenetic modifications and the exact sites of histone modification.

In addition to histone modification, DNA methylation has been a major factor in epigenetic processes, and methods of analysis of DNA methylation, and the DNMTs have been greatly improved in the past decade. There are now many different approaches to analysis of the exact methylation content of DNA, often involving bisulfite, which converts cytosine to uracil in single-stranded DNA but has negligible effects on 5-methylcytosine, the major product of DNA methylation in eukaryotic systems. Additional techniques include denaturing gradient gel electrophoresis and photo-crosslinking oligonucleotide hybridization assays for methylation analysis. The field of epigenetics, like most areas of molecular biology, will probably see a surge in microarray analysis and proteomics, techniques that hold great promise for elucidating the nature of the epigenome. These techniques, as well as advances in analysis of the DNMTs, are revealing the mechanisms for the establishment and modification of epigenetic processes and also for their stable inheritance from cell to cell and organism to organism.

2. Chromatin and Epigenetics

Chromatin structure regulates gene expression largely through posttranslational modifications of histones that include but are not limited to acetylation, methylation, and ADP ribosylation. These modifications are site-specific and occur during development, differentiation, tumorigenesis, and aging as well as in many other biological processes. These posttranslational modifications of histones impart a unique identity to the nucleosome that regulates the binding and activities of other proteins that interact with DNA and the histones. Methods designed to identify these specific modifications and their role in modulating the many interactions involved with chromatin remodeling hold considerable promise in revealing the fundamental molecular mechanisms by which epigenetic modifications regulate gene expression.

The amino-terminal region of histones is a hot spot for posttranslational modifications that affect the interactions of histones with DNA, each other, and chromatin remodeling proteins. The most studied of the posttranslational modifications of histones are acetylation and methylation of lysine residues in the amino-terminal tails of histones H3 and H4 *(3)*. In general, increased acetylation of the histones in gene control regions correlates with transcriptional activity, and methylation of histones is primarily found in transcriptionally silenced heterochromatin regions, although methylation of lysine 4 (K4) of histone H3 is often found in active chromatin regions. In contrast, methylation of H3-K9 usually leads to transcriptional repression and can inhibit acetylation of the H3 tail at several lysines, whereas H3-K4 methylation promotes acetylation of H3 *(4)*.

Local changes in chromatin are involved in the regulation of a large number of eukaryotic genes. The HATs and HDACs play major roles not only in allowing reversible changes in histones but also in maintaining chromatin configurations that allow stable inheritance of epigenetic traits. These enzymes affect the binding of many DNA sequence-specific transcription factors and, conversely, can be recruited to specific gene regions by transcription factors. Changes in chromatin are not confined to local regions of DNA but also affect domains of DNA (such as heterochromatin) and global regions of DNA (as seen in X-chromosome inactivation).

3. DNA Methylation and Epigenetics

The most thoroughly studied epigenetic modification is DNA methylation, which involves the addition of a methyl moiety to the cytosine-5 position in most eukaryotic organisms. This epigenetic process influences, most notably, gene expression, in that hypermethylation of promoter regions is associated with transcriptional repression and hypomethylation of control regions is generally associated with gene activity. However, the end results of DNA methylation go well beyond control of gene expression and extend to genomic imprinting, X-chromosome inactivation, and chromatin structure modifications. DNA methylation also appears to have a major role in complex and important biological processes such as cellular differentiation, embryonic development, tumorigenesis, and aging *(5)*.

DNA methylation is carried out by the DNMTs, and at least three functional DNMTs have been identified in eukaryotic systems. DNMT1 is the enzyme primarily involved in the maintenance of methylation patterns with each cell replication, and it preferentially methylates hemimethylated DNA *(6)*. Other known functional methyltransferases are DNMT3a and DNMT3b, which have significantly higher *de novo* methylation activity than DNMT1 and contribute to *de novo* methylation during embryogenesis *(7)*. DNMT2 is a methyltransferase that does not appear to have significant methylating activity and DNMT3L is likely to be specifically involved in germline development *(6)*.

4. Interactions Between Histone Modifications and DNA Methylation

The processes of histone modification and DNA methylation often involve dynamic interactions that can either reinforce or inhibit epigenetic changes. For example, methylation at H3-K9 can promote DNA methylation, and cytosine methylation stimulates both histone deacetylation of H3-K9 and methylation of H3-K9 *(8)*. The N-terminal domain of DNMT1 binds to the HDACs and can suppress gene transcription through facilitation of histone deacetylase activity *(9)*. DNMT3a and DNMT3b can also recruit the HDACs to silence genes *(10)*. In addition, there are links between the DNMTs and histone methylation since DNMT3a has recently been shown to localize with heterochromatin protein (HP)1, which binds to methylated histones *(11)*. Thus, the processes of histone modifications and DNA methylation are interdependent, and both contribute to the overall state of chromatin and its epigenetic control of gene expression.

5. Contents of This Book

5.1. Methods of Assessing Chromatin Remodeling

A major advance in assessing chromatin remodeling occurred with development of the ChIP assay. This technique provides a powerful in vivo tool for monitoring and evaluating DNA–protein interactions and allows determination of the chromatin architecture of specific DNA sequences. Chapter 2 details the protocols necessary for conducting conventional ChIP assays (crosslinked or xChIP) using various crosslinking agents such as formaldehyde. Through this method, the binding of proteins, such as most nonhistone proteins that interact with DNA at low affinity, can be analyzed. These assays have also recently been combined with DNA microarray techniques to assess global DNA protein interactions *(12)*. By contrast, nChIP (*see* Chapter 3) does not use formaldehyde crosslinking and is best suited for analysis of core histone modifications such as acetylation and methylation. Less strongly associated proteins are best assessed using xChIP. The nChIP method, when applicable, allows proteins to be recovered without charge modification. A new aspect of the ChIP assay is the application of quantitative polymerase chain reaction (Q-PCR), which, when used in combination with the ChIP assay (*see* Chapter 4), allows the amount of protein binding to a specific DNA region to be determined rapidly and accurately. Although there are additional ChIP assay procedures and modifications, those described in Chapters 2–4 should provide a basic set of tools for assessing the chromatin state of DNA and its interactions with various proteins.

5.2. Characterizing Chromatin Changes

Besides methods based on the ChIP assay, there are many other techniques to analyze and characterize chromatin changes during epigenetic processes.

For example, restriction endonuclease cleavage of chromosomal DNA (*see* Chapter 5) provides a method to assess general protein accessibility of a genomic region of interest and use of micrococcal nuclease (*see* Chapter 6) provides a simple means to identify the nucleosome positioning of any gene. The changes in chromatin structure associated with transcriptional activation can be readily detected with DNaseI hypersensitivity assays (*see* Chapter 7). Mapping of DNaseI hypersensitive sites has many useful applications; for example, it has been used to demonstrate chromatin changes associated with the transcription of specific genes during important biological processes such as cellular differentiation. Another means to assess chromatin structure and its role in epigenetic gene control is to intervene directly in the remodeling process and to monitor resulting changes in gene activity. A popular approach has been to inhibit the HDACs (*see* Chapter 8), leading to acetylation of the gene promoter and changes in gene activity if the gene is regulated by histone acetylation/deacetylation. This technique often employs trichostatin A (TSA), a hydoxamic acid that inhibits the HDACs at low concentrations. TSA is highly specific and can be used in vitro or in vivo. Ultimately, analysis of specific changes in histone methylation and acetylation is the goal of many investigations involving chromatin remodeling and epigenetic processes, and Chapter 9 provides protocols for site-specific analysis of these modifications.

5.3. Recently Developed Epigenetic Analyses

The spreading of chromatin changes in biological processes can affect many different genes within a particular region and lead to major changes in chromatin expression. For instance, the telomeric ends of each chromosome are surrounded by heterochromatin, and spreading of heterochromatin to new regions or the translocation of a gene near a telomere could lead to gene silencing. In Chapter 10, methods are described for the positioning of a transgene next to a newly formed telomere and analysis of the effects on the activity of the transgene. This procedure has numerous applications and could be especially important in cellular aging, in which the telomeres progressively shorten with each cell replication in the absence of telomerase, the enzyme that maintains telomeres in eukaryotic cells. Another recent advance in epigenetics has been the elucidation of the role of ADP ribosylation as a modifier of histones. *Hetero-* or *transmodification* is carried out by the enzyme poly(ADP-ribose) polymerase 1 (PARP-1). This enzyme adds poly(ADP-ribose) chains ($ADPR_n$) to proteins such as histone H1, octameric histones, and a variety of other nonhistone proteins including transcription factors. Analysis of ADP ribosylation has considerable potential in facilitating understanding of the role of this process in epigenetic control of gene expression and its changes during tumorigenesis, aging, and cellular differentiation. Yet another relatively new area in epigenetics is quantitative epigenetics (QE) (*see* Chapter 12). This procedure combines techniques for assessment of global quantitative trait loci (QTL) mapping analyses with epigenetic analysis, allowing determination of the positioning of epi-alleles of individual genes or chromosomal regions.

Although the fields of telomere position effects, ADP ribosylation, and quantitative epigenetics are relatively new to epigenetics, the techniques for analysis of these phenomena (*see* Chapters 10–12) appear to have considerable potential in further defining the mechanisms that affect epigenetic inheritance.

5.4. Determining Changes in DNA Methylation

There are many different ways to assess DNA methylation. Before the advent of DNA methylation sequencing methods, isoschizomers with different methylation sensitivities such as *Hpa*II and *Msp*I were frequently used to determine the methylation of DNA. The problem with methods such as this, however, is that less than about 5% of the methylated cytosines can be assessed in any given DNA sequence. A major breakthrough in DNA methylation analysis occurred in 1992 with the development of bisulfite methylation sequencing, which is described in Chapter 13. The advantages of bisulfite methylation sequencing are that it gives a positive display of methylated cytosines and provides the entire profile of methylation for a defined DNA sequence rather than assessment of just a few cytosines within a sequence. Several other methods have since been developed that are also based on bisulfite treatment of DNA. For example, methylation-sensitive single-strand conformation analysis (MS-SSCA; *see* Chapter 14) utilizes bisulfite treatment of DNA followed by PCR but leads to the methylation-dependent alteration of single-strand conformation. By mixing known ratios of methylated and unmethylated DNA sequences, the percentage of methylation can be directly compared as the ratio of intensity between the methylated and unmethylated bands.

Other techniques are also based on bisulfite treatment of DNA to assess the methylation status of a specific DNA sequence. For example, the single nucleotide primer extension (SNuPE) technique (*see* Chapter 15) involves extension of an oligonucleotide flanking the 5' end of a CpG site using either dideoxycytidine (ddCTP) or dideoxythymidine (ddTTP) for methylated and unmethylated templates, respectively. The reaction is quantitative, and several methylatable sites can potentially be assessed simultaneously. In addition, real-time PCR can be applied to analysis of DNA methylation in combination with bisulfite treatment (*see* Chapter 16) to provide quantitative information. It also allows for high throughput in 96-well plates, real-time analysis, and omission of post-amplification steps, which reduces the risk of contamination and the work load. Moreover, the melting differences between methylated and unmethylated DNA can give information about genomic methylation (*see* Chapter 17). Using denaturing gradient gel electrophoresis (DGGE), bisulfite-treated DNA sequences are determined based on changes in the T_m of the DNA fragments. Another application of this technique is to isolate DNA fragments containing a CpG island based on the reduced rate of strand dissociation of partly melted DNA fragments containing many CpG sites.

A relatively new technique applied to DNA methylation is the photo-crosslinking oligonucleotide hybridization assay (*see* Chapter 18). This technology is well suited for combining the high-throughput capacity of oligonucleotide hybridization with accurate measurement of relative gene dosage and can be applied to quantification of fractional resistance to methylation enzyme digestion. Another high-throughput approach capable of detecting DNA methylation in genes across several CpG sites is the methylation-specific oligonucleotide microarray assay (*see* Chapter 19). This technique uses short oligonucleotides corresponding to the methylated and unmethylated alleles as probes affixed to a solid support and products amplified from bisulfite-treated DNA as targets for hybridization. Methylation of DNA can also be assessed using *in situ* hybridization in the methylation-specific PCR *in situ* hybridization technique (*see* Chapter 20). The advantage of this procedure is that intact tissues or cell preparations can be analyzed for silencing of a given gene owing to hypermethylation of its promoter.

5.5. Analysis of the DNA Methyltransferases

Advances have also been made in analyzing not only methylated DNA, but also the DNMTs that carry out the methylation process. DNMT expression changes during many biological processes such as embryonic development, cancer, and aging (*5,6,13*). Real-time PCR has recently been applied to analysis of the expression of each of the functional DNMTs in mammalian cells (*see* Chapter 21). This is a widely available tool that is sensitive and specific and allows for rapid assessment of DNMT mRNA levels. In addition, newer methods have been developed for measuring DNMT activity. In the DNMT magnetic bead assay (*see* Chapter 22), a novel system has been developed in which DNMT activity is measured by the incorporation of tritiated methyl groups into biotinylated DNA oligonucleotides. The radioactive DNA can easily be separated from free radioactive substrate using a magnet after the DNA is immobilized onto magnetic beads with streptavidin covalently attached to the bead surface. This technique for measuring DNMT activity is simple and highly reproducible with very low background.

6. Conclusion

A broad analysis has been provided of techniques in current use for assessing epigenetic changes in DNA and its associated proteins. Procedures are presented in this book for analyzing chromatin and DNA methylation changes, the two most important processes in epigenetics. Often these processes are inter-dependent, and several methods used in conjunction will probably be neces-sary to unravel the mysteries of epigenetic modification. This book is intended to arm the reader with a set of contemporary and practical tools needed to study the rapidly developing field of epigenetics.

References

1. Brown, R. and Strathdee, G. (2002) Epigenomics and epigenetic therapy of can-cer. *Trends Mol. Med.* **8,** S43–S48.
2. Marks, P., Rifkind, R. A., Richon, V. M,, Breslow, R., Miller, T., and Kelly, W. K. (2001) Histone deacetylases and cancer: causes and therapies. *Nat. Rev. Can-cer* **1,** 194–202.
3. Fischle, W., Wang, Y., and Allis, C.D. (2003) Histone and chromatin cross-talk. *Curr. Opin. Cell Biol.* **15,** 172–183.
4. Wang, H., Cao, R., Xia, L., et al. (2001) Purification and functional characteriza-tion of a histone H3-lysine 4-specific methyltransferase. *Mol. Cell* **8,** 1207–1217.
5. Liu, L., Wylie, R. C., Andrews, L. G., and Tollefsbol, T. O. (2003) Aging, cancer and nutrition: the DNA methylation connection. *Mech. Ageing Dev.* **124,** 989–998.
6. Robertson, K. D. (2001) DNA methylation, methyltransferases and cancer. *Oncogene* **20,** 3139–3155.
7. Okano, M., Bell, D. W., Haber, D. A., and Li, E. (1999) Dnmt3a and Dnmt3b are essential for *de novo* methylation and mammalian development. *Cell* **99,** 247–257.
8. Fuks, F., Burgers, W. A., Brehm, A., Hughes-Davis, L., and Kouzarides, T. (2000) DNA methyltransferase Dnmt1 associates with histone deacetylase activity. *Nat. Genet.* **24,** 88–91.
9. Roundtree, M. R., Bachman, K. E., and Baylin, S. B. (2000) DNMT1 binds HDAC2 and a new co-repressor, DMAP1, to form a complex at replication foci. *Nat. Genet.* **25,** 269–277.
10. Fuks, F., Burgers, W. A., Godin, N., Kasai, M., and Kouzarides, T. (2001) Dnmt3a binds deacetylases and is recruited by a sequence-specific repressor to silence transcription. *EMBO J.* **20,** 2536–2544.
11. Bachman, K. E., Rountree, M. R., and Baylin, S. B. (2001) Dnmt3a and Dnmt3b are transcriptional repressors that exhibit unique localization properties to hetero-chromatin. *J. Biol. Chem.* **276,** 32,282–32,287.
12. Weinmann, A. S., and Franham, P. J. (2002) Identification of unknown target genes of human transcription factors using chromatin immunoprecipitation. *Meth-ods* **26,** 37–47.
13. Casillas, M. A., Lopatina, N., Andrews, L. G., and Tollefsbol, T. O. (2003) Tran-scriptional control of the DNA methyltransferases is altered in aging and neoplastically-transformed human fibroblasts. *Mol. Cell. Biochem.* **252,** 33–43.

2

Chromatin Immunoprecipitation Assays

Yan Yan, Haobin Chen, and Max Costa

Summary

Chromatin immunoprecipitation (ChIP) is a powerful tool to study protein–DNA interaction and is widely used in many fields to study proteins associated with chromatin, such as histone and its isoforms and transcription factors, across a defined DNA domain. Here, we show the step-by-step methods currently used in our lab to immunoprecipitate the formaldehyde crosslinked chromatin and further analyze the immuprecipitated DNA by semiquantitative PCR.

Key Words: Chromatin; immunoprecipitation; semiquantitative PCR.

1. Introduction

Chromatin immunoprecipitation (ChIP) assay refers to a procedure used to determine whether a given protein binds to a specific DNA sequence in vivo; in so doing, it allows one to determine the chromatin architecture of specific DNA sequences. Two approaches that differ primarily in how the chromatin is prepared have been employed. The first uses native chromatin prepared by standard micrococcal nuclease digestion of nuclei and is referred to as nChIP *(1,2)*. This method is used for the study of proteins that bind to DNA with high affinity, such as histones and their modified isoforms. The second method uses crosslinked chromatin prepared by adding formaldehyde to cells or exposing the cells to ultraviolet (UV) irradiation; the chromatin is then fragmented to small sizes by sonication *(3–6)*. This procedure is referred to as xChIP. This method is the only option when one is interested in proteins that bind to DNA with lower affinity, including most of the nonhistone proteins.

Among various crosslinking agents, formaldehyde (HCHO) is the most commonly used. It was shown that formaldehyde efficiently crosslinks protein–DNA, protein–RNA, and protein–protein in vivo by interacting between the amino and imino groups of lysine, arginine, and histidine and those of DNA

From: *Methods in Molecular Biology, vol. 287: Epigenetics Protocols*
Edited by: T. O. Tollefsbol © Humana Press Inc., Totowa, NJ

bases *(7,8)*. Furthermore, the chromatin structure is faithfully preserved by HCHO treatment, and the crosslinks can be readily reversed under mild conditions *(3)*. This technique was first applied to study DNA binding proteins *(6)*, and then its applications were broadened to include analysis of general transcription factors and protein complexes associated with chromatin remodeling and high-resolution mapping *(9,10)*. Recent advances include combining the ChIP assay with DNA microarray or cloning techniques to identify novel target genes or the DNA binding site of selected proteins in the global genome environments *(11,12)*. **Figure 1** outlines the main procedures of the xChIP assay. Briefly, living cells are first fixed by HCHO, and the crosslinked chromatin is then sheared and solubilized by sonication. This is followed by the selective immunoprecipitation of protein–DNA complexes utilizing specific protein antibodies. The crosslinks are then reversed, and the immunoprecipitated DNA is analyzed.

2. Materials

1. Cells to be tested.
2. Medium and supplements appropriate for the cells to be studied.
3. 37% Formaldehyde.
4. 2.5 M Glycine.
5. IB buffers: 10 mM Tris-HCl, pH 8.0, 3 mM CaCl$_2$, 2 mM MgCl$_2$, 1% NP-40.
6. Phosphate-buffered saline (PBS): 8 g NaCl, 0.2 g KCl, 1.15 g Na$_2$HPO$_4$ · 7H$_2$O, 0.2 g KH$_2$PO$_4$.
7. ChIP lysis buffer: 50 mM HEPES-KOH, pH 7.5, 140 mM NaCl, 1 mM EDTA, 1% Triton X-100, 0.1% sodium deoxycholate.
8. Complete protease inhibitor cocktails.
9. Branson 450 Sonifier.
10. Antibodies against proteins of interest.
11. Salmon sperm DNA/Protein-A agarose beads.
12. ChIP lysis buffer (high salt): lysis buffer containing 500 mM NaCl.
13. LiCl/detergent solution: 10 mM Tris-HCl, pH 8.0, 250 mM LiCl, 0.5% NP-40, 0.5% sodium deoxycholate, 1 mM EDTA.
14. TE buffer: 10 mM Tris-HCl, pH 8.0, 1 mM EDTA, pH 8.0.
15. DNase-free RNase A.
16. ChIP elution buffer: 1% sodium dodecly sulfate (SDS), 0.1 M NaHCO$_3$ (needs to be made fresh).
17. 10X Proteinase K buffer: 0.1 M Tris-HCl, pH 7.8, 50 mM EDTA, 5% sodium dodecyl sulfate (SDS).
18. 20 µg/µL Proteinase K in H$_2$O.
19. Ethanol.
20. Phenol/chloroform/isoamyl alcohol (25:24:1).
21. 3 M NaAc, pH 4.8.
22. Primers to amplify genes of interest.

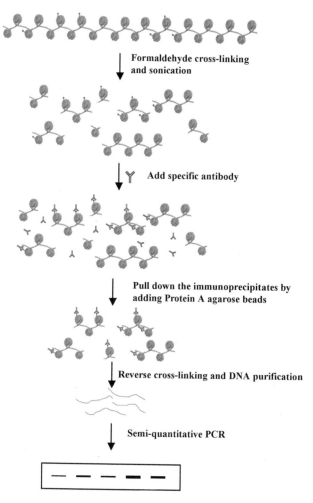

Fig. 1. Schematic procedures of chromatin immunoprecipitation (ChIP) assay. PCR, polymerase chain reaction.

23. 2.5 mM dNTP: 2.5 mM each deoxynucleoside triphosphate, dATP, dTTP, dGTP, and dCTP.
24. [α-^{32}P]dATP or [α-^{32}P]dCTP.
25. *Taq* DNA polymerase.
26. 10X *Taq* buffer: 100 mM Tris-HCl, pH 8.3, 15 mM MgCl$_2$, 500 mM KCl.
27. Thermocycler.
28. Agarose gel electrophoresis apparatus.
29. Ethidium bromide.
30. 6X DNA sample buffer: 0.25% bromophenol blue and 40% sucrose in water.

31. Vertical electrophoresis apparatus.
32. 30% Acrylamide/*bis*-acrylamide (37.5:1) solution.
33. 1 L: 5X TBE: 54 g Tris base, 27.5 g boric acid, and 20 mL 0.5 M EDTA (pH 8.0).
34. 10% Ammonium persulfate.
35. TEMED (*N,N,N,N*-tetramethylethelenediamine).
36. Kodak X-ray film or PhosphorImager system.

3. Methods

The methods described below outline (1) the preparation of soluble chromatin extract, (2) immunoprecipitation of crosslinked chromatin and (3) analysis of immunoprecipitated DNA by semiquantitative polymerase chain reaction (PCR).

3.1. Preparation of Soluble Chromatin Extract

3.1.1. Formaldehyde Crosslinking Protein–DNA Complexes In Vivo

1. Grow cells in appropriate medium and supplements.
   a. Collect cells by trypsinization followed by low-speed centrifugation.
   b. Resuspend 2.5×10^8 cells in 30 mL media (without serum) in a 50-mL conical tube.
   c. In a fume hood, add 0.81 mL of 37% formaldehyde solution directly to the cell suspension to a final concentration of 1%.
   d. Incubate the mixture at room temperature for 5–15 min, with occasionally shaking (*see* **Notes 1** and **2**).
   e. The cell numbers used here are enough for at least four immunoprecipitation.
2. Add 1.5 mL of 2.5 M glycine to a fixed cell suspension, arriving at a final concentration of 0.125 M to quench the crosslinks, and then incubate at room temperature for 5 min, with occasional shaking.
3. Centrifuge cells (5 min at 2000 rpm) and discard the supernatant. Wash the cells twice with 20–30 mL of ice-cold PBS, collect cells by centrifugation, and discard the supernatant. Maintain cells on ice (If you are collecting many samples, they may be frozen at –80°C).

3.1.2. Solubilization of Chromatin by Sonication

1. Resuspend cell pellet gently with 1 mL of ChIP lysis buffer supplemented with complete protease inhibitor cocktails and incubate on ice for 30 min. Transfer lysate to round-bottomed 3.5-mL Nunc cryotube vials (*see* **Note 3**). Put cryotube vials in glass beakers filled with crushed ice.
2. Using a Branson 450 Sonifier with a standard tip set at 40–50% output, 90% duty cycle; sonicate extracts for 8 s six times. In between pulses, let samples sit on ice for at least 2 min. This should shear chromatin to a final average size of 500–1000 bp (*see* **Fig. 2** and **Note 4**).
3. Centrifuge samples at the maximum speed for 15 min at 4°C. Transfer supernatant to a fresh 1.5-mL microcentrifuge tube and centrifuge samples again for 15

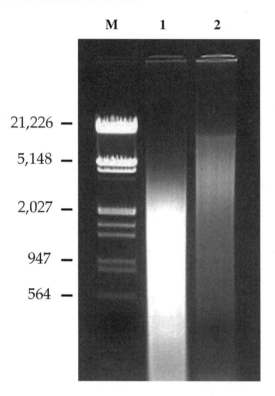

Fig. 2. The average size of the sheared DNA is dependent on the extent of crosslinking. *M* molecular weight markers; lane 1, chromatin with a bulk size of 1 kb; lane 2, the chromatin DNA has an average size of 2–5 kb, and a large size of chromatin DNA (20 kb) is noticed, indicating the chromatin is overcrosslinked.

    min at the maximum speed at 4°C. Collect the supernatant, which now contains the chromatin extract.

4. Add 80 µL salmon sperm DNA/protein A agarose beads to the cell lysate to preclear the chromatin extract, and incubate on a rotation wheel for 60 min at 4°C. Centrifuge samples at 8000 rpm for 2 min, and then transfer the supernatant to a fresh tube.

3.2. Immunoprecipitation and Purification of Crosslinked Chromatin

3.2.1. Immunoprecipitation of Crosslinked Chromatin

1. For quantifying the chromatin DNA, a fraction of the chromatin extract, usually 20–50 µL, was used to purify DNA using methods described in **Subheading 3.2.2.** or a DNA purification kit. The chromatin used for immunoprecipitation is standardized using the respective amount of DNA.
2. Add the primary antibody against the protein of interest to 300–400 µg chromatin extract (as DNA). Bring the volume to 500 µL with cold ChIP lysis buffer

     supplemented with protease inhibitor cocktails. Rotate the reaction at 4°C for 4 h to overnight (*see* **Notes 5** and **6**).

3. Equilibrate the salmon sperm DNA/protein A beads (*see* **Note 7**) with ChIP lysis buffer. Rotate at 4°C for 1 h.

4. Add 30 μL bed salmon sperm DNA/vol protein A agarose beads. Incubate on a rotating wheel for 1–3 h at 4°C. Centrifuge sample for 2 min at 8000 rpm at 4°C.

5. Keep 50 μL of supernatant, bring the volume to 500 μL with TE, add 20 μL 5 *M* NaCl, and discard the remainder. This is the unbound fraction. (If needed, a portion of 10% of that used for immunoprecipitation is saved as input fraction.) This will be needed as the input control for subsequent analyses.

6. Add 1 mL ChIP lysis buffer supplemented with the protease inhibitor cocktails to the beads to wash immunoprecipitates, incubate on ice for 5 min, with occasional inversion, and then centrifuge at 8000 rpm for 2 min. Discard the supernatant, and repeat this procedure once.

7. Wash the beads with 1 mL ChIP lysis buffer (high salt) supplemented with the protease inhibitor cocktails, and repeat once.

8. Wash the beads with 1 mL LiCl/detergent solution supplemented with protease inhibitor cocktails, and repeat once.

9. Add 1 mL TE to the beads and repeat incubation and centrifugation.

10. Suspend the beads in 200 μL TE, pH 8.0, containing 20 μg of DNase-free RNase A. Incubate at 37°C for 30 min. Add 1 mL TE, mix, and collect the beads.

11. Add 250 μL ChIP elution buffer, mix, and incubate at room temperature for 15 min. Vortex occasionally. Centrifuge briefly, transfer eluate to fresh tube and wash beads with 250 μL ChIP elution buffer again. Pool the supernatant.

3.2.2. Purification of Immunoprecipitated DNA (IP DNA)

1. Add 20 μL 5 *M* NaCl to the 500 μL eluent. Incubate the eluent and the input or unbound fraction for at least 6 h at 65°C to reverse crosslinks.

2. The immunoprecipitates are removed from the solution with the addition of 1 mL ethanol, followed by incubation at –70°C for at least half an hour. Centrifuge at the maximum speed for 15 min, and wash the pellet with cold 70% ethanol. Centrifuge again, discard the supernatant, and air-dry the pellet.

3. Dissolve the pellet in 178 μL TE. Add 20 μL 10X proteinase K buffer and 2 μL 20 μg/μL proteinase K. Incubate at 50°C for 30 min.

4. Extract with 200 μL 25:24:1 phenol/chloroform/isoamyl alcohol. Vortex vigorously for 1 min. Separate phases by centrifugation at the maximum speed for 5 min at room temperature. Repeat phenol/chloroform/isoamyl alcohol extraction once and chloroform extraction once. Back extract the organic phases sequentially with 150 μL TE. Pool the two aqueous solutions.

5. Add 35 μL 3 *M* NaAc, pH 4.8, 1 mL 100% ethanol. Precipitate the DNA by centrifugation and wash with 70% ethanol as described.

6. Resuspend IP DNA in 50 μL TE, and input or unbound DNA in 100 μL TE, and store at –20°C.

3.3. Semiquantitative PCR of IP DNA

IP DNA can be further analyzed by quantitative PCR, semiquantitative PCR, real-time PCR, or slot-blot hybridization, and other techniques. The steps described below are semiquantitative PCR (*see* **Note 8**). The final reaction volumes all are 50 µL.

3.3.1. Optimizing the PCR Conditions

1. Quantify the input or unbound DNA concentration using spectrometer.
2. Add 0.1–0.5 µg DNA into each 0.5-mL thin-walled PCR tube. The amount of DNA depends on the sensitivity of individual primers and genes amplified; we use higher amounts of DNA for the initial experiment.
3. Add 5 µL 10X *Taq* buffer, 2 µL 2.5 m*M* dNTP, and 2.5 µ *Taq* DNA polymerase.
4. Incubate the samples in a thermocycler. Ampilification parameters depend greatly on the primers and the thermocycler used; adjustment of the parameters might be necessary, and typically 25–30 cycles are used.
5. Separate PCR products using agarose gel electrophoresis and visualize with ethidium bromide.
6. If regular 10X *Taq* buffer doesn't work, a PCR Optimizer Kit (Invitrogen) can be used to choose optimal buffer according to the manufacturer's protocol.

3.3.2. Semiquantitative PCR

1. Serial dilute input or unbound DNA, starting from 0.1 µg/10 µL. Add 10 µL to each PCR tube.
2. Add appropriate amount (add [*n*+1] × each components for *n* samples) PCR buffer, primers, 2.5 m*M* dNTP, [α-^{32}P]dATP or [α-^{32}P]dCTP, *Taq* DNA polymerase and H$_2$O to a 1.5-mL Eppendorf tube, mix well, and separate equal amounts (40 µL) of the mixture into each PCR tube.
3. Incubate the samples in a thermocycler using the conditions decided on above. Separate the PCR products as described in **Subheading 3.3.3**.
4. Analyze the IP DNA in the same fashion, using 2.5–5 µL as a template. Make sure the signal falls into a linear dose–response range. If not, reduce the template or cycle number. Once the conditions are established, it is not necessary to amplify serial diluted input DNA every time for semiquantitative PCR, but an input DNA control is still needed for normalizing the signal.

3.3.3. Separation of PCR Products Using Native Polyacrylamide Gels

Most commercial vertical electrophoresis devices can be used; we use Bio-Rad Mini-PROTEIN II electrophoresis apparatus.

1. Prepare the glass plates and spacers according to the manufacturer's protocol.
2. Mix 3 mL 5X TBE buffer, 4 mL 30% acrylamide/*bis*-acrylamide (37.5:1) solution, 7.85 mL H$_2$O, 150 µL fresh made 10% ammonium persulfate, and 6 µL TEMED. This gel mixture is enough for casting two 1.5-mm-thick 8% polyacry-

lamide gels using Mini-PROTEIN II electrophoresis apparatus. The components of the mixture can be adjusted according to the different electrophoresis devices and gel concentrations.

3. Fill the space between the two glass plates to the top with the gel mixture, and insert the appropriate comb; we usually use a 10-well comb.
4. Allow the acrylamide to polymerize for at least 60 min at room temperature.
5. Attach the gels to the electrophoresis tank, fill with 1X TBE buffer, and carefully remove the comb.
6. Add 10 µL 6X DNA sample buffer to the PCR products, load 10 µL of the sample mixture, and run the gels at 100 V until the marker dyes have migrated the desired distance.
7. Move one glass plate, check that the gel remains attached to the other glass plate, and put a dry 3MM filter paper over the gel; the paper should be bigger than the gel. Detach the gel from the glass by lifting the paper; the gel should stick to the paper evenly. Expose to Kodak X-ray film at –70°C or screen of the PhosphorImager at room temperature. According to our experience, drying the gel is not necessary. Examples of ChIP assay results are given in **Fig. 3**.

4. Notes

1. The extent of crosslinking is critical and depends on the protein of interest. The conditions for crosslinking should be optimized. The concentration of formaldehyde, the length of crosslinking or the temperature of crosslinking should be adjusted for different cell types. Insufficient crosslinking may lead to incomplete fixation, and the average size of DNA fragments is less than 500 bp. Overcrosslinking may result in a substantial loss of material and prevent the production of small chromatin fragments, even by prolonged sonication *(13,14)*.
2. A nuclei isolation step can be included before crosslinking to keep the cytoplasmic proteins from interfering. This can be done by resuspending the cells in IB buffers and incubating them on ice for 15 min. For specific experiments, such as exposure of cells to hypoxia, crosslinking should be done as soon as the cells are moved out from the hypoxia culture conditions. Nuclei isolation can still be done after fixation, but a longer incubation time is needed.
3. The sonicator needs to be calibrated to yield the final desired average length of DNA. It is important to adjust the tip immersion depth. Violent motion on the surface and foaming results in a loss of energy. Small volumes of cell suspension in a 1.5 mL Eppendorf tube foam very easily; use a microtip if small volumes of samples are being used. We used a cell suspension of more than 1 mL in a 3.5-mL round-bottomed Nunc Cryotube vials, which reduced the possibility of foaming and possible sample loss. Variables such as processing time and output control settings can all be adjusted to produce optimal results. The addition of microglass beads (0.1–0.5 mm diameter) may improve the shearing efficiency. A ratio of one part glass beads to three to five parts liquid is recommended.
4. The size of the DNA fragments may be critical for high-resolution analysis. If the aim of the experiment is to show binding of a protein to a particular site, or a

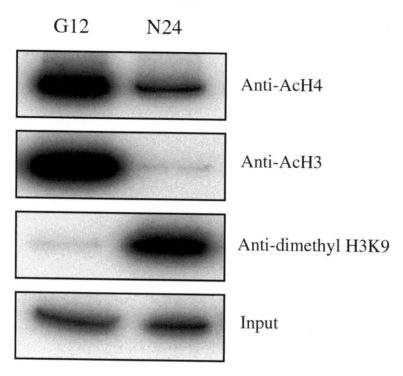

Fig. 3. Crosslinked chromatin of G12 and N24 (a derivate of G12 with an Ni silenced *gpt* gene) cells was immunoprecipitated with antiacetylated H3, antiacetylated H4, and antidimethyl H3K9 antibodies (Upstate Biotechnology). Immunoprecipitated DNA was analyzed by semiquantitative PCR using primers specific for the *gpt* gene *(17)*. Input shows the equal amount of chromatin used. The cycle conditions were 95°C 5 min, then 94°C 30 s, 55°C 30 s, 72°C 45 s for 30 cycles.

specific modification of histone in a particular site, fine tuning of the extent of crosslinking and sonication variables may be required. Another way is to prepare nucleosomes using micrococcal nuclease after mild crosslinking *(15,16)* or to perform nChIP if the target of interest is histone or its isoforms *(1,2)*. Otherwise, optimizing this parameter is not as important.

5. Preliminary immunoprecipitation experiments should be performed to determine the appropriate amount of antibody to be used. Excess antibodies results in higher overall DNA yields. Normally, 5 μg of antibodies will produce enough IP DNA from 300–400 μg chromatin (as DNA), but a lower specificity of antibody lowers the relative enrichment of IP DNA specifically.

6. It is very important to set a control to avoid nonspecific binding. Affinity-purified antibodies can reduce the amount of non-specific binding, but a mock IP (IP without antibody) is still needed. If polyclonal antisera are used, a control using unimmunized sera from the same species should be included. It is necessary to

include a control using non-crosslinked chromatin extract to avoid nonchromatin proteins and free DNA binding. This control allows one to monitor whether the high salt wash is efficient.

7. Antibodies from different species and different antibody subtypes have different binding properties with beads. When monoclonal antibodies are used, protein A beads are not efficient to bind the antibodies, then protein A/G beads or other specific beads (such as GammaBind [Pharmacia]) should be used.

8. It is essential to test the sensitivity and efficiency of the PCR before analyzing the immunoprecipitated DNA. The signal should be proportional to the amount of template DNA. It is recommended that ^{32}P be added in the reaction, because much less template DNA is then needed and the amount of the PCR product falls more easily into the linear dose–response range. Furthermore, multiple genes can be analyzed simultaneously.

References

1. Hebbes, T. R. Thorne, A. W., and Crane-Robinson, C. (1988) A direct link between core histone acetylation and transcriptionally active chromatin. *EMBO J.* **7,** 1395–1402.

2. Laura, P., Neill, O., and Turner, B. M. (2003) Immunoprecipitation of native chromatin: NChIP. *Methods* **31,** 76–82.

3. Jackson, V. and Chalkley, R. (1981) A new method for the isolation of replicative chromatin: selective deposition of histone on both new and old DNA. *Cell* **23,** 121–134.

4. Solomon, M. J., Larsen, P. L., and Varshavsky, A. (1988) Mapping protein–DNA interactions in vivo with formaldehyde: evidence that histone H4 is retained on a highly transcribed gene. *Cell* **53,** 937–947.

5. Dedon, P. C., Soults, J. A., Allis, C. D., and Gorovsky, M. A. (1991) A simplified formaldehyde fixation and immunoprecipitation technique for studying protein–DNA interactions. *Anal. Biochem.* **197,** 83–90.

6. Gilmour, D. S. and Lis, J. T. (1984) Detecting protein–DNA interactions in vivo: distribution of RNA polymerase on specific bacterial genes. *Proc. Natl. Acad. Sci. USA* **81,** 4275–4279.

7. McGhee, J. D. and von Hippel, P. H. (1975) Formaldehyde as a probe of DNA structure. I. Reaction with exocyclic amino groups of DNA bases. *Biochemistry* **14,** 1281–1296.

8. McGhee, J. D. and von Hippel P. H. (1975) Formaldehyde as a probe of DNA structure. II. Reaction with endocyclic imino groups of DNA bases. *Biochemistry* **14,** 1297–1303.

9. Orlando, V. and Paro, R. (1993) Mapping Polycomb-repressed domains in the bithorax complex using in vivo formaldehyde cross-linked chromatin. *Cell* **75,** 1187–1198.

10. Tomotsune, D., Shoji, H., Wakamatsu, Y., Kondoh, H., and Takahashi, N. (1993) A mouse homologue of the *Drosophila* tumour-suppressor gene l(2)gl controlled by Hox-C8 in vivo. *Nature* **365,** 69–72.

11. Weinmann, A. S. and Farnham, P. J. (2002) Identification of unknown target genes of human transcription factors using chromatin imunoprecipitation. *Methods* **26,** 37–47.
12. Wells, J. and Farnham, P. J. (2002) Characterizing transcription factor binding sites using formaldehyde crosslinking and immunoprecipitation. *Methods* **26,** 48–56.
13. Orlando, V., Strutt, H., and Paro, R. (1997) Analysis of chromatin structure by in vivo formaldehyde cross-linking. *Methods* **11,** 205–214.
14. Kuo, M. H. and Allis, C. D. (1999) In vivo cross-linking and immunoprecipitation for studying dynamic protein: DNA associations in a chromatin environment. *Methods* **19,** 425–433.
15. Kuhnert, P., Peterhans, E., and Pauli, U. (1992) Chromatin structure and DNase I hypersensitivity in the transcriptionally active and inactive porcine tumor necrosis factor gene locus. *Nucleic Acids Res.* **20,** 1943–1948.
16. Morrison, A., Sardet, C., and Herrera R. E. (2002) Retinoplastoma protein transcriptional repression through histone deacetylation of single nucleosome. *Mol. Cell. Biol.* **22,** 856–865.
17. Lee, Y. W., Pons, C., Tummolo, D. M., Klein, C. B., Rossman, T. G., and Christie, N. T. (1993) Mutagenicity of soluble and insoluble nickel compounds at the gpt locus in G12 Chinese hamster cells. *Environ. Mol. Mutagen.* **21,** 365–371.

3

Native Chromatin Immunoprecipitation

Alan W. Thorne, Fiona A. Myers, and Tim R. Hebbes

Summary

Chromatin immunoprecipitation (ChIP) is a technique widely used for determining the genomic location of modified histones and other chromatin-associated factors. Here we describe the methodology we have used in our laboratory for the immunoprecipitation of chromatin isolated from cells in the absence of crosslinking. Chromatin released from nuclei by micrococcal nuclease digestion is centrifuged through sucrose gradients to allow selection of mono- or dinucleosomes. This allows a protein or modification at a particular gene or locus to be mapped at higher resolution than in a crosslinked ChIP experiment. Two methods for the immunoprecipitation of chromatin are described: a large-scale fractionation by which it is possible to visualize the proteins of the immunoprecipitate by polyacrylamide gel electrophoresis, PAGE and a small-scale method that is more appropriate when the quantity of chromatin is limited. The sequence content of DNA extracted from the immunoprecipitated chromatin is analyzed by hybridization of Southern or slot blots, or by quantitative polymerase chain reaction. Enrichment of particular sequences in the immunoprecipitated fraction reveals the presence and extent of the modification at this location.

Key Words: Native chromatin immunoprecipitation; histone acetylation; active chromatin; chicken β-globin; human α-globin.

1. Introduction

The key features of a native chromatin immunoprecipitation (nChIP) experiment are the fragmentation of chromatin in the nuclei by micrococcal nuclease and the immunoselection of chromatin fragments bearing the protein, or modified protein, of interest using an appropriate antibody. Formaldehyde crosslinking is not used at any point during the preparation. The method is most frequently used to study the spatial or temporal location of posttranslational core histone modifications such as acetylation or methylation and has been developed from a method first described by Dorbic and Wittig (1,2). It is particularly suited for proteins such as core histones that are tightly bound to

From: *Methods in Molecular Biology, vol. 287: Epigenetics Protocols*
Edited by: T. O. Tollefsbol © Humana Press Inc., Totowa, NJ

chromosomes. Linker histones, transcription factors, and other less strongly associated proteins may relocalize or be lost from the chromatin during preparation, and an xChIP (crosslinked) is more suitable. The nChIP offers three major advantages:

1. High-resolution mapping, to mononucleosomal level, can be achieved by using sucrose gradient-purified, micrococcal nuclease-generated mononucleosomes as input chromatin for the experiment.
2. The protein content of the immunoprecipitate can be examined directly by Coomassie-stained polyacrylamide gel electrophoresis (PAGE) to check the efficiency of the immunoprecipitation. The absence of a formaldehyde crosslinking step allows proteins to be recovered without charge modification in a state suitable for analysis on acid–urea–Triton gels to detect enrichments in, for example, acetylated histones or primary sequence variants.
3. The loss of proteins during preparation of chromatin for an nChIP may also be advantageous in that nucleosomes bearing transcription factor-bound modified histones, which would be occluded by such proteins in xChIPs, should also be immunoprecipiataed.

The nChIP has been successfully used by several different groups in cells and tissues from a number of animals including chicken *(3–8)*, mouse *(9)*, and human *(10–14)* using a variety of antibodies.

The nChIP can be divided into three stages: chromatin preparation, immunoprecipitation, and finally analysis of DNA and protein. Conditions for chromatin preparation are largely governed by the particular experimental system; for example, buffers and conditions used for chicken erythrocyte cells are inappropriate for cultured human cells. nChIP experiments can be performed on a small or a large scale (15 or 400 µg chromatin) using either immune serum or affinity-purified antibodies dictated by the amounts of antibody or chromatin available. Analysis of the sequence content of chromatin bound by the antibody can be performed by a number of different methods such as hybridization or, more commonly, quantitative polymerase chain reaction (PCR). In the sections below we outline the different approaches we have used. As most of our studies have focused on histone acetylation, sodium butyrate is included in the buffers to inhibit the deacetylase enzymes and thereby preserve the acetylation pattern on the chromatin.

2. Materials

1. Phosphate-buffered saline (PBS)-butyrate: 135 mM NaCl, 2.5 mM KCl, 8 mM Na$_2$HPO$_4$, 1.5 mM KH$_2$PO$_4$, 10 mM Na-butyrate, 0.1 mM phenylmethylsulfonyl fluoride (PMSF), 0.1 mM benzamidine. Add protease inhibitors just prior to use and every 30 min to 1 h.
2. Erythrocyte lysis buffer: 80 mM NaCl, 10 mM Tris-HCl, pH 7.5, 10 mM Na-butyrate, 6 mM MgCl$_2$, 0.1 mM PMSF, 0.1 mM benzamidine, 0.1% w/v Triton X-100.

3. Nuclear wash buffer A: as in **step 2** but omitting Triton X-100.
4. Sucrose cushion: 30% w/w sucrose in wash buffer A.
5. Storage buffer: 80% v/v glycerol in wash buffer A.
6. Nuclei digest buffer A: 10 mM NaCl, 10 mM Tris-HCl, pH 7.5, 10 mM Na-butyrate, 3 mM MgCl$_2$, 1 mM CaCl$_2$, 0.1 mM PMSF, 0.1 mM benzamidine.
7. Nuclei lysis buffer: 10 mM Tris-HCl, pH 7.5, 10 mM Na-butyrate, 0.25 mM Na$_3$EDTA, 0.1 mM PMSF, 0.1 mM benzamidine.
8. Culture cell lysis buffer: 250 mM sucrose, 10 mM Tris-HCl, pH 7.4, 10 mM Na-butyrate, 4 mM MgCl$_2$, 0.1 mM PMSF, 0.1 mM benzamidine, 0.1% w/v Triton X-100.
9. Wash buffer B: 250 mM sucrose, 10 mM Tris-HCl, pH 7.4, 10 mM Na-butyrate, 4 mM MgCl$_2$, 0.1 mM PMSF, 0.1 mM benzamidine.
10. Sucrose cushion B: 30% w/v sucrose in wash buffer B.
11. Storage buffer B: 80% v/v glycerol in wash buffer B.
12. Dounce homogenizer with B pestle.
13. Sephadex C25-CM ion exchange resin.
14. nChIP buffer: 50 mM NaCl, 10 mM Tris-HCl, pH 7.5, 10 mM Na-butyrate, 1 mM Na$_3$ EDTA, 0.1 mM PMSF, 0.1 mM benzamidine.
15. Protein A Sepharose (Sigma).
16. Elution buffer: nChIP buffer containing 1.5% SDS.
17. Micrococcal nuclease (Worthington).

3. Method

In outline, cells from different sources are harvested and lysed with Triton X-100. Released nuclei are washed to remove cytoplasmic contaminants and stored in buffered glycerol at –80°C until required. Chromatin is fragmented in nuclei by micrococcal nuclease digestion, chromatin is released, and nucleosomal fractions are purified by centrifugation through sucrose gradients.

3.1. Preparation of Chromatin From Chicken Erythrocyte Cells

3.1.1. Nuclei Preparation

The quantities given below are suitable for up to 20 mL of adult or embryonic blood.

1. Collect the blood by venesection into ice-cold PBS-butyrate supplemented with 5 mM Na$_2$EDTA and filter through three layers of sterile gauze. Pellet erythrocytes by centrifugation at 1100g for 5 min at 4°C in a swingout rotor. If required, white cells can be removed from the preparation at this stage by carefully pipeting off the buffy coat (white blood cells) from the top of the erythrocyte pellet.
2. Resuspend the erythrocytes in PBS-butyrate (omitting the EDTA). Centrifuge as above.
3. Resuspend the cell pellet in a minimum volume of wash buffer A and add dropwise to 50 pellet vol of erythrocyte lysis buffer at 4°C while stirring rapidly.
4. Reduce the stirring speed and stir slowly for 20 min at 4°C to effect cell lysis.

5. Centrifuge at 1100g for 10 min to pellet nuclei, and discard the supernatant. A crude indicator of the efficiency of lysis is the color of the pellet. If it is straw colored, lysis has been effective, but if it remains red/pink, then further washing in lysis buffer is required. Monitor the removal of cytoplasmic tags using phase contrast microscopy.

6. Resuspend the nuclear pellet in 8 mL of wash buffer A, overlay 2 mL of the nuclei suspension onto each of four 4-mL 30% sucrose cushions in wash buffer A, and centrifuge at 2400g for 5 min in a swingout rotor at 4°C. Discard the supernatant.

7. Resuspend the nuclei in a minimum volume of wash buffer A, add an equal volume of storage buffer A, leave on ice for 15 min, freeze, and store at –80°C until required.

3.1.2. Chromatin Preparation

1. Thaw nuclei and dilute with an equal volume of digest buffer A, and centrifuge at 1100g for 5 min. For small quantities of nuclei, the centrifugation steps can be performed in a microcentrifuge at 12,000g for 6 s.

2. Wash the nuclei twice in digestion buffer, spinning at 1100g for 5 min. Prior to the final centrifugation step, estimate the DNA concentration by ultraviolet (UV) spectroscopy. Disperse 10 µL of the nuclei in 1 mL saturated salt urea (SSU), record the UV spectrum against an SSU blank, and use the reading at 260 nm to estimate the DNA concentration (1 AU at 260 nm = 50 µg/mL).

3. Resuspend the nuclei pellet in digest buffer at 5 mg/mL (DNA) and preincubate at 37°C for 3 min. Add micrococcal nuclease (Worthington) to a final concentration of 200 U/mL, vortex briefly, and incubate at 37°C. The length of the digest time is normally determined by the time-course but is usually 8–12 min. Terminate the digest by adding Na$_2$EDTA to a final concentration of 10 mM and transfer to ice.

4. Centrifuge the digested nuclei at 1100g for 5 min and retain the chromatin released in the supernatant S1, which is usually about 80–90% mononucleosomes. Resuspend the pellet in nuclei lysis buffer and incubate on ice for 1 h to allow the nuclei to lyse. (It may be necessary to sonicate briefly to encourage lysis.) Following incubation, centrifuge as above and collect the chromatin containing supernatant S2.

5. Combine the two supernatants S1 and S2. At this stage H1/5-containing chromatin can be selectively precipitated by salt fractionation (*see* **Subheading 3.3.**). Alternatively, the chromatin can be depleted of linker histones using C25 resin (*see* **Subheading 3.4.**). Mono-, di-, and trinucleosomes are then separated using sucrose gradient centrifugation (*see* **Subheading 3.5.**). Chromatin may be stored at –80°C at this point after the addition of sucrose to a minimum of 15% w/v.

3.2. Preparation of Chromatin From Cultured Human K562 Cells

Conditions used for the preparation of chromatin from tissue culture cells vary depending on the type of cells used. The stages below outline the methods we have found to be successful for K562 and HeLa. Other workers *(9,12,14)* have optimized the nuclei preparation/nuclease digest conditions to suit the individual systems.

3.2.1. Nuclei Preparation

1. Harvest the cells by centrifugation at 2500g for 20 min at 4°C.
2. Resuspend the cell pellet in ice-cold PBS-butyrate, and repeat the centrifugation as above.
3. Resuspend the pellet in cell lysis buffer B containing 0.1% w/v Triton X-100, and lyse with 10 strokes of the Dounce homogenizer.
4. Pellet the nuclei by centrifugation at 2000g for 10 min at 4°C. Discard the supernatant and resuspend the pellet in about 8 mL of wash buffer B.
5. Overlay 2 mL of the nuclei suspension onto each of four 4-mL 30% sucrose cushions in wash buffer B. Centrifuge at 2400g for 5 min in a swingout rotor at 4°C. Discard the supernatant.
6. Resuspend the nuclei in a minimum volume of wash buffer B, add an equal volume of storage buffer B, leave on ice for 15 min, freeze, and store at –80°C until required.

3.2.2. Chromatin Isolation

The preparation of chromatin from tissue culture cells follows essentially the same method as described for chicken erythrocytes with buffer and digestion conditions adapted to suit the particular cell type. For K562 cells we adjust the protocol described in **Subheading 3.1.** as follows:

1. Supplement the nuclear digest buffer with 250 mM sucrose.
2. Digest K562 nuclei at 5 mg/mL (DNA) using 300 U micrococcal nuclease (MNase)/mg DNA at 20°C for 2–5 min. The length of time and level of enzyme will vary considerably depending on cell type (*see* **Note 1**).

For some cell types it may be necessary to substitute 0.15 mM spermine and 0.5 mM spermidine for magnesium chloride in preparation and digestion buffers to stabilize the nuclei *(15)* and minimize endonuclease and protease digestion.

3.3. Salt Fractionation

Active sequences in a micrococcal nuclease-generated chromatin preparation can be enriched by salt precipitation of the H1/H5-containing chromatin *(16,17)*.

1. To the chromatin produced by micrococcal nuclease digestion (pooled S1 and S2), add 1 M NaCl to a final concentration of 100 mM and incubate on ice for 10 min.
2. Centrifuge at 10,000g for 5 min to pellet the H1/H5-containing chromatin. Retain the salt-soluble chromatin in the supernatant.

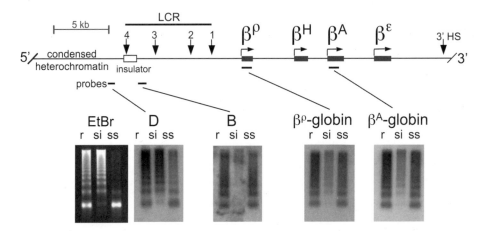

Fig. 1. Southern blot of DNA extracted following MNase digestion of 15-d chicken erythrocyte nuclei from (r) released, (si) salt-insoluble, and (ss) salt-soluble chicken chromatins. Blots were probed with sequences from inside and outside the β-globin domain; positions of the probes are indicated by the solid bars. LCR, locus control region.

The differing susceptibility to micrococcal nuclease (MNase) digestion of active and inactive chromatin is well documented *(10,18–21)* and the representation of different sequences in the input chromatin can vary significantly depending on the extent of digestion. **Figure 1** illustrates the differential digestion of inactive and active sequences from chicken erythrocyte nuclei. Ethidium bromide (EtBr) staining reveals the length distribution of bulk DNA in the released chromatin from a limited MNase digest. In this case the lengths vary from monomers to higher oligonucleosomes. The precipitated (salt-insoluble) fraction is predominantly higher molecular weight material, whereas most (~90%) of the salt-soluble chromatin is mononucleosomal in length. Southern blot analysis using a probe located in heterochromatin just outside the 5′ boundary of the β-globin locus, probe D, shows a similar pattern to the bulk DNA in that most of this chromatin is insoluble at 100 m*M* NaCl. In contrast, probes within the β-globin domain, β^r and β^A, show that these sequences are significantly depleted in the precipitated salt-insoluble fraction and are preferentially found in the soluble chromatin. Strikingly, a significant proportion of these sequences are not present in the mononucleosomal fraction but reside in the higher oligonucleosomes.

3.3.1. nChIP Sequence Representation in the Input Chromatin

The preceding data illustrate the importance of optimizing the MNase digestion for each cell type and testing the representation of the sequences of interest in the prepared chromatin prior to nChIP analysis. Clearly, for nChIP experiments using mononucleosomes, one must be sure that there *is* a nucleosome at the position of interest. If there is not, and the DNA is exposed, it will be rapidly digested by the MNase, and thus be substantially under-represented in the mononuclesome input material. Comparison of the input signal at each position with that from genomic DNA will check for possible under-representation. Typically, at the chicken globin locus using quantitative PCR methodologies (*see* **Subheading 3.6.2.**), the signal from the input mononucleosomes is about 30% of that obtained from an equal weight of genomic DNA. Enrichments achieved by the antibody are determined by calculating the ratio of the sequence content of the bound and input chromatin. This comparison normalizes for variations in the input signal that arise from differing susceptibilities to MNase at different points in the genome. We found no relationship between the amount of the target sequence in the input mononucleosomes and the enrichments observed (Bound/Input [B/I]) at the chicken β-globin locus. Provided there is an adequate number of a particular target nucleosome in the input sample, the nChIP experiment is viable, and the enrichment (B/I) obtained will reflect the level of (in our case) acetylation within those nucleosomes.

3.4. H1 Depletion

Linker histones (H1/H5) can cause nonspecific binding of the chromatin to the protein A Sepharose during the immunoprecipitation (*1*). To avoid such problems, we routinely deplete the chromatin of linker and nonhistone proteins using C25 ion exchange resin. This approach is also advantageous in that proteins binding to the modified histone tails, which if crosslinked would block the epitope and prevent its selection by the antibody, are probably removed from the chromatin.

1. Add 30 mg of dry C25-CM-type resin per mL of the prepared chromatin (pooled S1 and S2) and NaCl to a final concentration of 50 mM, and incubate for 2 h at 4°C, rolling end over end.
2. Following incubation, transfer the resin/chromatin slurry onto a column containing 0.25 g of C25 resin equilibrated in nChIP buffer. Allow the resin to settle, and collect the H1/H5-depleted chromatin in the eluent. Wash the column with one column volume of nChIP buffer to recover chromatin remaining on the column.

H1/H5-depleted chromatin can be used directly for nChIP experiments. Alternatively, if high-resolution mapping data are required, then mono- or tri-nucleosomes can be isolated by sucrose gradient centrifugation, as described below.

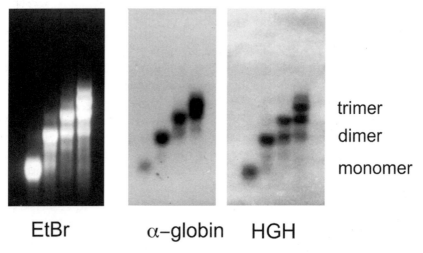

Fig. 2. Southern blot of DNA extracted from sucrose gradient-purified K562 mono-, di-, and tri-nucleosome fractions. Blots were probed with active α-globin and inactive (HGH) sequences.

3.5. Isolation of Chromatin Fragments by Sucrose Gradient Centrifugation

Defined-length chromatin fragments can be isolated using sucrose gradient centrifugation.

1. Construct 12-mL 5–30% exponential sucrose gradients in Beckman SW40 ultraclear tubes (volume of mixing chamber [V_m] = 10 mL, sucrose concentration in mixing chamber [C_m] = 5% w/w in lysis buffer, sucrose concentration in reservoir [C_R] = 40 % w/w in lysis buffer).
2. Overlay up to 1 mg of chromatin (measured as DNA) on each gradient.
3. Centrifuge for 20–24 h at 4°C in a Beckman SW40 rotor at 40,000 rpm (285,000*g*).
4. Fractionate the gradients and monitor the absorbance at 260 nm. Store nucleosome fractions at –80ºC for long term storage.

Figure 2 shows the distribution of active and inactive sequences within chromatin fragments purified by sucrose gradient centrifugation from H1-depleted, MNase-digested chromatin from K562 cells. In this example, the mononucleosomal fraction is depleted of active α-globin sequences, and dinucleosomes, which contain both α-globin (active) and HGH (inactive) sequences were used for nChIP analysis.

3.6. Antibody Purification

3.6.1. Antibody Generation

Antibodies against acetylated histones can be generated by immunization of animals with chemically acetylated purified histone fractions complexed with tRNA *(22)* or using synthetic N-terminal peptides (Alta Bioscience) modified at the appropriate residues and crosslinked to a suitable carrier (e.g. keyhole limpet hemacyanin [KLH] or ovalbumin) via a C-terminal cysteine residue. Immunogens are prepared in 0.9% w/v saline and mixed with up to 50% Freund's complete adjuvant (CFA) prior to immunization. Subsequent boosts utilize incomplete Freund's adjuvant (IFA). Typically, rabbits and sheep produce acceptable titers after three to four boosts.

3.6.2. Preparation of Serum

Obtain serum by allowing blood to clot for 1 h at room temperature and then at 4°C overnight. Remove the serum, centrifuge at 12,000*g* for 5 min, remove the supernatant, aliquot and store at –80°C.

3.6.3. Purification of Antibodies

Purification of total IgG from serum can be performed by protein A affinity chromatography using commercially available columns (e.g., Bio-Rad or Pharmacia) following the manufacturer's instructions or IgG using caprylic acid precipitation of serum proteins as described below in **Subheading 3.6.4.**

3.6.4. Purification of Total IgG From Serum by Caprylic Acid

1. Dilute 10 mL serum with 2 vol of 60 m*M* sodium acetate, pH 4.0. Stirring continuously, slowly add caprylic acid (Sigma) to a final concentration of 2.5%. Stir rapidly for a further 30 min.
2. Remove precipitated serum proteins by centrifugation at 2000*g* for 20 min at room temperature.
3. Recover the supernatant containing the IgG, filter through Whatman Grade 4 paper to remove particulate material, and dialyze overnight at 4°C against 2 L of 1X PBS.
4. Quantify IgG by UV spectrometry (1 mg/mL IgG gives 1.4 AU at ~275 nm in a 1-cm cuvette).

3.6.5. Antibody Purification

Specific antibodies are purified by affinity chromatography. Columns are most conveniently made using appropriately modified peptides synthesized on controlled pore glass (CPG) beads (Alta BioScience). Alternatively, partially acetylated histones are coupled to commercial resins (e.g., Bio-Rad Affi-Gel) following the manufacturer's instructions or to derivatized acrylamide resins *(22)*.

The method outlined below has been used for the purification of antitetraacetyl H4 antibodies. It should be generally applicable, although the elution buffer should be adjusted depending on the affinity of the particular antibody.

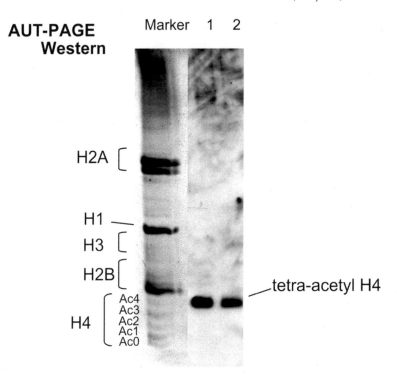

Fig. 3. Acid/urea/Triton X-100 polyacrylamide gel electrophoresis (AUT-PAGE) Western blot characterization of affinity-purified antitetraacetyl H4 antibody. Loading of total histone 60 µg and 30 µg from butyrate-treated HeLa cells as separated by AUT-PAGE. The histone marker lane was cut from the gel and stained with 0.1% Coomassie blue. Lanes 1 and 2: 30 µg and 15 µg, respectively, of histones extracted from butyrate-treated HeLa cells transferred onto nitrocellulose membrane. The membrane was probed with 200 ng/mL of affinity-purified antitetraacetyl H4 antibody and visualized using ECL (Amersham).

1. Dilute the IgG solution to 1–2 mg/mL and pass it through a 1-mL CPG peptide column with the synthetic peptide. Return the eluent to the top of the column and repeat the passage through the column two to four times.
2. Wash the column with 20 column volumes of 1X PBS.
3. Elute bound antibodies by addition of 3.5 M KSCN in 1-mL aliquots.
4. Immediately desalt the eluted antibodies using a 1.5×75-cm G25 column equilibrated with 10 mM sodium bicarbonate at 1 mL/min, collecting 8-mL fractions. Monitor the eluent continuously at 280 nm. Pool fractions containing antibody, which elutes at the void volume of the column.
5. Quantify the affinity-purified antibody by its UV absorbance, aliquot into 50-µg amounts, and lyophilize.
6. Characterize the affinity-purified antibody using enzyme-linked (ELISA) or Western blotting (*see* **Fig. 3**).

3.6.6. Characterization of Antibodies

Antibody titers in immunized animals are monitored by ELISA, and specificity is assessed by Western blotting using standard protocols.

3.7. Native Chromatin Immunoprecipitation (nChIP)

Different methodologies have been developed for nChIPs depending on the scale of the experiment. If quantities of chromatin and affinity-purified antibody are not limiting, the large-scale method allows recovered DNA to be quantified by UV spectroscopy. Proteins of the immunoselected (bound) fraction can also be analyzed to check that the antibody has enriched the modified histone. The smaller scale experiment can be used when chromatin or antibody is limited and is suitable when antibody is available only as serum.

3.7.1. Large-Scale ChIP Affinity Purified Antibody

In a large-scale nChIP we mix 100 µg of affinity-purified antibody with 400 µg of chromatin. Typically, sufficient bound chromatin is recovered from the immunoprecipitate to allow direct analysis of the histones by Coomassie-stained PAGE.

1. Remove sucrose from the chromatin using an Econo-column 10DG desalting column (Bio-Rad) equilibrated with nChIP buffer.
2. Reduce the volume of the chromatin to approx 700 µL in an Amicon C30 or C50 centricon concentrator.
3. Dissolve the freeze-dried antibody in 100 µL of nChIP buffer.
4. Mix the chromatin and antibody and incubate at 4°C for 2 h, rolling end over end.
5. Immobilize immunocomplexes by the addition of 50 mg protein A Sepharose, preswollen and washed twice in nChIP buffer. Incubate for 1 h at 4°C, rolling end over end.
6. Pellet the resin by centrifugation at 1300*g*, for 2 min. Retain the unbound supernatant fraction and add SDS to a final concentration of 0.5%.
7. Wash the resin with 1-mL aliquots of nChIP buffer five times by repeated suspension and centrifugation.
8. Release the bound material, by resuspending the resin pellet in 150 µL of nChIP elution buffer (contains 1.5% SDS) and incubate for 15 min at room temperature.
9. Pellet the resin and retain the supernatant (the bound fraction). Resuspend the resin in a further 150 µL of incubation buffer containing 0.5% SDS, centrifuge, and combine the supernatant with that recovered earlier.

Proteins and DNA are recovered from the input, unbound, and bound fractions by phenol/chloroform extraction. DNA is recovered in the normal way from the aqueous phase, and proteins are recovered by acetone precipitation from the phenol/chloroform phase.

10. Extract the input, unbound, and bound fractions using an equal volume of phenol/chloroform. Recover the DNA from the aqueous phase by ethanol precipitation following standard procedures.
11. Recover the proteins from the phenol/chloroform phase by the addition of 1/100th the volume of conc. HCl and NaCl to 100 mM followed by 12 vol of acetone. Mix and leave overnight at –20°C to precipitate the proteins.
12. Recover the proteins by centrifugation (2000g for 10 min) and transfer the pellets to 1.5-mL tubes by resuspending in freshly made acetone/100 mM HCl (9:1). Spin at 13,000g for 30 s and discard the supernatant. Resuspend the pellet in a further 1 mL of acetone/100 mM HCl and recentrifuge.
13. Wash the pellet in 1-mL aliquots of acetone three times by repeated suspension and centrifugation.
14. Vacuum-dry the pellets and analyze their protein content by PAGE.

Figure 4 shows acid/urea/Triton X-100 (AUT) PAGE analysis of histones recovered from ChIPs of chicken erythrocyte and human chromatin; a significant enrichment in acetylated histones in the fraction bound by the antibodies is seen.

3.7.2. Immunoprecipitation: Small-Scale ChIP Serum

For this type of nChIP the IgG fraction of the antibodies within the serum are first bound to protein A Sepharose, which is then mixed with the chromatin to perform the immunoprecipitation. Since antibody titers of different sera vary considerably it is important to optimize the serum and chromatin levels (*see* **Note 2**). As a guide, we use 20 µL of pan antiacetyl lysine serum to fractionate 15 µg of sucrose gradient-purified mono-/dinucleosomes (measured as DNA).

1. For each fractionation, dilute 20 µL of serum in 0.5 mL nChIP buffer. Add 100 mL of protein A Sepharose (50% suspension in nChIP buffer) and roll for 1 h at 4°C. Centrifuge at 6500g for 2 min and wash the resin-IgG three times in the same buffer to remove serum proteins.
2. Dilute 30 µg of chromatin in 400 µL of nChIP buffer. Divide the sample in half. Use one portion for the nChIP experiment and retain the other as the "input" fraction.
3. Adjust the volume of the input to 400 µL with nChIP buffer and leave on ice.
4. Add the chromatin to be fractionated to the resin-IgG, adjust the volume to 400 µL with nChIP buffer, and incubate overnight at 4°C, rolling end over end.
5. Pellet the resin by centrifugation at 6500g for 2 min. Remove and retain the unbound supernatant fraction (~400 µL).
6. Wash the resin pellet with 1-mL aliquots of nChIP buffer five times by repeated suspension and centrifugation.
7. Release the bound material by resuspending the resin pellet in 200 µL of nChIP elution buffer (contains 1.5% SDS) supplemented with 12.5 µg λ DNA (Gibco) to act as carrier. (For real-time PCR analysis, poly IC should be used as a carrier

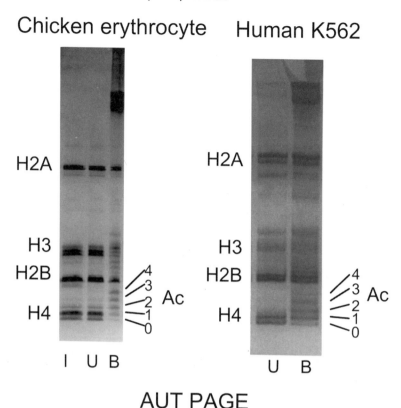

AUT PAGE

Fig. 4. Acid/urea/Triton X-100 polyacrylamide gel electrophoresis (AUT PAGE) analysis of the histones extracted from chicken erythrocyte and human K562 nChIP experiments. Input 8 µg; I) and unbound (U) histones together with *all* the bound (B) fraction from 400-µg scale ChIP were analyzed. Proteins were stained with Coomassie brilliant blue.

as λ DNA interferes with the TaqMan probe.) Incubate for 15 min at room temperature with occasional agitation.

8. Pellet the resin and retain the supernatant (bound fraction).
9. Re-extract the resin pellet by resuspension in 200 µL of nChIP buffer containing 0.5% SDS, pellet, and combine the supernatant with that recovered earlier. The procedure outlined above gives three fractions (input, unbound, and bound), each in a volume of 400 µL.
10. Add SDS to the input and unbound fractions to a final concentration of 0.5%.
11. Extract each fraction with an equal volume (400 µL) of phenol/chloroform.
12. Back-extract the phenol/chloroform phases with 100 µL of incubation buffer (no SDS) and combine with the aqueous phases from the first extraction.
13. To avoid DNA losses that can occur in ethanol precipitation, concentrate the samples to 100 µL using Amicon C30 Microcons. Separate equal volumes of

DNA from input, unbound, and bound fractions in an agarose gel prior to Southern blotting.

3.8. DNA Analysis of Immunoprecipitated Chromatin

The sequence content of the various fractions generated from the nChIP procedure can be assessed by hybridization of slot or Southern blots or by quantitative PCR.

3.8.1. Hybridization Analysis: Small- and Large-Scale nChIPs

DNA from the input, unbound, and bound fractions can be slot or Southern blotted onto nylon membranes. For large-scale nChIPs, we quantify the DNA recovered in each fraction and apply equal quantities (typically 0.5–2 μg) onto the membrane using a slot-blot manifold. For small-scale nChIP experiments, in which it is difficult to quantify the amount of DNA in the antibody-bound fraction, we load an equal volume of each fraction onto an agarose gel and then Southern blot it. Filters are probed with radiolabeled sequences corresponding to active and inactive chromatin using standard hybridization procedures. The method for applying the DNA onto the filters is as follows.

3.8.1.1. SLOT-BLOT ANALYSIS

1. Dissolve DNA samples from the nChIP in 0.1X saline sodium citrate (SSC). Estimate concentrations from UV spectra. Dilute 0.5 μg (for chicken) or 2 μg (for human) DNA in 200 μL 0.1X SSC. Add an equal volume of 1 M NaOH, 3 M NaCl.
2. Denature the DNA and hydrolyze any RNA present by incubating for 10 min at 37°C and then at 100°C for 1 min. Briefly centrifuge the samples.
3. Apply the samples to the prewetted nylon filters using a slot-blot manifold.
4. Transfer the membrane to denaturing solution (0.5 M NaOH, 1.5 M NaCl) for 5 min.
5. Transfer the membrane to neutralizing solution (2X SSC) for 1 min.
6. Allow the filter to air-dry on blotting paper before baking at 80°C for 30 min to fix the DNA

3.8.1.2. SOUTHERN BLOT ANALYSIS

1. Separate equal volumes of the concentrated DNA samples from each of the input, unbound, and bound fractions from a small-scale nChIP by agarose gel electrophoreseis.
2. Soak the gel in 200 mL of 0.5 M NaOH, 1.5 M NaCl for 30 min with constant agitation.
3. Southern transfer the DNA to a nylon membrane using 20X SSC.
4. Rinse the membranes in 2X SSC, blot dry, and bake at 80°C for 30 min.

Once applied to the membranes, the DNA is hybridized with [^{32}P] labeled DNA probes using conventional techniques. Filters are washed to a stringency of 10°C below the theoretical melting temperature of the probe. This is achieved by adjusting the SSC concentration in the stringent wash.

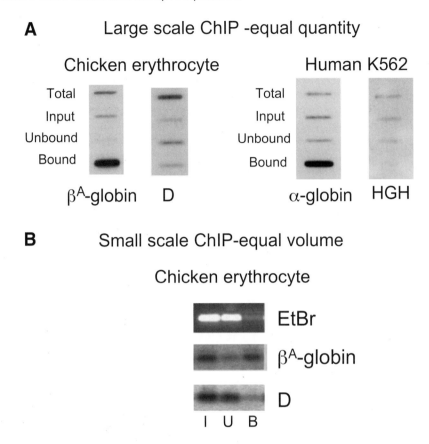

Fig. 5. (A) Slot-blot hybridization of DNA recovered from large-scale nChIPs of chicken erythrocyte mononucleosomes and K562 dinucleosomes immunofractionated with pan antiacetyl-lysine antibodies. Approximately 600 bp of sonicated genomic DNA (Total), Input, Unbound and antibody-Bound samples were blotted onto membranes and hybridized with $[\alpha^{32}P]dCTP$-labeled β^A-globin and a condensed chromatin probe (D) for chicken or α-globin and HGH sequences for K562. **(B)** Southern blot of DNA extracted from small-scale nChIP of chicken erythrocyte mononucleosomes. Chromatin was immunoprecipitated with pan antiacetyl-lysine serum. Equal volumes of the input (I), unbound (U), or antibody-bound (B) DNA were electrophoresed through 1.4% agarose-TBE gels and Southern blotted onto nylon membranes. The figure shows the ethidium bromide-stained gel (EtBr) and phosphorimages of the membranes probed with β^A-globin or a condensed heterochromatin (probe D) sequence.

Examples of each analysis method are shown in **Fig. 5. Figure 5A** shows analysis of a large-scale nChIP using a pan antiacetyl-lysine antibody with chromatin prepared from either 15-d embryonic chicken erythrocytes or human K562 tissue culture cells. Membranes were probed with sequences for active genes in each cell type, the β^A- and α-globin genes. Both show strong hybridization signals in the antibody-bound fractions. In contrast, probes from inactive regions D and HGH, respectively, show little or no enrichment in the bound compared with the input fraction. Hybridization signals can be quantified using a PhosphorImager to calculate enrichments (B/I ratios) achieved by the antibody. **Figure 5B** shows the analysis of a small-scale nChIP. Chromatin from 15-d chicken erythrocytes was immunoprecipitated with pan antiacetyl-lysine serum. Equal volumes of DNA from input, unbound, and antibody-bound fractions were Southern blotted and hybridized with active β^A-globin and inactive D probes. This reveals that the unbound fraction of chromatin is depleted in β^A-globin sequences. In contrast, sequences of the condensed heterochromatin (D) are found largely in the unbound fraction, which is comparable to that of the input. The DNA recovered from the bound fraction contains most of the β^A-globin and little or no D sequences, demonstrating the selectivity of the antibodies for active chromatin.

Using hybridization analysis, the spatial resolution achieved in mapping experiments is determined by the length of the chromatin and probe. If mononucleosomes are used for the ChIP, the resolution is determined by the size of the hybridization probes. To increase the spatial resolution to nucleosomal level, it is necessary to use quantitative PCR with amplicons shorter than the core particle DNA.

3.8.2. Manual Quantitative PCR

Establishing the sequence content of fractions from an nChIP can be achieved by PCR provided the reaction is within the exponential amplification phase. The inclusion of small quantities of α-[^{32}P] labeled dCTP in the PCR reaction allows quantification of the band intensity of PCR products in dried acrylamide gels using a PhosphorImager.

3.8.2.1. Primer Design

Design primers within sequences of interest (~300 bp) using suitable software. Avoid sequences that contain known repeated elements. Amplicons of up to approx 250 bp can be used, although for maximum spatial resolution they should be smaller than the core particle DNA (146 bp). For mapping across the β-globin locus, we used 60–100 bp amplicons with 18–21-bp forward and reverse primers and overall GC content of 45–65%. Sequences with high GC content (e.g., in CpG islands) will require significant alteration of PCR conditions *(6)*. Use a BLAST search (for short nearly exact matches) with the amplicon sequence to check for repeated sequences.

3.8.2.2. Primer Optimization

Optimize PCR conditions for each amplicon so that a single correctly sized product is produced. For the chicken system we optimize using genomic DNA in a final reaction volume of 50 µL as follows:

1. 100 ng Genomic DNA.
2. 0.5 µM Forward and reverse primers.
3. 1.5 mM MgCl$_2$.
4. 200 nM Each of the dATP, dGTP, dCTP, and dTTP, 1 unit of Prozyme DNA polymerase (BIOLINE) using the buffer provided.
5. Amplification conditions: 3-min denaturation at 94°C followed by N cycles of: denaturation (94°C for 1 min), annealing (temperature- and time-adjusted for each primer pair), and extension (72°C for 1 min).
6. Analyze the products in a 3% agarose-TAE gel staining with ethidium bromide.

3.8.2.3. Quantitative PCR

1. Quantify the DNA purified from input, unbound, and bound DNA fractions of the nChIP by UV spectroscopy in 0.1X SSC.
2. Optimize template concentrations for the input, unbound, and bound fractions and the number of cycles (N) for each primer pair so that the products are within the exponential phase of amplification. Include 5 µCi [^{32}P]dCTP in the PCR reaction mixture and analyze by 6–8% PAGE in TBE. Quantify band intensities using a PhosphorImager. Typically, for fractions from embryonic chicken erythrocyte nChIP assays, we use twofold serially diluted input and unbound templates from 8.0–0.5 ng and amplify for 26–28 cycles. Further serial dilution of the bound DNA will be required if high enrichments (possibly up to 50-fold) are obtained (*see* **Fig. 6**).
3. Plot signals from the correctly sized products from the Input (I) and Bound (B) samples as a function of template concentration to check for linearity. Determine the ratio of the slopes of the two plots in the linear region to derive the enrichment achieved by the antibody (calculated as B/I). **Figure 6** illustrates this process for an amplicon located at the 5′ hypersensitive site at the chicken β-globin locus. Results from input and bound templates are shown giving an enrichment of 35-fold. We also routinely amplify the unbound DNA at the same template levels as the input, and this should reveal a depletion compared with input (1.4-fold in this experiment; data not shown).

3.8.3. Quantitative PCR Using Real-Time PCR and TaqMan Probes

Sequence content of DNA from the nChIP fractions are more conveniently and accurately determined by real-time PCR. Several manufacturers produce suitable instruments; we use an Applied Biosystems 7900HT. The method is

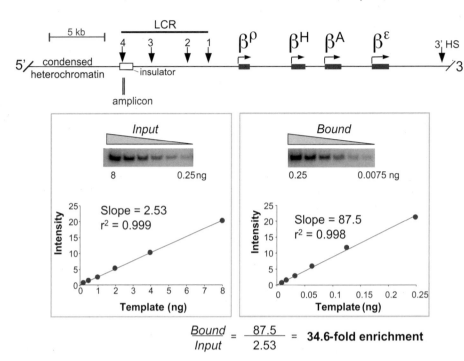

Fig. 6. Manual quantitative PCR analysis of DNA recovered from large-scale nChIP of chicken erythrocyte mononucleosomes fractionated with antihyperacetylated H4 antibodies. Input and bound DNAs were serially diluted (input 8–0.25 ng, bound 0.25–0.0075 ng), and amplified, and products were quantified by phosphorimage analysis of the band intensities shown.

dependent on cleavage of a specifically annealed fluorescently labeled oligo-nucleotide (the TaqMan probe) by the exonuclease activity of the polymerase, resulting in a fluorescent signal. The TaqMan probe, labeled at its 5′ end with a reporter dye (FAM) and a quencher (TAMRA) at its 3′ end, anneals to one of the strands between the forward and reverse primers. As the polymerase extends from the forward primer and reaches the TaqMan probe, it displaces and cleaves nucleotides, releasing FAM from the proximity of the TAMRA quencher and causing an increased fluorescent signal. The accumulation of PCR products is detected and quantified by monitoring the fluorescence increase throughout the PCR.

3.8.3.1. Primer and Probe Design

1. Use Primer Express software to generate primer and TaqMan probes within selected target sequences applying design guidelines as directed by Applied Biosystems. The software selects primer and probe sequences to allow the same reaction conditions and temperature profile to be used for all amplicons. Locate

TaqMan probes as close to the forward primer as possible. Typically, forward and reverse primers are 15–30 bp and have (theoretical) melting temperatures (T_m) of approx 60°C. TaqMan probes are generally longer (~30 bp) and have T_ms 10°C higher than that of the primers. As discussed earlier, use short (60–80 bp) amplicons to give maximal resolution in mapping experiments.

2. Optimize primer and TaqMan probe concentrations to compensate for possible T_m errors using Applied Biosystem's protocols as necessary. For most amplicons tested, the preferred concentration of forward and reverse primers is 900 nM, with a probe concentration of 200 nM.

3. Amplify the templates in a real-time PCR machine using the TaqMan Universal PCR Master Mix protocol (Applied Biosystems) with the following temperature profile: 50°C for 2 min and 95°C for 10 min, followed by 40 cycles of 95°C for 15 s and 60°C for 1 min.

4. For each amplicon, generate standard curves using a twofold serially diluted gDNA template from 100 to 0.36 ng in the reaction mix (90 µL final volume), amplifying 25-µL aliquots in triplicate by real-time PCR.

5. PCR reactions to quantify input, unbound, and bound fractions from the nChIP should be carried out simultaneously in the same plate, also in triplicate. Typically, we use 20 ng of input and unbound DNA (in a 90 µL reaction mix) and separately amplify three 25-µL aliquots. Lower quantities of bound DNA (1–10 ng) may be amplified depending on enrichments.

3.8.3.2. Data Analysis

A detailed description of the analysis of the real-time PCR data is given in Litt et al. *(7)*. Once sufficient cycles have been completed, the fluorescence signal from the TaqMan probe will be above the noise and will increase exponentially (**Fig. 7A**); initially a log amplification plot (log of fluorescence intensity (ΔRn) vs cycle number) is linear (**Fig. 7B**).

As reactants are depleted in later cycles, linearity is lost and the log plot will show a plateau (**Fig. 7B**). Typically, we define baseline noise between 3 and approx 20 cycles and set the threshold above the baseline noise but as low as possible in the linear region of this plot (**Fig. 7B**).

1. Obtain crossing values (Ct) of the fluorescence intensity curves generated from known amounts of serially diluted genomic DNA template (typically 100, 50, 12.5, 3.12, 0.78, and 0.39 ng by serial dilution). These represent the cycle at which a significant increase in fluorescence intensity is first detected. For example, for an amplicon from the β^A-globin promoter, 100 ng of chicken gDNA template gives a Ct value of approx 25 (**Fig. 7B**). Precise Ct values are determined by the Sequence Detection software of the 7900HT.

2. Generate a standard curve for each amplicon by plotting the Ct value vs amount of genomic DNA template (**Fig. 7C**).

3. Obtain the crossing values from known amounts of input, unbound, and bound DNA and hence the sequence content of the particular amplicon from the stan-

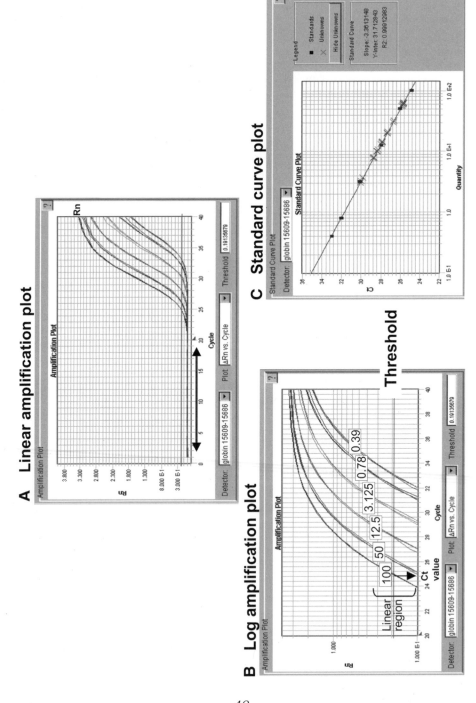

A Linear amplification plot

B Log amplification plot

C Standard curve plot

dard curve, adjusting for the quantity of template. Sequence contents are obtained directly from the sequence analysis software of the 7900HT device.

4. Determine the enrichment of a given target sequence achieved by the antibody by the ratio of the sequence content of the bound to input fractions (B/I). When the bound signal is lower than input, calculate the depletion (I/B). Calculate B/I errors as the sum of the fractional errors obtained for the bound and input samples. Note that the signal from the unbound fraction in **Fig. 8A** is depleted compared with the input fraction.

Figure 8 shows the standard curve and log amplification plots generated from input, unbound, and bound DNA recovered from a tetraacetyl H4 nChIP analyzed for the content of heterochromatin and β^A promoter sequences. Ct values fall within the range of the standards analyzed. For the β^A promoter (**Fig. 8B**), the Ct value of the input DNA is approx 26 and approx 28 for the bound, i.e., about a four-fold difference in sequence content. (One cycle represents a twofold difference in sequence content.) The software calculates the precise target sequence content (B = 59.35 and I = 14.62, giving a ratio of 4.06). The true B/I ratio is calculated by adjusting for the eightfold lower amount of bound DNA template, which gives an enrichment of 32.5-fold achieved by the antibody.

Figure 8A shows that the signal from 20 ng input DNA exceeds that from 10 ng bound DNA for the amplicon in the heterochromatin and gives a depletion of 1.6-fold. Sequence analysis by real-time PCR is more accurate than hybridization or manual quantitative PCR, and such depletions are meaningful. Typical B/I errors obtained from real-tme PCR are about two-fold lower than from manual quantitative PCR, but maps obtained of modified histone distributions are similar.

4. Notes

1. Optimization of the digest conditions is an important and necessary part of the chromatin preparation. This is a two-stage process. In general, we digest the nuclei at a DNA concentration of 5 mg/mL DNA. The first stage is to perform a concentration course digest using MNase over a range of 20–500 U/mL for a fixed time interval at 37°C. At each point, terminate the digest and analyze the DNA from the released chromatin by Southern blot, or quantitativePCR analysis,

---

Fig. 7. *(opposite page)* Standard curve generation in real-time PCR analysis of an amplicon from the chicken β^A-globin promoter with a gDNA template. Amplifications were performed in triplicate using serially diluted gDNA. (**A**) Linear amplification plot (cycle no. against Rn [fluorescence signal]) with the baseline defined from 3 to 20 cycles (double-headed arrow). (**B**) Log amplification plot (cycle no. against log Rn) with the threshold adjusted to 0.19 from which Ct values for the standards are defined. (**C**) Standard curve (Ct values against template amount).

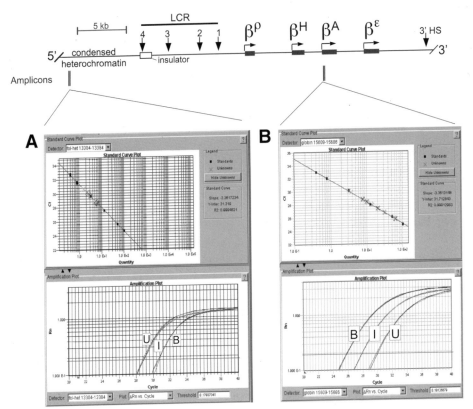

Fig. 8. Standard curve and log amplification plots from real-time PCR analysis of input unbound and bound fractions from an antitetraacetyl H4 nChIP performed with 15-d embryo erythrocyte mononucleosomes using TaqMan probes. **(A)** An amplicon from heterochromatin approx 7 kbp upstream of the β-globin locus; 20 ng of input and unbound was analyzed with 10 ng of bound. A depletion in the bound is observed by its lower *C*t value compared with the input (approximately two cycles). **(B)** An amplicon from the β^A-globin promoter (20 ng input and unbound DNA) was amplified alongside 2.5 ng of bound DNA. Enrichments are calculated as the B/I ratio. Adjusting the B/I ratio calculated from the software (4.06) to compensate for the eightfold lower amount of bound DNA reveals a 32.5-fold enrichment of this sequence in the bound fraction.

testing the representation of sequences from active and inactive chromatin regions. Southern blots can be helpful in that they show the size class of the released chromatin. After the enzyme level is determined the second stage is to perform a time-course digestion and analyze in the same way. The combination of time and concentration courses should identify suitable digest conditions for a particular system. It may also be necessary to alter the nuclei concentration and/or the temperature of digestion to maximize recovery of some sequences.

Chromatin regions that are either particularly susceptible, or indeed resistant, to MNase can be recovered by performing a number of separate digests, optimizing for each sequence as outlined above. Mononucleosomes from such digests can be isolated by centrifugation through sucrose gradients and pooled to obtain an input chromatin that contains a good representation of both susceptible and resistant sequence classes.

2. As titers of antibody vary in different batches of sera in the small-scale nChIP, it is important to optimize amounts of serum and chromatin used. Perform a series of nChIP experiments reducing the quantity of chromatin and keeping the serum levels constant. As the chromatin level is reduced, the relative proportion of active chromatin precipitated by the antibody will increase and deplete active sequences from the unbound DNA. Using this approach with a pan antiacetyl-lysine serum, it is possible to precipitate >60% of active chromatin sequences while leaving the inactive chromatin in the unbound fraction.

Acknowledgments

The authors would like to thank D. Evans, A. Pelling, and W. Chong for illustrative data. This work was supported by the Wellcome Trust and BBSRC.

References

1. Dorbic, T. and Wittig, B. (1986) Isolation of oligonucleosomes from active chromatin using HMG17-specific monoclonal antibodies. *Nucleic Acids Res.* **14,** 3363–3376.
2. Dorbic, T. and Wittig, B. (1987) Chromatin from transcribed genes contains HMG17 only downstream from the starting point of transcription. *EMBO J.* **6,** 2393–2399.
3. Hebbes, T. R., Thorne, A. W., and Crane-Robinson, C. (1988) A direct link between core histone acetylation and transcriptionally active chromatin. *EMBO J.* **7,** 1395–1402.
4. Hebbes, T. R., Thorne, A. W., Clayton, A. L., and Crane-Robinson, C. (1992) Histone acetylation and globin gene switching. *Nucleic Acids Res.* **20,** 1017–1022.
5. Hebbes, T. R., Clayton, A. L., Thorne, A. W., and Crane-Robinson, C. (1994) Core histone hyperacetylation co-maps with generalized DNase I sensitivity in the chicken beta-globin chromosomal domain. *EMBO J.* **13,** 1823–1830.
6. Myers, F. A., Evans, D. R., Clayton, A. L., Thorne, A. W., and Crane-Robinson, C. (2001) Targeted and extended acetylation of histones H4 and H3 at active and inactive genes in chicken embryo erythrocytes. *J. Biol. Chem.* **276,** 20,197–20,205.
7. Litt, M. D., Simpson, M., Recillas-Targa, F., Prioleau, M. N., and Felsenfeld, G. (2001). Transitions in histone acetylation reveal boundaries of three separately regulated neighboring loci. *EMBO J.* **20,** 2224–2235.
8. Litt, M. D., Simpson, M., Gaszner, M., Allis, C. D., and Felsenfeld, G. (2001). Correlation between histone lysine methylation and developmental changes at the chicken beta-globin locus. *Science* **293,** 2453–2455.

9. Madisen, L., Krumm, A., Hebbes, T. R., and Groudine, M. (1998). The immuno-globulin heavy chain locus control region increases histone acetylation along linked c-myc genes. *Mol. Cell Biol.* **18,** 6281–6292.

10. Clayton, A. L., Hebbes, T. R., Thorne, A. W., and Crane-Robinson, C. (1993). Histone acetylation and gene induction in human cells. *FEBS Lett.* **336,** 23–26.

11. Pelling, A. L., Thorne, A. W., and Crane-Robinson, C. (2000). A human genomic library enriched in transcriptionally active sequences (aDNA library). *Genome Res.* **10,** 874–886.

12. O'Neill, L. P., Keohane, A. M., Lavender, J. S., et al. (1999). A developmental switch in H4 acetylation upstream of Xist plays a role in X chromosome inactivation. *EMBO J.* **18,** 2897–2907.

13. Elefant, F., Cooke, N. E., and Liebhaber, S. A. (2000). Targeted recruitment of histone acetyltransferase activity to a locus control region. *J. Biol. Chem.* **275,** 13,827–13,834.

14. Elefant, F., Su, Y., Liebhaber, S. A., and Cooke, N. E. (2000). Patterns of histone acetylation suggest dual pathways for gene activation by a bifunctional locus control region. *EMBO J.* **19,** 6814–6822.

15. Hewish, D. R. and Burgoyne, L. A. (1973). Chromatin sub-structure. The digestion of chromatin DNA at regularly spaced sites by a nuclear deoxyribonuclease. *Biochem. Biophys. Res. Commun.* **52,** 504–510.

16. Ridsdale, J. A. and Davie, J. R. (1987). Chicken erythrocyte polynucleosomes which are soluble at physiological ionic strength and contain linker histones are highly enriched in beta-globin gene sequences. *Nucleic Acids Res.* **15,** 1081–1096.

17. Ridsdale, J. A. and Davie, J. R. (1987). Selective solubilization of beta-globin oligonucleosomes at low ionic strength. *Biochemistry* **26,** 290–295.

18. Sung, M. T. and Dixon, G. H. (1970). Modification of histones during spermiogenesis in trout: a molecular mechanism for altering histone binding to DNA. *Proc. Natl. Acad. Sci. USA* **67,** 1616–1623.

19. Wood, W. I. and Felsenfeld, G. (1982). Chromatin structure of the chicken beta-globin gene region. Sensitivity to DNase I, micrococcal nuclease, and DNase II. *J. Biol. Chem.* **257,** 7730–7736.

20. Stratling, W. H., Dolle, A., and Sippel, A. E. (1986). Chromatin structure of the chicken lysozyme gene domain as determined by chromatin fractionation and micrococcal nuclease digestion. *Biochemistry* **25,** 495–502.

21. Leuba, S. H., Zlatanova, J., and van Holde, K. (1994). On the location of linker DNA in the chromatin fiber. Studies with immobilized and soluble micrococcal nuclease. *J. Mol. Biol.* **235,** 871–880.

22. Hebbes, T. R., Turner, C. H., Thorne, A. W., and Crane-Robinson, C. (1989). A "minimal epitope" anti-protein antibody that recognises a single modified amino acid. *Mol. Immunol.* **26,** 865–873.

4

Q-PCR in Combination With ChIP Assays to Detect Changes in Chromatin Acetylation

Ryan A. Irvine and Chih-Lin Hsieh

Summary

Quantitative polymerase chain reaction (Q-PCR) allows for the accurate and reproducible determination of the amount of target DNA in a sample through the measurement of PCR product accumulation in "real time." This method determines starting target DNA quantity over a large assay dynamic range and requires no post-PCR sample manipulation. When used in combination with the method of chromatin immunoprecipitation (ChIP), the amount of protein binding to a specific region of DNA can be accurately and rapidly determined. A method for quantifying the presence of acetylated histones H3 and H4 on different regions of a target locus using Q-PCR after ChIP is described.

Key Words: Quantitative PCR; chromatin immunoprecipitation; histone acetylation; and chromatin structure.

1. Introduction

This chapter details a method for using quantitative polymerase chain reaction (Q-PCR) in combination with chromatin immunoprecipitation (ChIP) to determine the extent of histone acetylation at discrete regions of nucleosomal DNA. This method was used in a recent study assessing the impact of DNA methylation on gene transcription and local chromatin structure (1). In that study, it was shown that although acetylated histones are largely absent from patches of methylated DNA, they are strongly associated with adjacent unmethylated DNA regions within the same gene. Although the described method was optimized for the analysis of DNA sequences on a replicating episome in human cells, it is generally applicable to the analysis of genomic loci.

The ChIP technique provides a powerful in vivo tool for detecting protein-DNA interactions through formaldehyde crosslinking of proteins to DNA, fol-

From: *Methods in Molecular Biology, vol. 287: Epigenetics Protocols*
Edited by: T. O. Tollefsbol © Humana Press Inc., Totowa, NJ

lowed by immunoprecipitation with specific antibodies (*see* Chapter 1 and **ref. 2**). Theoretically, any protein and its in vivo binding site can be directly detected by this technique. After immunoprecipitation of crosslinked chromatin, the formaldehyde crosslinks are reversed and the DNA is purified. Determination of the amount of immunoprecipitated DNA from a specific genomic or extrachromosomal region by Q-PCR provides a direct assessment of the frequency of protein association with that region. In this way, not only can a detailed "map" of protein binding to a particular gene or region be generated, but the relative amount of protein binding among different samples can also be assessed.

In addition to its application to ChIP, Q-PCR has been used successfully to quantify gene expression, gene copy number, viral load, and minimal residual disease in cancer patients *(3,4)*. The Q-PCR strategy used in the described method employs a dual-labeled fluorescent TaqMan probe that anneals to the target sequence within the PCR amplicon *(5)*. During the extension phase of PCR, the 5′ exonuclease activity of *Taq* polymerase cleaves the probe, liberating the 5′-fluorescent reporter molecule from the linked 3′-quencher moiety. With successive rounds of PCR amplification, the reporter fluorescence in the reaction increases. This change in fluorescent emission over time (or cycle number) is detected and measured by a charge-coupled device (CCD) camera equipped with filters that absorb light at the appropriate wavelength. Importantly, during the exponential phase of PCR amplification, a linear relationship exists between the log of the amount of starting template DNA and the cycle at which the reporter fluorescence significantly exceeds background levels (i.e., the threshold cycle). Consequently, using a standard curve of known amounts of the target sequence (e.g., a dilution series of a plasmid that contains the sequence), the quantity of target DNA in an unknown sample can be accurately determined from its threshold cycle.

Q-PCR is a highly reproducible and sensitive technique that offers clear advantages over traditional PCR, semiquantitative PCR, and Southern blotting methods. Traditional PCR is not quantitative and is primarily used for endpoint analysis by assaying the amplified product from the "plateau phase" of the reaction. By amplifying a dilution series of template DNA over a limited number of cycles, some degree of quantification has been achieved with so-called semiquantitative PCR. Q-PCR, on the other hand, provides a direct measurement of amplified product at every PCR cycle and therefore ensures that template quantification occurs during the exponential phase of the reaction. Q-PCR, furthermore, requires no postamplification handling of the reaction products. Southern blotting is another method that provides semiquantification of target DNA, although it is generally less preferable than the PCR methods owing to the relatively large amounts of starting material that are required.

2. Materials

2.1. Chromatin Immunoprecipitation

1. Phosphate buffered saline (PBS), pH 7.2.
2. Dulbecco's modified Eagle's medium (DMEM) containing 10% fetal bovine serum and hygromycin (200 μg/mL).
3. Trypsin/EDTA solution: 0.5 g trypsin, 0.2 g EDTA per liter (Irvine Scientific, cat. no. 9340).
4. TE: 10 mM Tris-HCl, 1 mM EDTA, pH 8.0.
5. 37% Formaldehyde solution (JT Baker, cat. no. 2106-02).
6. 10% Sodium dodecyl sulfate (SDS).
7. Radioimmunoprecipitation assay (RIPA) buffer: 10 mM sodium phosphate, pH 7.2, 2 mM EDTA, 150 mM NaCl, 50 mM NaF, 0.2 mM Na$_3$OV$_4$, 1% sodium deoxycholate, 1% Nonidet P40, 0.1% SDS. RIPA buffer is stable for up to 1 y at 4°C. The sodium orthovanadate should be added immediately before use from a 0.2 M stock solution.
8. Mammalian protease inhibitor cocktail tablets (Roche, cat. no. 1836170). One tablet is dissolved in 10 mL of RIPA buffer or PBS immediately before use.
9. Antiacetyl-histone H3/H4 antibodies (Upstate Biotechnology, cat. nos. 06-599 and 06-598).
10. 10 mg/mL salmon sperm DNA (Gibco-BRL, cat. no. 15632-011).
11. Protein G Sepharose (Amersham Biosciences, cat. no. 17-0618-03). The Sepharose beads are equilibrated in TE, pH 8.0, through repeated washing steps. A final 50% (v/v) slurry is prepared for use.
12. Proteinase K (Roche, cat. no. 1092766). A 20 mg/mL stock solution is prepared in H$_2$O.
13. Elution buffer: 0.1 M NaHCO$_3$, 1% SDS.
14. 3 M Sodium acetate, pH 5.2.
15. 20mg/mL glycogen (Roche, cat. no. 901393).
16. Phenol (TE, pH 8.0 buffered, saturated).
17. Chloroform.

2.2. Quantitative PCR

1. 10X PCR buffer: 150 mM Tris-HCl, pH 8.0, 500 mM KCl.
2. 10X PCR stabilizer: 0.5% gelatin, 0.1% Tween-20.
3. 40% Glycerol solution.
4. 350 mM MgCl$_2$ stock solution.
5. 2.5 mM Deoxyribonucleotide triphosphate (dNTP) mix.
6. AmpliTaq Gold DNA polymerase (PE Applied Biosystems, cat. no. 4311816).
7. Fluorophore-labeled TaqMan probe (5'-FAM [6-carboxyfluorescein] labeled, 3'-Black Hole Quencher [BHQ]-1 labeled; Biosearch Technologies. Fluorogenic probes are dissolved in H$_2$O or TE, stored at –20°C, and protected from direct light exposure.
8. Oligonucleotide primers (Operon Technologies).

3. Methods

3.1. Chromatin Immunoprecipitation

This ChIP protocol is derived from previously published methods (6,7).

1. Grow human 293/EBNA1 cells (a human embryonic kidney carcinoma cell line that expresses the viral replication factor EBNA1 [8]) transfected with replicating episomes, in DMEM that contains 10% FBS and 200 μg/mL hygromycin.
2. Wash exponentially growing cultures that are 70–80% confluent (approx 3×10^6 cells per 10-cm dish; see **Note 1**) once with warm PBS and then trypsinize with 1 mL trypsin/EDTA solution for 10 min at room temperature (RT).
3. To neutralize the trypsin, add 3 mL of media to the dish and transfer the resulting 4-mL cell suspension to a 14-mL culture tube (Applied Scientific, cat. no. AS-2263).
4. To fix the cells, add 108 μL of 37% formaldehyde solution to the cell suspension (i.e., 1% working concentration) followed by gentle rotory mixing for exactly 10 min at RT (see **Note 2**).
5. Collect fixed cells by centrifugation at 2000g in a Beckman GS-6KR swinging bucket centrifuge) for 5 min at 4°C.
6. Resuspend the cell pellet in 4 mL of ice-cold PBS and collect by centrifugation as in **step 5**.
7. Repeat **step 6**.
8. Following complete removal of the second PBS wash, snap freeze the cell pellet in liquid nitrogen and store at –80°C until use (see **Note 3**).
9. Thaw the cell pellet on ice, thoroughly resuspend in 1 mL of RIPA buffer that contains mammalian protease inhibitors, and transfer to a 1.9-mL Eppendorf tube.
10. Perform sonication with a Branson Sonifier 450, equipped with a microtip, using an output power setting of 5 and a constant duty cycle (i.e., 100%). Subject the cell suspension to 20 consecutive 10-s bursts with cooling on a dry ice/ethanol bath between each sonication event. The cell lysate must be kept cool throughout the sonication procedure, as high temperatures can denature proteins. It cannot be overstated that the sonication regimen is critical to the success of the ChIP technique and must be empirically determined for each study (see **Note 4**). In our hands, this procedure produces average chromatin fragment sizes of about 1 kb or less for 293/EBNA1 cells fixed in 1% formaldehyde for 10 min at RT.
11. Following sonication, centrifuge the lysate at 16,000g in a microcentrifuge for 15 min at 4°C to pellet insoluble material. The supernatant is the soluble chromatin sample.
12. Remove a 50 μL aliquot of the soluble chromatin, mix with 50 μL TE, and store as the total chromatin fraction (TCF) at –20°C until use (see **step 23**).
13. Divide the remainder of the soluble chromatin sample into two 475-μL fractions in 1.9-mL Eppendorf tubes on ice: fraction 1, antiacetyl H3/H4 and fraction 2, no antibody (Ab).
14. To the antiacetyl H3/H4 tube only, add 5 μg each of antiacetylated histone H3 and antiacetylated histone H4 IgG. Add nothing to the no-Ab tube.
15. Incubate both tubes for 5 h at 4°C with gentle rotory mixing.

16. To both tubes, add 40 μg of sheared salmon sperm DNA and 100 μL of the 50% slurry of protein G Sepharose (prepared in TE).
17. Incubate the samples overnight at 4°C with mixing as before.
18. Collect the Sepharose beads by centrifugation at 2000g in a microcentrifuge for 2 min at 4°C, and then transfer the unbound soluble chromatin to a new tube and store at –20°C.
19. Wash the Sepharose beads sequentially for 10 min each at 4°C, once with 0.5 mL of ice-cold RIPA buffer and twice with 0.5 mL of ice-cold PBS. Both the RIPA buffer and PBS should contain protease inhibitors.
20. Elute immunocomplexes from the protein G Sepharose in 0.5 mL of elution buffer by incubation for 30 min at RT with rotory mixing.
21. To each eluate, add 25 μL of 5 M NaCl and then incubate at 65°C for 5 h to reverse the formaldehyde crosslinks.
22. Ethanol-precipitate the released DNA, wash with 70% ethanol, and dissolve the DNA pellet in 100 μL TE.
23. To the 100 μL antiacetyl H3/H4, no Ab, and TCF (*see* **step 12**) samples, add 10 μL of 10% SDS and 2.5 μL of proteinase K solution (20 μg/mL), and then incubate at 55°C for 2 h.
24. Extract the samples with 1 vol of phenol/chloroform (1:1), ethanol-precipitate the DNA in the presence of 20 μg of glycogen, wash with 70% ethanol, and dissolve in 50 μL TE.

3.2. Quantitative PCR

1. Design TaqMan probes and primers using the Primer Express (v 1.5) software package from PE Applied Biosystems. This program facilitates the selection of probe/primer sets that result in high-efficiency target amplification using a simple two-step cycling program. In general, a TaqMan probe should be selected that is less than 40 nucleotides in length, has a G/C content in the 20–80% range, has a melting temperature (T_m) near 70°C that is 8–10°C higher than the primers, has no runs of four or more of an identical nucleotide (especially G), and does not have a G at the 5′ end. Primers should be 10–20 nucleotides in length and designed as close as possible to the probe without overlapping it so that the amplicon is between 50 and 150 bp in size. Small amplicon size serves to maximize PCR efficiency. In addition, to avoid nonspecific amplification, primers should not be rich in G and/or C bases at their 3′ ends. A general guideline is that primers should not have more than two G and/or C bases in the last five nucleotides at the 3′ end. All TaqMan probes used in our studies were synthesized with a 5′-FAM reporter fluorophore and a 3′-BHQ-1 quencher (Biosearch Technologies). All primers were synthesized by Operon Technologies.
2. Amplify ChIP DNA samples (*see* **Subheading 3.1.** above) in 25 μL reactions that contain 1 μL of DNA template (*see* **Note 5**), 15 mM Tris-HCl, pH 8.0, 50 mM KCl, 3.5 mM MgCl$_2$, 200 μM dNTPs, 0.05% gelatin, 0.01% Tween-20, 8% glycerol, 50 nM TaqMan probe, 300 nM of each primer, and 1 U of AmpliTaq Gold DNA polymerase (*see* **Note 6**). Prepare reactions at RT in iCycler iQ PCR 96-

well plates (Bio-Rad, cat. no. 223-9441) and then seal them with iCycler iQ Optical Quality Sealing Tape (Bio-Rad, cat. no. 223-9444). Perform PCR cycling and fluorescence detection with a Bio-Rad iCycler using the following two-step program after an initial 10-min incubation at 95°C to activate the polymerase: 95°C for 15 s and 60°C for 1 min for 40 cycles. In general, the PCR conditions and cycling parameters listed here produced high-efficiency amplification of the target DNA sequences used in our studies. It should be recognized, however, that probe and primer concentrations might need to be optimized for the efficient amplification of other target sequences (*see* **Note 7**).

3. To quantify the amount of target DNA in a given ChIP sample, simultaneously amplify a standard curve consisting of titrations of a known amount of the target sequence on the same Q-PCR plate. A fivefold dilution series of the 12-kb pCLH22 episome, from 100 to 0.00128 pg, served as the standard curve in our experiments *(1)*. This range of input target DNA is compatible with the known dynamic range of linear response for the iCycler. The efficiency of a particular Q-PCR reaction is inferred from the slope of the standard curve graph (log of input DNA [pg] vs threshold cycle) generated by the iCycler (v 2.3) software package. Q-PCR reactions with standard curve slopes of –3.0 to –3.7 were arbitrarily accepted for our experiments (a slope of –3.32 indicates 100% efficiency). Standard curve slopes outside of this range are indicative of either inefficient Q-PCR reactions or of reactions generating substantial nonspecific products, both of which must be optimized before continuing with ChIP sample analysis. It should be stated that some Q-PCR applications may require more stringent efficiency parameters (e.g., absolute mRNA quantification via reverse-transcriptase Q-PCR). The standard curve is a critical feature of Q-PCR as the amount of DNA in all unknown samples is extrapolated from it. Therefore, it must be empirically validated before reliable quantitative results can be attained.

4. Perform all Q-PCR reactions (unknown ChIP samples and standards) in duplicate and use mean quantities for all subsequent data analyses. The fraction of immunoprecipitated DNA was calculated by subtracting the amount of DNA in the no-Ab control from that in the antiacetyl H3/H4 sample and dividing by the amount of DNA in the corresponding TCF sample. Using this calculation, we determined the amount of acetylated histones H3 and H4 that were associated with different regions of the pCLH22 episome in 293/EBNA1 cells.

4. Notes

1. For our experiments, the target DNA sequences for immunoprecipitation (IP) were on episomes that were maintained at 10–100 copies per cell. Therefore, the sensitivity of target DNA detection in our assays was greater than that for standard ChIP experiments, in which targets are endogenous genomic sequences with two copies per cell. Consequently, only about 3×10^6 cells were required for each IP described here, compared with approx 10^8 cells recommended for other ChIP strategies (e.g., **ref. 9**).

2. It is our experience that the duration of formaldehyde fixation is a critical parameter of this technique. Modest variations in fixation times can have a significant,

negative impact on assay reproducibility. Thus, once a fixation time has been validated for a particular cell type and ChIP experiment, it should be used consistently. In general, crosslinking times of 10 min or less are suitable for ChIP analyses of nucleosomal proteins; longer times (i.e., 30 min to 1 h) may be required for other DNA binding factors. It should be mentioned that in the study of histone modifications, some protocols omit the formaldehyde crosslinking step, using native chromatin directly for IP. This is a reasonable variation of the ChIP protocol in this context, as core histones are tightly bound to DNA. The potential advantages of skipping the crosslinking step include shorter processing times and the avoidance of epitope masking by formaldehyde crosslinks, which can result in suboptimal IP efficiency. The potential disadvantages of skipping the crosslinking step, however, include lowered IP efficiency owing to potentially significant core histone dissociation from target chromatin. In the study of DNA binding proteins other than core histones, formaldehyde fixation is almost always required.

3. Usually, several dishes of cells are collected simultaneously for a single ChIP experiment. Thus, freezing and storing the fixed cell pellets at this step in the protocol may be convenient. We have noticed no negative impact on results by freezing the fixed pellets, although the protocol can be continued without this step.

4. The reproducible fragmentation of formaldehyde crosslinked chromatin into approx 500–1000-bp fragments by sonication depends on several factors including, the type of sonicator, the cell type used in the experiment, and the duration of formaldehyde crosslinking. The fixation and sonication parameters detailed above should be used only as a starting point for new ChIP experiments. It is highly recommended that a formaldehyde fixation time course be run and that the intensity and duration of sonication be fully investigated with each new ChIP assay. A small amount of soluble chromatin should be electrophoresed on a 1% agarose gel to assess chromatin fragment size after sonication.

5. Theoretically, 1 μL of a given TCF sample contains about 36 ng of genomic DNA (i.e., [3×10^6 cells][12 pg genomic DNA per tetraploid human 293/EBNA1 cell][1/20 total sample volume] = 18×10^5 pg DNA per 50 μL TCF sample). For an autosomal target gene, 36 ng of genomic DNA contains about 12,000 gene copies (i.e., 4 copies per tetraploid genome or 12 pg). For our experiments, target genes were on replicating episomes, which were maintained at high, although variable copy numbers in 293/EBNA1 cells. On average, 35 pg (i.e., 2.6×10^6 copies; nearly 90 copies/cell) of target DNA were detected in 1 μL of a given TCF sample. Immunoprecipitations are carried out on 475 μL (47.5%) of the total DNA sample (i.e., about 17 μg of genomic DNA). Again, for an autosomal target gene, 17 μg of genomic DNA contains about 5.7×10^6 gene copies. Assuming 100% IP efficiency and a 150-bp target PCR amplicon, about 0.85 pg of target DNA should be obtained in a given antiacetyl H3/H4 sample. For our experiments, 0.1–5 pg of target DNA (i.e., 1.4×10^5 copies on average; nearly 5 copies/cell) were detected in 1 μL of each antiacetyl H3/H4 sample, depending on the histone acetylation status of the episomal target gene. Background levels of target DNA, detected in the no-Ab control samples, were routinely 10–100-fold

lower than experimental values. Obviously, the histone acetylation status of the target chromatin largely determines the background level. Thus, if the target gene contains mostly deacetylated histones, background and experimental values will be similar. Finally, since we were detecting different target genes on episomes maintained at different copy numbers within cells, it was important to verify that IP efficiencies were similar across ChIP samples (*1*). This was achieved by quantifying the amount of an endogenous target locus (i.e., XRCC1) in all samples.

6. We prefer to make and use our own PCR reaction buffer. Certainly, the 10X PCR Gold Buffer (cat. no. L0026-01) provided by PE Applied Biosystems for use with AmpliTaq Gold DNA polymerase can also be used.

7. PE Applied Biosystems recommends varying probe and primer concentrations within the 50–250-nM and 50–900-nM ranges, respectively, to optimize Q-PCR efficiencies (resources available at appliedbiosystems.com). As with all other quantitative assays, reactions need to be set up in a consistent manner in order to maximize accuracy and reproducibility. Although the detection system allows for the precise measurement of the amplified product, it cannot overcome manual errors introduced into the reaction during setup.

References

1. Irvine, R. A. and Hsieh, C.-L. (2002) DNA methylation has a local effect on transcription and histone acetylation. *Mol. Cell. Biol.* **22,** 6689–6696.
2. Orlando, V. (2000) Mapping chromosomal proteins in vivo by formaldehyde-crosslinked-chromatin immunoprecipitation. *Trends Biochem. Sci.* **25,** 99–104.
3. Ginzinger, D. G. (2002) Gene quantification using real-time quantitative PCR: An emerging technology hits the mainstream. *Exp. Hematology* **30,** 503–512.
4. Stevens, S. J., Verschuuren, E. A., Pronk, I., van Der Bij, W., Harmsen, M. C., The, T. H., Meijer, C. J., van Den Brule, A. J., and Middeldorp, J., M. (2001) Frequent monitoring of Epstein-Barr virus DNA load in unfractionated whole blood is essential for early detection of posttransplant lymphoproliferative disease in high-risk patients. *Blood* **97,** 1165–1171.
5. Heid, C. A., Stevens, J., Livak, K. J., and Williams, P. M. (1996) Real Time Quantitative PCR. *Genome Res.* **6,** 986–994.
6. Solomon, M. J., Larsen, P. L., and Varshavsky, A. (1988) Mapping protein-DNA interactions in vivo with formaldehyde: evidence that histone H4 is retained on a highly transcribed gene. *Cell* **53,** 937–947.
7. Braunstein, M., Rose, A. B., Holmes, S. G., Allis, C. D., and Broach, J. R. (1993) Transcriptional silencing in yeast is associated with reduced nucleosome acetylation. *Genes Dev.* **7,** 592–604.
8. Hsieh, C.-L. (1994) Dependence of transcriptional repression on CpG methylation density. *Mol. Cell. Biol.* **14,** 5487–5494.
9. Chen, H., Lin, R. J., Xie, W., Wilpitz, D., and Evans, R. M. (1999) Regulation of hormone-induced histone hyperacetylation and gene activation via acetylation of an acetylase. *Cell* **98,** 675–686.

5

Restriction Endonuclease Accessibility as a Determinant of Altered Chromatin Structure

William M. Hempel and Pierre Ferrier

Summary

Active genes in eukaryotic genomes are typically found in open, nuclease-sensitive regions of chromatin. This chapter presents an overview of the techniques used to assay restriction endonuclease cleavage of chromosomal DNA as an approach to assess general accessibility at a genomic region of interest. We describe protocols to (1) prepare nuclei templates, (2) treat chromosomal DNA with a restriction enzyme(s), and (3) visualize and quantify chromosomal cleavage(s), with an emphasis on ligation-mediated (LM) PCR techniques.

Key Words: Chromatin; accessibility; restriction endonuclease; ligation-mediated PCR.

1. Introduction

With the realization that epigenetic phenomena play a critical role in normal and pathological cell processes in eukaryotes *(1–3)* , numerous approaches have been utilized to decipher changes in chromatin structure at given chromosomal locations. Because active genes and associated regulatory elements are typically found in open, nuclease-sensitive regions of chromatin *(4)*, techniques that monitor restriction enzyme cleavage within chromosomal DNA can provide information on general accessibility at a genomic region of interest *(5–7)*. Indeed, numerous studies have used these techniques to analyze changes in chromatin structure at a discrete site(s) during cell differentiation/activation processes in organisms ranging from yeast to human *(5–18)*. Along these lines, the use of ligation-mediated polymerase chain reaction LM-PCR *(19,20)* has proved to be instrumental in generating restriction endonuclease accessibility data from chromatin templates available in limited quantity. Recent examples notably include the analysis of coding sequences and flanking promoter/enhancer regions within the interleukin *IL-12 p40* gene *(11)*, or the antigen receptor gene loci *(14–16)* in cells of the immune system. The changes in restriction endonu-

From: *Methods in Molecular Biology, vol. 287: Epigenetics Protocols*
Edited by: T. O. Tollefsbol © Humana Press Inc., Totowa, NJ

clease cleavage that are observed at discrete sites within the *TCR* β locus during T-lymphocyte early differentiation events are used here to illustrate these methods.

2. Materials

1. Cultured cell line(s) and/or primary cells from animal tissues.
2. Phosphate-buffered saline (PBS).
3. Sucrose buffer: 32 m*M* sucrose, 3 m*M* CaCl$_2$, 2 m*M* MgOAc, 0.1 m*M* EDTA, 10 m*M* Tris-HCl, pH 7.4.
4. Dithiothreitol (DTT).
5. Phenylmethylsulfonyl fluoride (PMSF).
6. Trypan blue.
7. Nonidet P-40 (NP-40).
8. Nuclei buffer: 20 m*M* HEPES, pH 7.4, 2 m*M* MgCl$_2$, 70 m*M* KCl, 0.1 m*M* EDTA, 1 m*M* DTT, 0.5 m*M* PMSF, 25% (v/v) glycerol.
9. Restriction enzymes.
10. 2X Restriction endonuclease digestion buffer: 20 m*M* Tris-HCl, pH 7.9, 100 m*M* NaCl, 20 m*M* MgCl$_2$, 4% (v/v) glycerol.
11. 2X DNA extraction buffer: 20m*M* Tris-HCl, pH 8.0, 200m*M* NaCl, 2 m*M* EDTA, 1.0% sodium dodecyl sulfate (SDS).
12. Proteinase K.
13. Oligonucleotides for preparation of the unidirectional linker (*BW-1*: GCGGTGACCCGGGAGATCTGAATTC; *BW-2*: GAATTCAGATC) *(19)*.
14. Linker ligation mix: 66 m*M* Tris-HCl, pH 7.5, 5 m*M* MgCl$_2$, 1 m*M* DTT.
15. T4 DNA ligase.
16. PCR-lysis buffer: 10 m*M* Tris-HCl, pH 8.3, 50 m*M* KCl, 0.5% NP-40, 0.5% Tween-20.
17. Oligonucleotide primers for PCR: including the distal and proximal (locus-specific) primers, the anchor (linker-specific) primer *BW-1H*: CCGGGAGAT CTGAATTCCAC *(19)*, and a third locus-specific internal oligonucleotide.
18. 10X PCR buffer: 100 m*M* Tris-HCl, pH 8.3, 15 m*M* MgCl$_2$, 450 m*M* KCl, 2 m*M* dNTP (of each dGTP, dATP, dTTP, dCTP).
19. *Taq* DNA polymerase.
20. Agarose, NuSieve, and DNA electrophoresis gel equipment.
21. 5X DNA loading buffer: 100 m*M* Tris-HCl, pH 7.4, 100 m*M* EDTA, 0.1% SDS, 50% (v/v) glycerol, 0.1 mL/10 mL saturated xylene cyanol, 0.1 mL/10 mL saturated bromophenol blue.
22. 20X TAE buffer (20X): 0.8 *M* Tris-acetate, 1 *M* NaOAc, 20 m*M* EDTA.
23. Membrane and filter paper for Southern blot.
24. 20X SSCPE: 2.4 *M* NaCl, 300 m*M* NaOAc, 2 m*M* KH$_2$PO$_4$, 20 m*M* EDTA; pH adjusted to 7.2 with NaOH.
25. 50X Denhardt's reagent: 1% bovine serum albumin (BSA), 1% polyvinylpyrrolidone, 1% Ficoll, 0.1% sodium azide.
26. T4 polynucleotide kinase.

3. Methods

Previously, we have used restriction endonuclease assays and LM-PCR to analyze changes in chromosomal accessibility at discrete regions within normal and/or enhancer-deleted TCRβ loci during T-lymphocyte development in the mouse thymus *(14,21)*. The methods described below outline the successive steps used in this approach, including (1) purification of cell nuclei; (2) digestion of chromosomal DNA with a restriction enzyme(s), followed by the preparation of genomic DNA; (3) amplification of the DNA sequence of interest using LM-PCR; and (4) characterization of the amplified DNA fragments by Southern blot analysis and quantification of the data. As an example, we describe the differential behavior—in terms of accessibility to restriction enzyme cleavage—that can be observed at the TCRβ locus between the 5' distal Vβ5 gene and the 3' proximal Vβ14 gene, as lymphocyte precursors develop from early pro-T to late pre-T cells *(21)*.

3.1. Purification of Cell Nuclei

In the aforementioned experiments, cell nuclei have generally been obtained from primary mouse thymocytes and (as a nonlymphoid cell control), from cultured NIH-3T3 fibroblasts.

1. To prepare primary thymocytes, dissect the thymus from a 4-wk-old mouse into ice-cold DMEM medium Gibco-BRL) and then disrupt it into a single cell suspension by shearing between frosted microscope slides and filtering through a nylon mesh.
2. Centrifuge the cells (5×10^7 to 1×10^8 thymocytes; *see* **Note 1**) (for 5 min, at 120g 4°C) and wash twice in ice-cold PBS. Afterwards, resuspend the cell pellet in 5 mL of ice-cold sucrose buffer supplemented with 1 mM DTT and 0.5 mM PMSF.
3. Working on ice, further dilute the above solution by addition of 5 mL sucrose buffer containing 0.5% NP-40. Cell disruption is improved by pipeting up- and -down several ($\geq$10) times. The extent of cell lysis can be evaluated microscopically by staining of an aliquot with trypan blue (typically, >90% of the cells must be permeable to the dye).
4. Then centrifuge the released nuclei at 450g. 4°C for 10 min. (Pelleted nuclei should be noticeably whiter than the original cell pellet.) After aspiration of the supernatant, resuspend the nuclei gently in 5 mL of ice-cold sucrose buffer (supplemented with DTT and PMSF, as above; without NP-40). Then count the nuclei using trypan blue. (Nuclei should stain with trypan blue and appear large and perfectly round.)
5. Once again centrifuge the nuclei at 450g, at 4°C for 10 min, and finally, resuspend the pellet gently in ice-cold nuclei buffer, at a concentration of 5×10^7 nuclei/mL (50,000 nuclei/mL). Aliquot the nuclei (10 μL/5×10^5 nuclei), freeze in liquid nitrogen, and store at –80°C.

3.2. Restriction Enzyme Cleavage and Preparation of Genomic DNA

1. For restriction enzyme digests, treat nuclear templates (~10^5 nuclei; prepared as above) with a mix containing 12.5 μL of 2X digestion buffer, increasing concentrations of a restriction endonuclease (typically from 0.1 to 10 U of enzyme; also *see* **Note 2**), and enough water to bring up the final volume to 25 μL. For most enzymes, perform digestion on ice for 1 h (*see* **Note 2**). For convenience during the next step of LM-PCR, we have a preference for restriction endonucleases producing blunt-ended DNA extremities (e.g., *Rsa*I, *Hae*III, *Pvu*II, *Eco*RV, *Msc*I, *Xmn*I, and others, but the utilization of restriction enzymes producing asymmetric DNA cleavage is equally possible (*see* **Note 3**).
2. Stop restriction enzyme cleavage (and the nuclei lysed) by the addition of 25 μL 2X DNA extraction buffer, in the presence of proteinase K (final concentration of 0.4 mg/mL), followed by incubation on a thermomixer at 56°C for 2 h.
3. Finally, extract the DNA (we use 1X phenol/chloroform and, then 1X chloroform), precipitate with isopropanol, and resuspend in 25 μL of H_2O. At this step, the restricted DNA can be stored at –20°C, before it is used in a linker-ligation reaction to carry out LM-PCR, as described below in **Subheading 3.3**. For normalization purposes during quantitation analysis of restriction enzyme sensitivity data from hybridized Southern blots (*see* **Subheading 3.4.2.**), the deproteinized DNA can be cleaved to completion with a second enzyme as an internal reference (using standard recombinant DNA methods *[22]*), thus allowing presentation of the data as the ratio of nuclear cleavage to in vitro cleavage (e.g., **refs**. *9–11,13,18*). Alternatively, especially when using LM-PCR, nuclear cleavage can also be normalized relative to the digestion efficiency at a homologous site within a known accessible locus (e.g., **ref**. *15*; **Fig. 1**).

Fig. 1. *(opposite page)* Accessibility to restriction enzyme cleavage of the Vβ5.2/ Vβ8.3- and Vβ14-containing regions within the TCRβ locus in developing mouse thymocytes. **(A)** Structural organization of the Vβ5.2/Vβ8.3- and Vβ14-containing DNA regions (located on, respectively, the 5′ and 3′ sides of the TCRβ locus). **(B)** Relative location of the *Rsa*I sites that have been analyzed, and the schemes of the LM-PCR assays used to visualize chromosomal cleavages. Bold lines in (A) indicate the ligated anchor; arrowheads indicate the relative location of the PCR primers. Nuclei purified from either early (pro-T; first set of lanes on the left) or late (pre-T; middle set of lanes) developing mouse thymocytes, and nuclei from NIH-3T3 fibroblasts (Fibro.; last set of lanes), were treated with increasing amounts of *Rsa*I (0.1, 0.3, 1, 3, and 10 U). Enzyme cleavage at the indicated site(s) was revealed by LM-PCR and Southern blotting. Quantitation of restriction enzyme sensitivity was obtained by analysis of the hybridizing bands with a phosphorImager® (BAS 1000; Molecular Dynamics) and MacBAS software. **(C)** Results in pre-T cells and fibroblasts are given as percentage of residual accessibility relative to that in the pro-T cells, to which the 100% value was attributed. LM-PCR signals for *Rsa*I digests were normalized for DNA content (assessed by parallel PCR amplification of linker-ligated DNA for a fragment within the Cβ2 constant region gene), and for digestion efficiency at *Rsa*I sites in the accessible

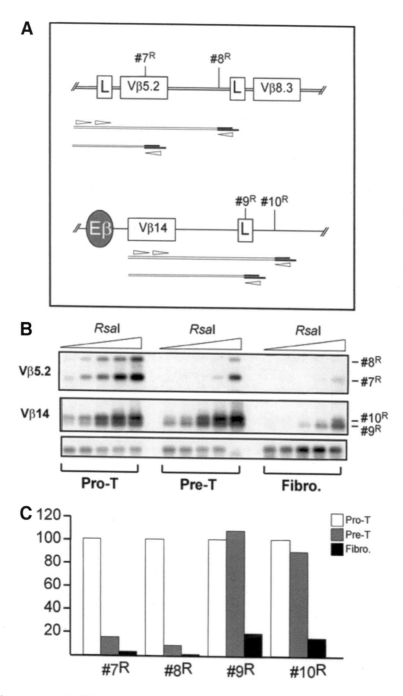

Fig. 1. *(continued)* CD3ε locus (data not shown). Similar percentages were obtained in separate restriction enzyme cleavage/LM-PCR experiments. The results demonstrate that, upon pro-T- to pre-T-cell development, the Vβ5 chromosomal region becomes resistant to enzyme cleavage (and presumably acquires an altered, repressed chromatin structure), whereas the Vβ14 region remains in an open, nuclease-sensitive state.

3.3. LM-PCR

The steps described in **Subheadings 3.3.1., 3.3.2.** and **3.3.3.** outline the procedure for LM-PCR in a manner that yields restriction endonuclease accessibility data even when starting from a minimal number of nuclear templates (also *see* **Notes 1 and 4**). These steps comprise preparation of the unidirectional linker (*BW*), followed by ligation of the *BW* linker to enzyme-restricted, blunt-ended DNA and PCR amplification (*see* **Note 5** for primer design considerations). These three steps are common to protocols focusing on the analysis of changes in restriction enzyme accessibility as a determinant of altered chromatin structure (as described here), and the determination of in vivo footprinting profiles and, more generally, of DNA double-strand break cleavage at a sequence of interest (e.g., **refs. *20* and *23–31***).

3.3.1. Preparation of the Unidirectional BW Linker

1. Bring oligonucleotides *BW-1* (16 µg) and BW-2 (7 µg) to 100 µL in 250 m*M* Tris-HCl, pH 7.7.
2. Denature at 95°C for 5 min.
3. Transfer to a heat block prewarmed to 70°C, allow to cool to RT for 1 h, and keep overnight at 4°C.
4. Prepare 10-µL aliquots and store at –20°C.

3.3.2. Ligation of the BW Linker to Genomic DNA

1. Mix 10 µL of enzyme-restricted DNA (~0.2 µg of genomic DNA, prepared as described in **Subheading 3.2.**) with 37.5 µL of linker ligation. Mix, 1 µL each of 20 p*M*/µL BW linker and T4 DNA ligase (2.5 U/µL), and 0.5 µL 1 m*M* ATP; incubate overnight at 16°C.
2. Add an equal volume (50 µL) of PCR-lysis buffer, incubate at 95°C for 15 min (on a thermal cycler), and then place on ice (at this stage, it is possible to store the linker-ligated DNA at –20°C).

3.3.3. Nested LM-PCR Amplification

1. Prepare 20 µL PCR mix per sample based on the following proportions: 2.5 µL of PCR buffer; 0.1 µL of the *BW-1H* anchor primer (0.25 µg/µL); 0.1 µL of the distal locus-specific primer (0.25 µg/µL); 0.1 µL of *Taq* DNA polymerase; 17.2 µL H$_2$O.
2. Transfer 5 µL of linker-ligated DNA (prepared as described in **Subheadings 3.3.2.**) into PCR tubes, and add 20 µL of the PCR mix to each tube.
3. Amplify by PCR for 12 cycles (cycling profile: 1X 94°C, 1 min; 12X [94°C, 1 min and 66°C, 2 min]; 1X 72°C, 5 min).
4. Prepare a second PCR mix of 24 µL per sample based on the following proportions: 0.25 µL of 50 m*M* MgCl$_2$; 0.1 µL of the *BW-1H* primer (0.25 µg/µL); 0.1 µL of the proximal locus-specific primer (0.25 µg/µL); 0.1 µL of *Taq* DNA polymerase; 20.95 µL H$_2$O.

5. Transfer 24 μL of the second PCR mix into PCR tubes, and add 1 μL of the first PCR reaction to each tube.
6. Amplify by PCR for 27 cycles (cycling profile: 1X 94°C, 1 min; 12X [94°C, 1 min and 66°C, 2 min]; 1X 72°C, 5 min).
7. Add 5 μL of standard DNA loading buffer (5X), before gel separation of LM-PCR products and Southern blotting (the samples can also be frozen here).

3.4. Gel Separation of LM-PCR Products and Data Analysis

Described below are the steps dedicated to the separation of the LM-PCR products by gel electrophoresis and quantitation of the restriction endonuclease sensitivity data by Southern blot and phosphorimager scanning analysis.

3.4.1. Gel Electrophoresis and Southern Blotting Procedures

1. For analysis of the generated restriction endonuclease cleavages, first electrophorese the PCR products through mixed 1% agarose/0.5% NuSieve gels in 1X TAE buffer.
2. Transfer onto nylon membranes (e.g., Gene Screen Plus; NEN Life Science Products) under alkaline conditions using standard Southern blotting procedures.
3. Hybridize with an end-labeled, [γ^{32}P]ATP locus-specific oligonucleotide (probe) internal to the amplifying primers.
4. Visualize by autoradiography.
5. Southern blotting and hybridization/washing procedures are performed by standard recombinant DNA methods *(22)* and are not described in detail here because of space limitations (also *see* **Note 6**). The quality of the analyzed DNA templates and normalization for sample loading can be assessed by parallel PCR amplification of linker-ligated DNA using forward and reverse primers specific for a locus region that does not contain the restriction endonuclease site tested in the particular assay *(14,16)*.

3.4.2. Quantitation of Restriction Endonuclease Sensitivity Data

Quantitation of image data from restriction endonuclease sensitivity assays is generally accomplished by phosphorimager analysis with the help of an appropriate software (e.g., MacBAS; ImageQuant). By comparing profiles of LM-PCR products from nuclei in various situations (e.g., **Fig. 1**), the relative level of restriction enzyme cleavage at a given site can be evaluated and is a reflection of chromosomal access/alteration in chromatin structure within the region of interest. To this end, LM-PCR signals must be normalized for (1) DNA content (assessed by parallel PCR amplification of linker-ligated DNA, as stated above), (2) the digestion efficiency at an homologous site within a known accessible locus and, possibly, (3) substrate copy number (for example, when distinct transgenic lines containing different copy numbers of the analyzed region are studied) *(15)* (*see* **Fig. 1** and **Note 7**).

4. Notes

1. We have routinely prepared nuclei starting from a lesser amount of primary thymocytes ($3–5 \times 10^6$ cells; microscale protocol). In this case, cells are pelleted in a microfuge at 6800g for 15 s, washed in 1 mL ice-cold PBS, centrifuged as above, and gently resuspended in 0.5 mL of ice-cold sucrose buffer. The next steps comprise the addition of 0.5 mL ice-cold sucrose buffer with 0.5% NP-40 to the cell pellet with up and down pipetting (≥ 10 times), a 15-s spin at 6800g in a cold microfuge, a wash of the nuclei in 1 mL ice-cold sucrose buffer followed by another 15-s spin at 6800g in a cold microfuge, and finally, gentle resuspension of the nuclei pellet in 50 mL of nuclei buffer. (Nuclei are counted on 1 μL.)

2. The amount of restriction endonuclease required for the assay will be a function of the activity of the enzyme at the selected temperature and the inherent accessibility of the site tested. It may thus be important first to perform titration assays and determine the conditions (optimal concentrations) under which specific cutting is achieved, e.g., by assaying control nuclei in which the particular site is expected not to be cleaved (in our case, nuclei from a nonlymphoid, NIH-3T3 fibroblast origin). Along these lines, we have found—with several restriction enzymes—that reduced temperature reaction conditions minimize nonspecific cleavage observed at room (or higher) temperatures.

3. When utilizing restriction endonucleases that produce asymmetric DNA cleavages, a first-strand synthesis reaction (using a locus-specific primer) is required to generate a family of blunt-ended duplex molecules, which are substrates for T4 DNA ligase-catalyzed addition of the anchor primer, as originally described for LM-PCR protocols *(19,20)* (also *see* **refs. *11*** and ***16***).

4. Instead of using LM-PCR, restriction endonuclease sensitivity analysis can also be performed by standard Southern blotting of the restricted DNA and indirect end-labeling techniques *(9,13,18)*. One advantage of directly analyzing restriction fragments in the absence of a PCR amplification step is that the magnitudes of differences in cleavage efficiency between the various samples will not be artificially amplified. However, a higher number of cells may be required when the PCR step is omitted ($2–5 \times 10^6$ cells/~2 μg of genomic DNA per tested point according to **ref. *18***; compared with an estimated ~$2–5 \times 10^3$ cells per point in the LM-PCR protocol), although this number can probably be reduced by also adapting the Southern protocol to a smaller number of cells. A more sophisticated approach has also recently been described, based on real-time PCR analysis (referred to as chromatin accessibility by real-time PCR [CHART]; *[12,17,32]*). Accordingly, a potential advantage of the latter assay may be that it probably requires fewer cells than all the other methods. However, as CHART monitors the reduced intensity of a PCR product in response to chromatin remodeling, as opposed to the increased intensity of the product monitored by the other assays, it may be somewhat less sensitive. Also, because of its still limited utilization, it remains to be determined, whether this technique can be generalized (to address changes in chromatin structure).

5. Locus-specific primers are generally 25 nucleotides in length with a 52% GC content and are positioned in the sequence such that the internal locus-specific primer used in the second PCR amplification reaction gives rise to an approx 200-bp product (i.e., it is positioned about 200 bp upstream of the restriction endonuclease cleavage site).

6. Using standard protocols *(22)*, the oligonucleotide probe (0.1 μg) is labeled with [γ32P]ATP (7000 Ci/mM) to a specific activity of 1×10^9 to 2×10^9 cpm/μg of DNA. We generally hybridize overnight at 56°C (in 6X SSCPE, 0.2% SDS, 5X Denhardt's reagent) using 1×10^6 cpm/mL of the labeled probe. With these conditions, a 20–30-min exposure of the washed membrane on a phosphorimager screen, or 1–2 h on a film, is usually sufficient to obtain a good signal.

7. When a second restriction enzyme has been used to digest the deproteinized DNA (in vitro cleavage), normalization of the LM-PCR/Southern results is typically performed as a ratio of nuclear cleavage to in vitro cleavage [*(9–11,13)*]. In the CHART protocol, quantitation (by real-time PCR) is based on the assumption that the amount of PCR product generated is inversely proportional to the amount of restriction endonuclease digestion occurring across the region amplified by the primers *(12,17)*.

Acknowledgments

This work was supported by institutional grants from INSERM and the CNRS and by specific grants from the Association pour la Recherche sur le Cancer (ARC), the Commission of the European Communities, and the Fondation Princesse Grace de Monaco.

References

1. Henikoff, S. (2003) Position effect variegation after 60 years. *Trends Genet.* **6,** 422–426.

2. Hendrich, B. D. and Willard, H. F. (1995) Epigenetic regulation of gene expression: the effect of altered chromatin structure from yeast to mammals. *Hum. Mol. Genet.* **4,** 1765–1777.

3. Jones, P. A. and Baylin, S. B. (2003) The fundamental role of epigenetic events in cancer. *Nat. Rev. Genet.* **3,** 415–428.

4. Felsenfeld, G. (1996) Chromatin unfolds. *Cell* **86,** 13–19.

5. Loo, S. and Rine, J. (1994) Silencers and domains of generalized repression. *Science* **264,** 1768–1771.

6. Wallrath, L. L. and Elgin, S. C. R. (1995) Position effect variegation in *Drosophila* is associated with an altered chromatin structure. *Genes Dev.* **9,** 1263–1277.

7. Beato, M. and Eisfeld, K. (1997) Transcription factor access to chromatin. *Nucleic Acids Res.* **25,** 3559–3563.

8. Aronow, B. J., Ebert, C. A., Valerius, M. T., et al. (1995) Dissecting a locus control region: facilitation of enhancer function by extended enhancer-flanking sequences. *Mol. Cell. Biol.* **15,** 1123–1135.

9. Gong, Q. H., McDowell, J. C., and Dean, A. (1996) Essential role of NF-E2 in remodeling of chromatin structure and transcriptional activation of the ε-globin gene in vivo by 5′ hypersensitive site 2 of the β-globin locus control region. *Mol. Cell. Biol.* **16**, 6055–6064.

10. Brown, S. A. and Kingston, R. E. (1997) Disruption of downstream chromatin directed by a transcriptional activator. *Genes Dev.* **11**, 3116–3121.

11. Weinmann, A. S., Plevy, S. E., and Smale, S. T. (1999) Rapid and selective remodeling of a positioned nucleosome during the induction of IL-12 p40 transcription. *Immunity* **11**, 665–675.

12. Rao, S., Procko, E., and Shannon, M. F. (2001) Chromatin remodeling, measured by a novel real-time polymerase chain reaction assay, across the proximal promoter region of the IL-2 gene. *J. Immunol.* **167**, 4494–4503.

13. Carr, A. and Biggin, M. D. (2000) Accessibility of transcriptionally inactive genes is specifically reduced at homeoprotein-DNA binding sites in *Drosophila. Nucleic Acids Res.* **28**, 2839–2846.

14. Mathieu, N., Hempel, W. M., Spicuglia, S., Verthuy, C., and Ferrier, P. (2000) Chromatin remodeling by the T cell receptor (TCR)-β gene enhancer during early T cell development: implications for the control of TCR-β locus recombination. *J. Exp. Med.* **192**, 625–636.

15. Sikes, M. L., Meade, A., Tripathi, R., Krangel, M. S., and Oltz, E. M. (2002) Regulation of V(D)J recombination: a dominant role for promoter positioning in gene segment accessibility. *Proc. Natl. Acad. Sci. USA* **99**, 12,309–12,314.

16. Chowdhury, D. and Sen, R. (2003) Transient IL-7/IL-7R signaling provides a mechanism for feedback inhibition of immunoglobulin heavy chain gene rearrangements. *Immunity* **18**, 229–241.

17. Holloway, A. F., Rao, S., Chen, X., and Shannon, M. F. (2003) Changes in chromatin accessibility across the GM-CSF promoter upon T cell activation are dependent on nuclear factor κB proteins. *J. Exp. Med.* **197**, 413–423.

18. Jackson, D. A., McDowell, J. C., and Dean, A. (2003) β-Globin locus control region HS2 and HS3 interact structurally and functionally. *Nucleic Acids Res.* **31**, 1180–1190.

19. Mueller, P. R. and Wold, B. (1989) *In vivo* footprinting of a muscle specific enhancer by ligation mediated PCR. *Science* **246**, 780–786.

20. Garrity, P. A. and Wold, B. J. (1992) Effects of different DNA polymerases in ligation-mediated PCR: enhanced genomic sequencing and *in vivo* footprinting. *Proc. Natl. Acad. Sci. USA* **89**, 1021–1025.

21. Mathieu, N., Spicuglia, S., Gorbatch, S., et al. (2003) Assessing the role of the T cell receptor beta gene enhancer in regulating coding joint formation during V(D)J recombination. *J. Biol. Chem.* **278**, 18,101-18,109.

22. Sambrook, J., Fritsch, E. F., and Maniatis, T. (1989) *Molecular Cloning: A Laboratory Manual*, 2nd ed. Cold Spring Harbor, NY: Cold Spring Harbor Laboratory Press.

23. Zhu, C. and Roth, D. B. (1995) Characterization of coding ends in thymocytes of *scid* mice: implications for the mechanism of V(D)J recombination. *Immunity* **2**, 101–112.

24. Zhu, C. M., Bogue, M. A., Lim, D. S., Hasty, P., and Roth, D. B. (1996) Ku86-deficient mice exhibit severe combined immunodeficiency and defective processing of V(D)J recombination intermediates. *Cell* **86**, 379–389.

25. Stanhope-Baker, P., Hudson, K. M., Shaffer, A. L., Constantinescu, A., and Schlissel, M. S. (1996) Cell type-specific chromatin structure determines the targeting of V(D)J recombinase activity in vitro. *Cell* **85**, 887–897.

26. McPherson, C. E., Shim, E.-Y., Friedman, D. S., and Zaret, K. S. (1993) An active tissue-specific enhancer and bound transcription factors existing in a precisely positioned nucleosomal array. *Cell* **75**, 387–398.

27. Spicuglia, S., Payet, D., Tripathi, R. K., et al. (2000) TCRα enhancer activation occurs via a conformational change of a pre-assembled nucleo-protein complex. *EMBO J.* **19**, 2034–2045.

28. Schlissel, M. S., Constantinescu, A., Morrow, T., Baxter, M., and Peng, A. (1993) Double-strand signal sequence breaks in V(D)J recombination are blunt, 5′-phosphorylated, RAG-dependent, and cell cycle regulated. *Genes Dev.* **7**, 2520–2532.

29. Hempel, W. M., Stanhope-Baker, P., Mathieu, N., Huang, F., Schlissel, M. S., and Ferrier, P. (1998) Enhancer control of *V(D)J* recombination at the TCRβ locus: differential effects on DNA cleavage and joining. *Genes Dev.* **12**, 2305–2317.

30. Papavasiliou, F. N. and Schatz, D. G. (2000) Cell-cycle-regulated DNA double-stranded breaks in somatic hypermutation of immunoglobulin genes. *Nature* **408**, 216–221.

31. Papavasiliou, F. N. and Schatz, D. G. (2002) The activation-induced deaminase functions in a postcleavage step of the somatic hypermutation process. *J. Exp. Med.* **195**, 1193–1198.

32. Rao, S., Gerondakis, S., Woltring, D., and Shannon, M. F. (2003) c-Rel is required for chromatin remodeling across the IL-2 gene promoter. *J. Immunol.* **170**, 3724–3731.

6

Measuring Changes in Chromatin Using Micrococcal Nuclease

Nicolas Steward and Hiroshi Sano

Summary

This chapter documents a simple protocol to identify the nucleosome positioning of any given genes. The procedure includes partitioning 200-bp DNA fragments constituting the nucleosomal core region by micrococcal nuclease digestion and semiquantitative polymerase chain reaction amplification using multiple sets of primers covering arbitrary regions of approximately 150 bp in the gene. If the nuclease-digested 200-bp DNA is efficiently amplified, the region is inside the core. If the amplification is poor, the region spans the linker region. By a combination of this method with direct methylation mapping, the core region of a maize gene, *ZmMI1*, was shown to be less methylated than the linker region. The potential usefulness of the technique is discussed.

Key Words: 5-Methylcytosine; micrococcal nuclease; nucleosome; *Zea mays*.

1. Introduction

In the DNA of higher eukaryotes 5-methylcytosine (m^5C) accounts for up to 30% of the total cytosines. In vertebrates, m^5C is located almost exclusively in CpG, whereas in plants it occurs in both CpG and CpNpG *(1)* and also in nonsymmetrical cytosines *(2)*. The distribution within the genome is nonrandom and varies depending on the tissue and the developmental stage. A major physiological function of m^5C is to silence gene expression, which is important for host DNA defenses against incorporation of parasitic DNA *(3)*. Intensive studies on animal cells have revealed distinct examples, including inactivation of the X -chromosome, imprinting of genes, and silencing of parasitic DNA such as retroelements and transposons *(4)*. In plants, mobilization of transposons is also reported to be repressed by DNA methylation *(5)*.

The molecular mechanism is considered to involve changes in DNA structure caused by m^5C. Two possibilities have been proposed. One is direct

From: *Methods in Molecular Biology, vol. 287: Epigenetics Protocols*
Edited by: T. O. Tollefsbol © Humana Press Inc., Totowa, NJ

repression owing to methylated promoter regions blocking binding of transcriptional machinery, and the other is indirect repression owing to altered nucleosome structures affecting the chromatin conformation *(3)*. Recent studies have indicated that the latter occur frequently and play an essential role in controlling global gene expression *(6)*. For example, various disorders have been found to be the result of abnormal chromosome structures caused by defective DNA methylation *(7)*. It is also known that, in cancer cells, chromosomal DNA is locally hypermethylated and globally hypomethylated *(8)*. Despite its importance, information on the exact positioning of nucleosomes in a given gene and its relationship to m^5C is limited. This chapter describes methodology to identify core and linker regions of nucleosomes in a particular gene, using a combination of micrococcal nuclease, which preferentially cleaves the linker but not the core regions, and semiquatitative polymerase chain reaction (PCR). The method was successfully applied to correlate methylation status with nucleosome structure.

2. Materials

2.1. Plant Materials

1. Maize seeds (*Zea mays* L. cv. Golden Arrow).
2. Murashige and Skoog medium (Nihon Seiyaku).
3. Temperature-, light-, and humidity-regulated growth cabinet.
4. Nucleon Phytopure kit (Amersham) for DNA extraction.

2.2. Nucleosome Isolation

1. Grinding medium (NGM): 20 mM Tris-HCl, 0.5 mM spermidine, 10 mM mercaptoethanol, 40% glycerol, 5 mM sodium butyrate.
2. Brinkmann/KINEMATICA POLYTRON benchtop homogenizer (model PTA 20S).
3. Miracloth (Calbiochem) filter.
4. Percoll (Pharmacia, Piscataway, NJ).
5. Swing rotor ultracentrifuge.
6. Glass Pasteur pipete.
7. Ultraviolet (UV) spectrophotometer.
8. Sodium dodecyl sulfate (SDS).
9. 10X TBS buffer: 0.1 M Tris-HCl, 30 mM $CaCl_2$, 20 mM $MgCl_2$, 50 mM Na-butyrate.
10. 15–30 U/µL Micrococcal nuclease (Takara, cat. no. 2910A).
11. NuSieve 3:1 agarose (BioWhittaker Molecular Applications).
12. 4′,6-Diamidino-2-phenylindole (DAPI; Sigma, cat. no. D-9542).

2.3. DNA Extraction and PCR

1. Prep-A-Gene DNA extraction kit (Bio-Rad).
2. 50 µM of Primers sets: 2.50 mM each 10X ExTaq PCR buffer (Takara), ExTaq enzyme (Takara), PCR nucleotide mix.
3. Thermal cycler.

2.4. Bisulfite Modification

1. Restriction endonucleases: *Xba*I and *Alu*I.
2. Salmon sperm DNA.
3. 3 *M* Sodium acetate, pH 7.0.
4. 0.2 *N* and 5 *N* NaOH.
5. 0.5% Acrylamide aqueous solution.
6. Sodium bisulfite (Sigma, cat. no. S1516).
7. Hydroquinone (Sigma, cat. no. H9003).
8. pGEM-T easy vector (Promega).
9. Competent *E. coli* JM109 (Stratagene).
10. ABI PRISM BigDye™ Terminator DNA sequencing kit (Applied Biosystems).
11. 3100 Genetic Analyser automated sequencer (Applied Biosystems).

3. Methods

The methods described below pertain to nucleosome localization using micrccocal nuclease digestion followed by semiquantitative PCR. This allows nucleosome mapping on differentially methylated DNA sequences to indicate alternative nucleosome positions.

3.1. Plant Culture and DNA Extraction

1. Germinate maize seeds (*Zea mays* L. cv. Golden Arrow) on a wet paper towel for 3 d in an incubator at 30°C in the dark.
2. Transfer approx seven young seedlings onto a net fixed on the top of a 150-mL cup, so that roots are immersed in a 1:5 diluted Murashige and Skoog medium *(9)*.
3. Culture seedlings further hydroponically in a growth cabinet at 70% relative humidity and 23°C under continuous light for 13 d *(10)*.
4. Perform cold pulses transferring 13-d old seedlings to an incubator at 4°C for several days and then returning samples to 23°C for further periods. Maintain light and humidity conditions constant throughout the experimental periods.
5. Extract genomic DNA using a Nucleon Phytopure Kit (Amersham).

3.2. Nucleosome Isolation

3.2.1. Extraction of Nuclei From Maize Tissues

Harvest roots from 13-d-old seedlings and obtain pure preparations of nuclei by centrifugation on a 30% Percoll cushion *(11)*.

All steps should be performed at 4°C unless otherwise noted.

1. Prepare 250 mL of fresh nucleus grinding medium (NGM) containing 20 m*M* Tris-HCl, 0.5 m*M* spermidine, 10 m*M* mercaptoethanol, 40% glycerol, 5 m*M* sodium butyrate. Keep on ice.
2. Chop 2–3 g of roots freshly harvested from 15-d old seedlings into small pieces (1 cm long). Place them into a 15-mL Falcon tube, and add 10 mL chilled NGM.
3. Release the nuclei from the tissues using a Brinkmann/KINEMATICA POLYTRON benchtop homogenizer (model PTA 20S) set at level 1 with 5–7 pulses of 2 s each.

4. Filter the homogenized sample through a Miracloth (Calbiochem) filter.
5. Prepare 10 mL of a 30% Percoll (Pharmacia) solution with NGM buffer in a 50-μL Falcon tube.
6. Load the sample carefully on the top of the Percoll cushion.
7. Spin for 20 min at 2500g using a swing rotor and recover the nuclei fraction from the layer at the boundary between the NGM buffer and the Percoll cushion using a Pasteur pipet.
8. Dilute the recovered nuclei with 2-vol of NGM buffer and spin again under the same conditions.
9. Resuspend the nuclei pellet in 10 mL NGM buffer and repeat **steps 5–8**.
10. Resuspend the nuclei pellet in 1 mL NGM buffer, which can be kept at –30°C (*see* **Note 1**).
11. Mix 20 μL of the nuclei solution with 380 μL of 0.1% SDS by a quick vortex. Incubate for 5 min at 37°C and measure the DNA concentration with a spectrophotometer. The DNA concentration should be around 300 μg/mL with a 260/280-nm ratio of 1.4–1.6.

3.2.2. Nucleus Digestion With Micrococcal Nuclease

Digest a 60-μg aliquot of nuclei suspension with 4 U of micrococcal nuclease (Takara) at 37°C for 4 min, and fractionate on a 2.5% NuSieve 3:1 agarose gel (BioWhittaker Molecular Applications). Extract a fraction containing approx 200 bp corresponding to mononucleosomal DNA using a Prep-A-Gene kit (Bio-Rad) (**Fig. 1**).

1. Prepare 10X TBS buffer solution containing 0.1 M Tris-HCl, 30 mM CaCl$_2$, 20 mM MgCl$_2$, 50 mM Na-butyrate.
2. Spin an aliquot of nuclei solution containing 60 μg DNA (~200 μL) at 5000g for 3 min.
3. Resuspend the pellet in 1 mL 1X TBS and spin at 15,000g for 3 min.
4. Resuspend the pellet in the micrococcal digestion buffer according to the manufacturer's instructions with a final DNA concentration of 500 μg/mL.
5. Add 4 U of the micrococcal nuclease and incubate for 4–5 min (do not incubate further, to avoid overdigestion) at 37°C (*see* **Note 2**).
6. Stop the reaction by adding EDTA to a final concentration of 5 mM and place the sample on ice for 5 min.
7. Spin the sample at 15,000g for 5 min and collect the supernatant into a new tube.
8. Add SDS to the sample at a final concentration of 0.1% in order to strip the shorter oligonucleotides from the histones.
9. Load onto a 2.5% NuSieve 3:1 high-grade agarose gel (BioWhittaker Molecular Applications).
10. Visualize the oligonucleosome ladder by ethidium bromide staining (*see* **Note 3**) and collect the 145–200-bp fraction using a Prep-A-Gene extraction kit (Bio-Rad).

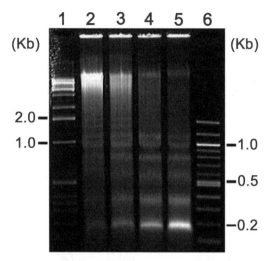

Fig. 1. Time-course of nuclei digestion by micrococcal nuclease. Maize nuclei were subjected to nuclease digestion for 1 min (lane 2), 2 min (lane 3), 4 min (lane 4), and 6 min (lane 5) and subjected to agarose gel electrophoresis. Size marker (lanes 1 and 6) were also electrophoresed in parallel.

3.3 Nucleosome Mapping: PCR Amplification and Quantification

To determine the nucleosome arrangement in a given sequence, PCR can be used with a series of primer sets designed from the sequence of concern. In each set, the forward and reverse primers are designed to cover approx 145 bp on the template sequence, which theoretically constitutes the core region of a nucleosome. Primers should essentially possess similar characteristics such as *T*m and not form dimers. Successive series of primers are designed after the sequence by shifting approx 15 bp from the initial position, so that a set of 145 bp can be amplified from arbitrary positions if the template is available (**Fig. 2**).

Optimal cycle conditions should be determined to ensure an exponential range of amplification, and the loading amount of amplified DNA to agarose gel should also be selected to ensure a linear range of signal intensity after ethidium bromide staining (*see* **Note 3**). Amplified DNA is quantified by densitometric Image Gauge V3.3 software (Fuji Film Science Lab and Kohshin Graphic Systems). Alternatively, the product can be quantified by measuring ^{32}P incorporation into the PCR products or by using the SYBR green technique in a light cycler.

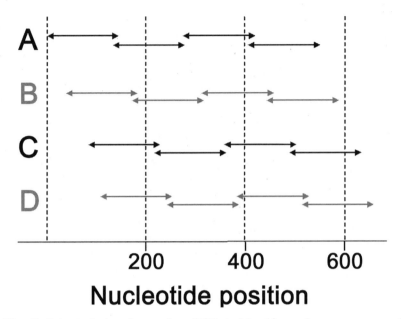

Fig. 2. Primer design for random PCR to identify nucleosome core and linker regions. Series (A–D) of forward and reverse primers (arrows), each approx 145 bp from another, can be designed on an arbitrary gene (indicated on the horizontal axis in bp). Successive series of primers are designed after the positions of the preceding primer set each shifting by approx 15 bp.

3.4. A Case Study: Methylation Mapping on Nucleosomes

The method is applied to determine the relationship between m^{5}C and the nucleosome structure of a particular maize gene, *ZmMI1* *(10)*. The position of m^{5}C is first identified by bisulfite modification followed by cloning and sequencing.

3.4.1. Bisulfite Modification

Digest total genomic DNA with appropriate restriction enzymes that do not cut the sequence of interest (*Xba*I was used in this case) and perform bisulfite modification by the method described *(12)*, with modification.

1. Digest 5 µg of genomic DNA with 35 U of *Xba*I for 16 h.
2. Add 10 µg of salmon sperm DNA as the carrier prior to precipitation with ethanol/sodium acetate (24:1), spin, and recover pellets.
3. Dissolve the pellet in 53 µL distilled water, mix with 2 µL 5 *N* NaOH, and incubate at room temperature for 10 min.
4. Mix the sample quickly with 1 mL of a freshly prepared bisulfite solution, cover the surface with mineral oil, and incubate at 50°C for 4 h. Prepare the bisulfite solution by mixing the reagents in the following order:

    a. Dissolve 1.9 g of sodium bisulfite (Sigma, cat. no. S1516) in 2.2 mL distilled water in a 15-mL Falcon tube to saturation by vigorous mixing (use a vortex).

    b. Add 280 μL of 5N NaOH and mix.

    c. Add 950 μL of a solution containing 55 mg of hydroquinone (Sigma, cat. no. H9003) completely dissolved in 920 μL distilled water.

    d. Mix well and adjust the final volume to 4 mL with distilled water.

5. Chill on ice for 5 min, and successively add 2430 μL of distilled water, 530 μL of 3 M sodium acetate, pH 7.0, 40 μL of 0.5% acrylamide aqueous solution, and 4055 μL of isopropanol. Mix the solution and spin at 7500g for 10 min at room temperature.

6. After washing with 70% ethanol and drying, dissolve the pellet in 400 μL of distilled water and transfer it into a 1.5-μL tube.

7. Add 40 μL of 3 M sodium acetate, pH 7.0, and 800 μL ethanol, and spin at 15,000g for 10 min at room temperature.

8. After washing with 70% ethanol and drying, dissolve the pellet in 350 μL of 0.2N NaOH and incubate 15 min at room temperature.

9. Add 175 μL 7.5 M ammonium acetate and 1050 μL ethanol, leave the sample at room temperature for 15 min, and then spin at 15,000g for 10 min at room temperature.

10. After washing with 70% ethanol and drying, dissolve the pellet in 250 μL TE buffer.

3.4.2. DNA Amplification, Selection, Cloning, and Sequencing

1. Perform PCR on the modified DNA using *ZmMI1*-specific primers (5'-GAGGAAGAGAAAGGGAGAG-3' and 5'-AAATCCATTTTCTATTCATTTA TTC-3'), ExTaq enzyme (Takara), 250 μM (*see* **Note 4**) each of dATP and TTP, and 125 μM each of dGTP and dCTP.

2. Amplification is as follows: 35 cycles of 96°C for 20 s, 52°C for 25 s, and 72°C for 1.1 min.

3. To remove partially and nonmodified sequences, digest the PCR products with *Alu*I (Takara), for which sites were confirmed to be rarely or never methylated by a preliminary methylation mapping.

4. Isolate a 1015-bp *Alu*I-resistant fraction after 1.2% agarose gel electrophoresis, ligated to the pGEM-T easy vector (Promega), and cloned in *E. coli* JM109 (Stratagene).

5. Determine the sequence with an ABI PRISM BigDye Terminator DNA sequencing kit (Applied Biosystems) and a 3100 Genetic Analyser automated sequencer (Applied Biosystems).

6. The results reveal that m^{5}C does not occur uniformly but rather periodically within approx 200 bases (**Fig. 3A**). The heavily methylated region, in which up to 100% of the methylatable sites are saturated with m^{5}C, comprises approx 45 bases. The relatively undermethylated region, in which only approx 60% of methylatable sites are m^{5}C, comprises approx 145 bases. The two alternate, forming a periodic oscillation pattern in terms of DNA methylation level, suggesting an association with the nucleosome structure.

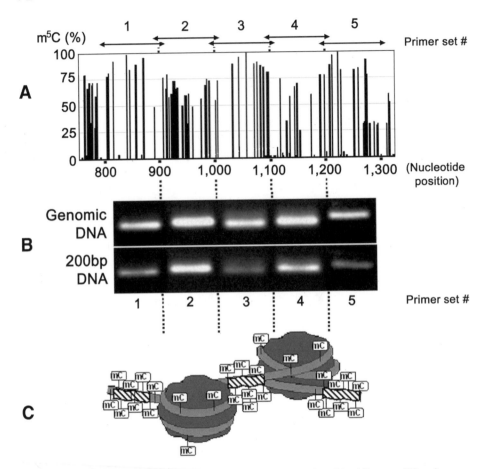

Fig. 3. Methylation profile in nucleosomes. (**A**) After bisulfite modification, an 886-bp region of the *ZmMI1* locus was amplified with PCR, cloned, and the sequence was determined. The position of cytosine in the *ZmMI1* genomic sequence is indicated on the horizontal axis, and the frequency of m⁵C in the total cytosines at the indicated position is expressed on the vertical axis (%). The number of examined clones was 64, and the average methylation frequency was 38.2% *(10)*. The position of PCR amplification is illustrated: fragments 1, 3, and 5 are expected to be amplified from hypermethylated regions; fragments 2 and 4 are from hypomethylated regions. (**B**) Template efficiency. To determine positioning of nucleosomal DNA, PCR was performed with 5 ng of mononucleosomal approx 200-bp fragments, or of total genomic DNA as the control in a reaction mixrure containing 0.5 U ExTaq (Takara), 10 m*M* Tris-HCl, pH 8.3, 50 m*M* KCl, 1.5 mM MgCl₂, 250 μ*M* dNTPs. Five sets of primers were designed after the *ZmMI1* sequence: set 1 forward, 5'-CTTGGCAAGGGTGCG AGTAC-3', reverse 5'-CGTGAATCTGGGCGCAATC-3'; set 2 forward 5'-CTGCGTGAACCATGTTGATTGC-3', reverse 5'-GGCACCATACAGGTGATTGG

3.4.3. Differential PCR

To assess this possibility, micrococcal nuclease-digested approx 200-base fragments were subjected to PCR in parallel with control undigested genomic DNA. Primers were designed to amplify independently five approx 150-base fragments, each containing either hypermethylated or hypomethylated regions (**Fig. 3A**). When genomic DNA was used as the template for PCR with five sets of primers, corresponding fragments were equally well amplified (**Fig. 3B**). When nuclease-digested 200-base DNA fragments were employed, fragments containing hypomethylated regions were more efficiently amplified than those containing hypermethylated regions (**Fig. 3B**). This finding suggested that micrococcal nuclease preferentially cleaved DNA around the hypermethylated regions. In other words, approx 145 base regions enriched with hypomethylated cytosines were resistant to nuclease and hence corresponded to the core, whereas approx 45-base regions enriched with hypermethylated cytosines were sensitive to nuclease and hence corresponded to the linker regions. We concluded therefore that DNA in the core and linker regions of nucleosomes was hypo- and hypermethylated, respectively (**Fig. 3C**).

3.5. Concluding Remarks

The present method is potentially useful to identify the nucleosome positioning of any gene of interest. Two points are unique. The first is the use of micrococcal nuclease, which selectively cleaves the linker region of a nucleosome, producing a 200-bp unit fragment containing the core region. The second is the use of multiple sets of PCR primers covering arbitrary regions of approximately 150–200 bp in the gene. If nuclease-digested 200 bp is ampli-

---

Fig. 3. *(continued)* ATTTC-3′; set 3 forward 5′-CCAATCACCTGTATGGTGCCTC-3′, reverse 5′-ATGCCACACGCTGGTCATC-3′); set 4 forward 5′TTGGATGAC CAGCGTGTGG-3′; reverse 5′-CTATGGCTCCTAAGTCGCGTGG-3′), set 5 forward 5′-GAGCGGTCACCGTGCGATC-3′ reverse 5′GCACAACTGGCAATCCA AGGTC-3′). Amplification was performed with 35 cycles of 95°C for 20 s, 63°C for 25 s, and 72°C for 10 s. The optimal cycle number was determined to ensure an exponential range of amplification, and the loading amount of amplified DNA to agarose gel was determined to ensure a linear range of signal intensity after ethidium bromide staining. Amplified samples from total genomic DNA (upper panel) or mononucleosomal 200-bp DNA fragments (lower panel) as the template were subjected to agarose gel electrophoresis and visualized with ethidium bromide staining. (**C**) Image of nucleosomes based on the above results. Regions 2 and 4 constitute the core, and 1, 3, and 5 constitute the linker. The positions of m^5C are indicated by the flags; m^5C distributes densely in the linker region.

fied, the region is inside the core. In contrast, if amplification is poor, the region spans the linker region. The procedure is simple, and reproducible. To our surprise, however, the nucleosome positioning in the *ZmMI1* gene, which is silent under normal growth conditions, appears to be fixed among individual seedlings. Since we used multiple seedlings from different cultures for one assay, it is significant that all of them exhibited the same nucleosome positioning, suggesting a common rule for nucleosome organization. Although it remains to be determined whether this is also the case in mammalian cells, it is attractive to examine and compare the nucleosome arrangement in, for example, normal and tumor cells. Furthermore, if the method is developed to handle only a few cells, correlations between gene expression and nucleosome structure could be analyzed in much more detail.

4. Notes

1. Using a microscope supplied with an HBO lamp set at 461 nm, the nuclear suspension is checked with 0.3% (w/v) DAPI staining. The suspension composed of nuclei (bright blue) is often surrounded by cell debris (unstained). A fraction of the nuclei looks damaged owing to the grinding step, but this does not affect the quality of the mononucleosomal fraction isolated.
2. To determine the optimal time period for micrococcal nuclease digestion, it is recommended to perform a time-course analysis first, with sampling every minute for 2–8 min. The optimal digestion time can be estimated from the production of a clear and intensive 146-bp fragment after gel electrophoresis.
3. **Caution:** ethidium bromide is highly toxic and must be handled with appropriate care.
4. Bisulfite modification results in particularly AT-rich sequences, of which PCR often causes a depletion of dATP and dTTP. This appears not to disturb the DNA amplification itself, but strongly inhibits the template-independent terminal transferase activity that adds a single deoxyadenosine residue to the 3'-end of synthesized DNA fragments, hampering the following T-vector ligation. To avoid this and to improve the ligation efficiency, an increase in the concentration of dATP and dTTP is highly recommended for PCR of the modified DNA amplification.

Acknowledgments

This work was supported by a grant from the Research for the Future Program (JSPS-RFTF00L01604) from the Japan Society for the Promotion of Science.

References

1. Gruenbaum, Y., Naveh-Many, T., Cedar, H., and Razin, A. (1981) Sequence specificity of methylation in higher plant DNA. *Nature* **292**, 860–862.
2. Oakeley, E. J. and Jost, J.-P. (1996) Non-symmetrical cytosine methylation in tobacco pollen DNA. *Plant Mol. Biol.* **31**, 927–930.

3. Bird, A. P. and Wolffe, A. P. (1999) Methylation-induced repression—belts, braces, and chromatin. *Cell* **99,** 451–454.
4. Yoder, J. A., Walsh, C. P., and Bestor, T. H. (1997) Cytosine methylation and the ecology of intragenomic parasites. *Trends Genet.* **13,** 335–340.
5. Miura, A., Yonebayashi, S., Watanabe, K., Toyama, T., Shimada, H., and Kakutani, T. (2001) Mobilization of transposons by a mutation abolishing full DNA methylation in Arabidopsis. *Nature* **411,** 212–214.
6. Bird, A. P. (2002) DNA methylation patterns and epigenetic memory. *Genes Devel.* **16,** 6–21.
7. Robertson, K. D. and Wolffe A. P. (2000) DNA methylation in health and disease. *Nature Rev. Genet.* **1,** 11–19.
8. Ehrlich, M. (2000) DNA hypomethylation and cancer, in *DNA Alteration in Cancer* (Ehrlich, M., ed.), Eaton Publishing, Natick, MA, pp. 273–291.
9. Murashige, T. and Skoog, F. (1962) A revised medium for rapid growth and bioassays with tobacco tissue cultures. *Physiol. Plant.* **15,** 473–497.
10. Steward, N., Ito, M., Yamaguchi, Y., Koizumi, N., and Sano, H. (2002). Periodic DNA methylation in maize nucleosomes and demethylation by environmental stress. *J. Biol. Chem.* **277** , 37,741–37,746.
11. Yamaguchi, J., Lim, P. Y., Aratani, K., and Akazawa, T. (1992). Isolation and characterization of nuclei from rice embryos. *Cell Struct. Func.* **17,** 87–92.
12. Raizis, A. M., Schmitt, F., and Jost, J. P. (1995) A bisulfite method of 5-methylcytosine mapping that minimizes template degradation. *Anal. Biochem.* **226,** 161–166.

7

DNaseI Hypersensitivity Analysis of Chromatin Structure

Qianjin Lu and Bruce Richardson

Summary

Transcriptionally inactive DNA is packaged into condensed chromatin such that it is unavailable to the transcription initiation complex. Activation of the silenced genes during processes such as differentiation first requires that the chromatin structure be remodeled into a transcriptionally permissive configuration, with the DNA "exposed" and accessible to transcription factors. The change in chromatin structure associated with transcriptional competence can be detected as increased sensitivity of the exposed DNA to digestion with DNaseI. This increased susceptibility is referred to as DnaseI-hypersensitivity. DNaseI hypersensitive sites are often located in the recognition sites for transcription factors, including promoters and enhancers. This chapter describes the protocols necessary to perform and analyze DNaseI hypersensitivity assays, a technique becoming increasingly important given the rapid advances in our understanding of the chromatin remodeling processes.

Key Words: DnaseI; hypersensitivity; chromatin structure; gene transcription.

1. Introduction
1.1. Background

Eukaryotic DNA is packaged as chromatin, the basic unit of which is the nucleosome, consisting of DNA wrapped twice around a core of four histone pairs and connected by the DNA strand; the nucleosomes are further assembled into higher order structures. The structure of chromatin in or near promoters and enhancers has profound effects on gene expression. In general, a condensed structure makes the DNA inaccessible to transcription factors, preventing gene expression, whereas a more open configuration is associated with transcription factor binding, resulting in gene expression *(1)*. For transcription factors to bind their recognition sequences, condensed chromatin must first be remodeled into an "open" configuration permitting interactions between the DNA

From: *Methods in Molecular Biology, vol. 287: Epigenetics Protocols*
Edited by: T. O. Tollefsbol © Humana Press Inc., Totowa, NJ

and transcription factors and allowing the transcription initiation complex to assemble *(2)*. This open configuration also makes the DNA accessible to the endonuclease DNaseI. The localized accessibility of transcriptionally permissive DNA to DNaseI digestion forms the basis of the DNaseI hypersensitivity assay, in which limited digestion reveals the accessible sites.

Consistent with the idea that DNA in transcriptionally active regions is in a configuration accessible to transcription factors, DNaseI-hypersensitive sites often map at or near recognition sequences for promoter-specific DNA binding proteins. Studies performed over more than 20 yr have shown that DnaseI-hypersensitive sites are most commonly located within 1 kb 5′ to the transcription start site. However, the relationship is not strict, and hypersensitive sites have been found quite distant, as well as downstream, of the start site or within introns *(3–5)*. An excellent example is provided by the β-globin gene cluster: the locus control region is located approx 120 kb 5′ to the gene cluster, and DNaseI hypersensitivity was used to identify the region *(6)*. The sites have been mapped to a large number of functional DNA segments, including promoters, enhancers, locus control elements, transcriptional silencers, origins of replication, recombination elements, and structural sites within or around telomeres *(7,8)*. Mapping of DNaseI-hypersensitive sites and monitoring their kinetics of appearance has been used successfully to demonstrate changes in chromatin structure around specific genes occurring during differentiation, correlating with the acquisition of transcriptional competence *(9)*.

Advances made in the last several years demonstrate persuasively that gene expression states are determined by epigenetic mechanisms including DNA methylation and a variety of histone modifications such as methylation and acetylation; many if not all of these affect chromatin structure. The rapid development of this field has stimulated new interest in the venerable DNaseI hypersensitivity assay as a tool to identify regions of the genome with the potential for gene transcription that may be caused by localized alterations in the chromatin structure, making reviews of this technique timely. In eukaryotes, DNA methylation refers to the methylation of deoxycytosine (dC) bases in CG pairs to form deoxymethylcytosine (d^mC). Methylcytosine binding proteins such as MeCP2 bind d^mC and attract chromatin inactivation complexes including histone deacetylases, which remove acetyl groups from histones and promote chromatin condensation into an inactive configuration *(10)*. Methylation of histone H3 lysine 9 creates a binding site for HP1 *(12)*. Recruitment of HP1 to euchromatin can also establish a silenced state *(12)*. DNaseI assays have been used by our group to demonstrate that perforin expression in primary CD4+ and CD8+ T cells involves the demethylation and development of a DNaseI-hypersensitive site in an enhancer 5′ to the *PRF1* gene *(13)*. We also reported a similar association among DNA hypomethylation, DNaseI hypersensitivity, and gene expression in the promoter of the *ITGAL* (CD11a) gene *(14)*.

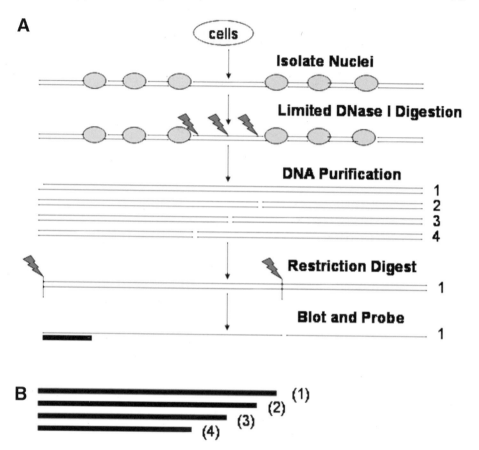

Fig. 1. (A). Schematic diagram of the DNaseI hypersensitivity assay. Nucleosomes are represented by filled circles and DNA by the double line. Nuclei are isolated from cells, and then incubated with limiting amounts of DNaseI, producing on average less than one cut per DNA strand. DNA is then purified, and digested with an appropriate restriction endonuclease, and the resulting fragments are analyzed by Southern blotting, probing with a labeled DNA fragment complementary to sequences at the end of the restriction fragment. **(B).** Mapping of DNaseI hypersensitive sites. Line 1 represents the restriction fragment without DNaseI digestion. Lines 2, 3, and 4 represent fragments resulting from limited cleavage at the indicated DNaseI-hypersensitive sites.

Others have used DNaseI hypersensitivity assays to demonstrate the consequences of altering histone acetylation and methylation on chromatin structure (*15–17*).

1.2. Strategy

The general strategy for DNaseI hypersensitivity assays is shown in **Fig. 1A**. Treating chromatin briefly and with limiting amounts of DNaseI will cleave exposed hypersensitive sites. It is important to note that longer digestions or

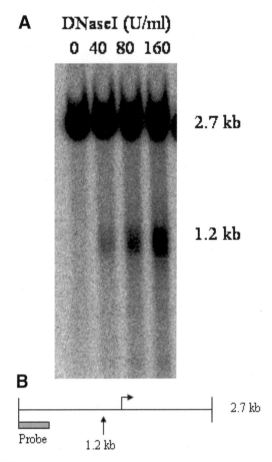

Fig. 2. DNaseI hypersensitive site in the *PRF1* promoter. CD4+ T-lymphocyte nuclei were treated with the indicated amounts of DNaseI, DNA isolated and digested with *Eco*RI, hybridized to a nylon filter, and hybridized with α^{32}P-labeled probe complementary to the 3' end of the fragment. (**A**) Autoradiogram. (**B**) Schematic diagram showing the *Eco*RI sites, the probe, the transcription start site (bent arrow), and the location of the DNaseI site producing the 1.2-kb fragment.

greater amounts of the enzyme will cleave the DNA of active genes at multiple sites, referred to as general DNaseI sensitivity *(8)*. Detection of the hypersensitive sites thus requires treating nuclei, containing intact chromatin, with limited amounts of DNaseI for a short period such that partial digestion is achieved, and then halting the digestion to prevent further DNA degradation. To map the cleavage sites, the DNA is isolated, digested with an appropriate restriction endonuclease, and analyzed by traditional Southern blotting. The hypersensitive sites are revealed by indirect end-labeling, using a short probe comple-

Table 1
DNaseI Buffer

Component	Stock	Final	Amount for 50 mL
HEPES, pH 8.0	1 M	10 mM	500 μL
KCl	3 M	50 mM	833 μL
MgCl$_2$	500 mM	5 mM	500 μL
CaCl$_2$	1 M	3 mM	150 μL
NP40	100%	0.1%	50 μL
Glycerol	100%	8%	4 mL
Dithiothreitol (DTT)	1 M	1 mM	50 μL

Add DTT μL/mL just prior to use.

Table 2
DNaseI Digestion Stop Buffer

Component	Stock	Final	Amount for 15 mL
EGTA	50 mM	20 mM	6 mL
Sodium dodecyl sulfate (SDS)	10%	1%	1.5 mL
DNase-free H$_2$O			7.5 mL

mentary to sequences near, or at the end of, the predicted restriction fragment. This produces a series of fragments similar to those shown in **Fig. 1B** and permits mapping of the cleavage sites to specific regions. An example of a DNaseI-hypersensitive site in the *PRF1* promoter is shown in **Fig. 2**. In this figure DNaseI digestion produces a 1.2-kb band that maps to a postion approx 200 bp 5′ to the transcription start site.

2. Materials

2.1. Isolation of Nuclei

1. 1-mL Dounce homogenizer (Wheaton).
2. Phosphate-buffered saline (PBS): 8 g/L NaCl, 0.2 g/L KCl, 1.44 g/L Na$_2$HPO$_4$, 0.24 g/L KH$_2$PO$_4$, pH 7.4.
3. Trypsin-EDTA: 0.5 g/L trypsin, 0.2 g/L EDTA (Invitrogen).
4. *See* **Table 1**.

2.2. DNaseI Treatment (see Table 2)

1. DNaseI buffer (*see* **Subheading 2.1.**, item 4).
2. DNaseI (molecular biology grade, Worthington).

2.3. DNA Purification

1. 10 mg/mL, DNase-free ribonuclease A (Invitrogen).
2. 10 mg/mL, Proteinase K (Invitrogen).

3. 3 M Sodium acetate.
4. Phenol/chloroform/isoamyl alcohol (25:24:1).
5. Isopropanol.
6. 70% Ethanol.
7. TE: 10 mM Tris-HCl, pH 7.5, 0.1 mM EDTA.

2.4. Restriction Enzyme Digestion

1. Gene-appropriate restriction enzyme with suitable 10X reaction buffer.

2.5. Gel Electrophoresis, Southern Blotting, and Hybridization.

1. Agarose, electrophoresis grade.
2. 1X TAE: 20 mM Tris-acetate, pH 8.0, 1 mM EDTA.
3. 10X Loading buffer: 65% (w/v) sucrose, 10 mM Tris-HCl, pH 7.5, 10 mM EDTA, 0.3% (w/v) bromphenol blue.
4. 1-kb Ladder (Invitrogen).
5. [α^{32}P]dCTP (Perkin Elmer).
6. Random primers DNA labeling system (Invitrogen).
7. PhosphorImager storage plates (Molecular Dynamics) or X-ray film.

3. Methods

3.1. Isolation of Nuclei

1. Harvesting Cells
   a. Adherent Cells. 1. For each 100×20-mm dish (1.5–2.0×10^7 cells), remove culture medium, rinse plate twice with PBS, add 1 mL trypsin-EDTA, and incubate at 37°C for 3–5 min. 2. Dislodge the cells with gentle shaking, and then immediately add back culture medium to quench the trypsinization. 3. Transfer the cells to a centrifugation tube, collect by sedimenting at 200g for 5 min at 4°C, and then wash twice with cold PBS.
   b. Suspension Cells. 1. Harvest the cells ($\sim 2 \times 10^7$) from the flask by sedimenting at 200g for 5 min at 4°C, and then wash twice with cold PBS.
2. Isolation of Nuclei. 1. Resuspend the cell pellet in 1.2 mL ice-cold DNaseI buffer, and then disrupt cells on ice using a Dounce homogenizer (~ 10 strokes). 2. Make four aliquots (280 µL each), keeping the aliquots at 4°C on ice (*see* **Notes 1** and **2**).

3.2. DNaseI Treatment of Nuclei

1. Reconstitution of Enzyme: Reconstitute vial with DNaseI buffer and glycerol according to the manufacturer's instructions, mix by gentle inversion, gently centrifuge to remove the liquid from the lid, and store aliquots (5 U/µL) at –80°C.
2. DNA Digestion: Incubate the four 280-µL aliquots with 0, 40, 80, and 160 U/mL of DNaseI (0, 2.2, 4.4, and 9.0 µL, respectively) at 25°C in a controlled temperature water bath for 3 min (*see* **Notes 3** and **4**). Add 300 µL DNaseI stop buffer to terminate the reaction (*see* **Note 5**).

3.3. DNA Purification

1. Add 5.8 μL DNase-free ribonuclease A (10 mg/mL) to each sample, incubate the mixture at 37°C for 2 h, and then add 11.6 μL proteinase K (10 mg/mL) and incubate the mixture overnight at 55°C.
2. The next day add 60 μL 1 3 *M* sodium acetate, pH 5.4, extract each sample twice with 1 vol of phenol/chloroform/isoamyl alcohol, centrifuge at 20,800*g* at room temperature in a microfuge for 5 min, transfer the aqueous phase to fresh tubes, precipitate the DNA with 0.7 vol of isopropanol, mix by inverting the tubes at least twice, incubate at –20°C for 1–2 h or overnight, sediment the DNA by centrifugation at 20,800*g* 4°C for 10 min, and rinse with ice-cold 70% ethanol.
3. Resuspend the DNA pellets in 31 μL TE.
4. To check the size distribution of the cleavage products, electrophorese 1 μL of sample through a 1% agarose gel in 1X TAE with 0.5 μL/mL ethidium bromide (*see* **Note 6**).

3.4. Restriction Endonuclease Digestion

Restriction enzyme digestion reactions are performed as follows.
1. Using 1.5-mL microcentrifuge tubes, add 5 μL of the appropriate 10X restriction enzyme buffer, 30 μL DNA (*see* **Subheading 3.3.**), and DNase-free H_2O to a final volume of 50 μL.
2. Add an appropriate amount of the restriction enzyme and incubate at 37°C overnight (*see* **Note 7**).

3.5. Gel Electrophoresis, Southern Blotting, and Hybridization

1. Fractionate digested DNA (50 μL from **Subheading 3.4.**) by electrophoresis through a 25-cm 1.2–1.5% agarose/TAE gel, using 2.0 v/cm (40 v) until the bromphenol blue tracking dye has migrated across approx 80% of the gel. This is often done overnight (*see* **Note 8**).
2. Transfer the DNA to a nylon filter using standard methods *(18)*.
3. Hybridze the immobilized DNA with an $\alpha^{32}P$-labeled fragment from the region of interest, labeled by random priming (*see* **Note 9**), and visualized bands by autoradiography, using PhosphorImager plates or X-ray film.

3.6. Mapping Cleavage Sites

Autoradiography frequently reveals multiple bands reflecting multiple cleavage sites in the chromatin. Each band corresponds to a DNA fragment with the reference restriction site at one end and either the second restriction cleavage site or a DNaseI cut at the other end. The length of the band allows calculation of the distance of the DNaseI cut from the restriction site (*see* **Figs. 1B** and **2** for examples).

4. Notes

1. Endogenous nucleases may create artifacts in the analysis of chromatin from some tissues and cell lines. It is therefore advisable to process the samples quickly during the nuclear isolation and keep the temperature of the solutions as close to 4°C as possible. A useful control is to include a sample incubated in DNaseI digestion buffer under the same conditions, but without added DNaseI. Nucleases also sometimes demonstrate sequence specificity. This may be controlled for by digesting naked DNA with the nuclease and analyzing the digest alongside the chromatin digestion to determine whether the cleavage is really caused by chromatin structure.

2. The methods for cellular disruption described work well in our hands for T cells, natural killer cells, and fibroblasts. However, variations exist, and it is important to establish the optimal method of disruption and nuclear isolation.

3. It is often necessary to establish first the optimal amount of DNaseI for digestion, since the appropriate concentration is likely to vary for different cell types. To avoid under- or overdigestion, some authorities recommend first performing a test series of DNaseI hypersensitivity analyses, using a wide range of DNaseI concentrations, before selecting the range to be used.

4. An alternative strategy for identifying optimal DNaseI concentrations, which works well in our hands, is to treat the nuclei first with graded concentrations of DNaseI, varying enzyme levels in twofold steps over the desired range. The DNA is then isolated, fractionated by electrophoresis, and stained with ethidium bromide. **Figure 3** shows an example of a digest, with progressive increases in the amount of smaller DNA fragments with higher DNaseI concentrations.

5. It is important to make certain that each sample is treated with DNaseI for the same amount of time. When working with multiple samples, add DNaseI to each sample in 15-s intervals. When the digestion is complete, add the stop buffer to each sample in 15-s intervals.

6. Using the numbers of cells and volumes described will produce DNA at concentrations suitable for this protocol. If necessary, the DNA may be quantitated by diluting the DNA 1:20 in TE and measuring absorbance at 260 and 280 nm, assuming 1 OD unit = 50 μg/mL DNA and correcting for the dilution.

7. The relative amounts of DNA and restriction enzyme may vary according to the enzyme, and appropriate conditions should be used for each enzyme.

8. DNaseI digestion is suitable for comparing the chromatin structure of two (or more) different cell lines or cells in two (or more) different states (e.g., before or after treatment with inhibitor of histone deacetylase, before and after differentiation, and so on). When comparing multiple samples, all should be run on the same gel and all procedures carried out simultaneously to minimize experimental variability.

9. It is important to avoid selecting a probe hybridizing with either a restriction site or a DNaseI-hypersensitive site. The best way to avoid this is to design the probe to hybridize with the end of a fragment, referred to as indirect end labeling. A hypersensitive site close to one end of the fragment and within the probe hybrid-

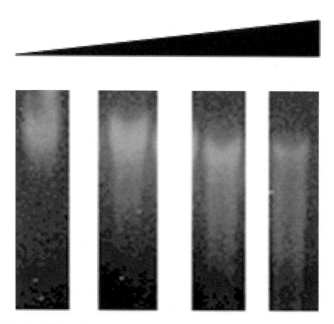

Fig. 3. Testing DNaseI enzyme concentrations. Chromatin was treated with 0, 40, 80, and 160 U/mL of DNaseI for 3 min. Then the reaction was stopped, and DNA was isolated, fractionated by electrophoresis, and stained with ethidium bromide. Increasing amounts of DNaseI generate progressively smaller DNA fragments.

izing area can be verified by hybridizing with a short probe to the other end of the fragment. Stripping the blot and hybridizing with a probe to the other end of the fragment is also a good way to verify the location of a hypersensitive site. We recommend generating probes by cutting subcloned DNA fragments and using fragments of approx 200 bp as probes. Alternatively, similarly sized DNA sequences can be directly amplified from plasmid DNA or genomic DNA using PCR and specific primers. To control for the specificity of probe hybridization, and to exclude effects of endogenous nucleases, a sample of total genomic DNA should always be analyzed without DNaseI digestion.

References

1. King, I. F. and Kingston, R. E. 2001. Specifying transcription. *Nature* **414,** 858–861.
2. Ahmad, K. and Henikoff, S. 2002. Epigenetic consequences of nucleosome dynamics. *Cell* **111,** 281–284.
3. Bier, E., Hashimoto, Y., Greene, M. I., and Maxam, A. M. 1985. Active T-cell receptor genes have intron deoxyribonuclease hypersensitive sites. *Science* **229,** 528–534.
4. Elgin, S. C. 1981. DNAase I-hypersensitive sites of chromatin. *Cell* **27,** 413–415.

5. Kok, K., Snippe, L., Ab, G., and Gruber, M. 1985. Nuclease-hypersensitive sites in chromatin of the estrogen-inducible apoVLDL II gene of chicken. *Nucleic Acids Res* **13**, 5189–5202.

6. Orkin, S. H. 1995. Regulation of globin gene expression in erythroid cells. *Eur. J. Biochem.* **231**, 271–281.

7. Reeves, R. 1988. Active chromatin structure, in *Chromosomes and Chromatin*, (Adolph, K., ed.), CRC, Boca Raton FL, pp.110–125.

8. Wolffe, A. P. 1998. *Chromatin: Structure and Function*. Academic, San Diego, CA, pp.199–212.

9. Agarwal, S. and Rao, A. 1998. Modulation of chromatin structure regulates cytokine gene expression during T cell differentiation. *Immunity* **9**, 765–775.

10. Bird, A. P. and Wolffe, A. P. 1999. Methylation-induced repression—belts, braces, and chromatin. *Cell* **99**, 451–454.

11. Lu, Q., Ray, D., Deng, C., et al. (2003) DNA methylation and chromatin structure regulate T cell perforin gene expression. *J Immunol.* **170**, 5124-5132.

12. Lachner, M. O'Carroll D, Rea S, Mechtler K, Jenuwein T. (2001) Methylation of histone H3 lysine 9 creates a binding site for HP1 proteins. *Nature* **410**, 116–120.

13. Ayyanathan, K., Lechner M.S., Bell, P., et al. (2003) Regulated recruitment of HP1 to a euchromatic gene induces mitotically heritable, epigenetic gene silencing: a mammalian cell culture model of gene variegation. *Genes Dev.* **17**, 1855–1869.

14. Lu, Q., Ray, D., Gutsch, D., and Richardson, B. 2002. Effect of DNA methylation and chromatin structure on ITGAL expression. *Blood* **99**, 4503–4508.

15. Gregory, R. I., O'Neill, L. P., Randall, T. E., et al. (2002) Inhibition of histone deacetylases alters allelic chromatin conformation at the imprinted U2af1-rs1 locus in mouse embryonic stem cells. *J. Biol. Chem.* **277**, 11,728–11,734.

16. Schubeler, D., Lorincz, M.C., Cimbora, D.M., et al. 2000. Genomic targeting of methylated DNA: influence of methylation on transcription, replication, chromatin structure, and histone acetylation. *Mol. Cell. Biol.* **20**, 9103–9112.

17. Stimson, K. M. and Vertino, P. M. 2002. Methylation-mediated silencing of TMS1/ASC is accompanied by histone hypoacetylation and CpG island-localized changes in chromatin architecture. *J. Biol. Chem.* **277**, 4951–4958.

18. Brown, T. 1993. Analysis of DNA sequences by blotting and hybridization, in *Current Protocols in Molecular Biology*, (Ausubel, B.R., Kingston, F., Moore, R., Seidman, D., Smith, J., and Struhl, K., eds.) John Wiley & Sons, New York. pp.2.9.1–2.9.15.

8

Inhibition of Histone Deacetylases

Cheng Liu and Dawei Xu

Summary

Reversible histone acetylation, governed dynamically by histone acetyltransferases (HATs) and histone deacetylases (HDACs), plays a pivotal role in regulation of gene expression through remodeling chromatin structure. Manipulation of the equilibrium between acetylation and deacetylation of histones by specific HDAC inhibitors is thus a useful tool to study functional role(s) for histone hyper-/hypoacetylation in controlling gene transcription and many other cellular activities. By using the *trans*-activating effect of trichostatin A (TSA), a widely used HDAC inhibitor, on the telomerase reverse transcriptase (hTERT) gene as an example, we summarize various aspects of HDAC inhibitors and provide a general strategy for their in vitro application in studies of gene regulation.

Key Words: Histone deacetylases (HDACs); histone acetyltransferases (HATs); trichostatin A (TSA); chromatin remodeling; gene regulation.

1. Introduction

Acetylation/deacetylation of proteins influences protein properties and thus modifies their ability to recognize DNA and their protein–protein interaction. In this protein family are histones that, together with DNA, are compacted to form chromatin in eukaryotic cells. Acetylation of lysine residues on the amino-terminal tails of the histones promotes destabilization of histone–DNA interaction in the nucleosome, resulting in open chromatin, easier access to corresponding promoter regions of genes by transcription factors, and subsequent *trans*-activation of specific genes *(1,2)* (*see* **Notes 1** and **2**). The dynamic interplay between histone deacetylases (HDACs) and histone acetyltransferases (HATs) has been shown to be a key mechanism in this form of regulation. Manipulation of the balance between acetylation and deacetylation of histones by specific HDAC inhibitors is thus a useful tool to delineate functional role(s) for histone hyper-/hypoacetylation in various cellular activities. According to their structures, HDAC inhibitors fall into five categories: (1) short-chain fatty

From: *Methods in Molecular Biology, vol. 287: Epigenetics Protocols*
Edited by: T. O. Tollefsbol © Humana Press Inc., Totowa, NJ

acids (e.g., sodium butyrate *[3]*); (2) hydroxamic acids (e.g., trichostatin A [TSA] *[4]* or suberoylanilide hydroxamic acid [SAHA] *[5]*); (3) cyclic tetrapeptides containing a 2-amino-8-oxo-9,10-epoxy-decanoyl moiety (e.g., trapoxin A *[4]*); (4) cyclic peptides lacking the 2-amino-8-oxo-9,10-epoxy-decanoyl moiety (e.g., apicidin *[6]*); and (5) benzamides (e.g., MS-27-275 *[7]*) (*see* **Note 3**). To date, HDAC inhibitors have been shown to affect numerous biological processes such as cell differentiation *(8,9)*, proliferation *(10,11),* and apoptosis *(9,12)* through their specific regulation of a variety of genes. For instance, TSA induces the cyclin-dependent kinase inhibitor p21$^{WAF1/Cip1}$, thereby causing either G1 and/or G2/M arrest of the cell cycle in many types of cells *(13,14)*.

TSA, a potent and highly specific HDAC inhibitor, has been widely used in histone acetylation studies in vitro and in vivo. It reversibly binds the active site in the catalytic site of HDACs and interacts with a zinc metal ion within the catalytic pocket, thereby causing acetylated histones to accumulate in cells *(15)*. In addition to a direct inhibition of HDAC catalytic activity, TSA has recently been shown to accelerate degradation of HDAC1 *(16)*. Through these different mechanisms, significant inhibition of HDACs by TSA can occur at nanomolar concentrations. However, the efficacy of TSA treatment on histone acetylation and gene activation in vitro is affected by a variety of factors, including types of cells, culture media, confluence of cultured cells, time of incubation, concentrations of TSA, and so on. Multiple experiments should be performed to achieve desirable results. **Table 1** summarizes various conditions for in vitro TSA treatment of different cell lines reported in the literature.

The *trans*-activation of the human telomerase reverse transcriptase (hTERT) gene in resting T lymphocytes by TSA treatment will be used as a model to illustrate a general strategy for inhibition of HDACs. hTERT mRNA is very low or undetectable in resting T lymphocytes, and TSA treatment of T cells results in dramatic upregulation of hTERT expression in a time- and dose-dependent manner owing to the increased level of acetylated histones in the *hTERT* promoter region *(17,31)* (*see* **Note 4**).

2. Materials

2.1. Time and Dose-Course Studies of TSA Treatment

1. Normal human T lymphocytes isolated from peripheral blood of healthy individuals.
2. Cell culture medium: RPMI-1640 (Life Technologies) containing 10% fetal calf serum (FCS), 100 U/mL penicillin, and 2 m*M* L-glutamine.
3. TSA (7-[4-(dimethylamino) phenyl]-*N*-hydroxy-4,6-dimethyl-7-oxo-2,4-heptadienamide; Sigma) dissolved in 100% ethanol at a concentration of 2 m*M*, stored at –20°C, and diluted as required.

Table 1
Cell Culture Conditions and TSA Concentrations for Different Cell Lines

Cell line	TSA conc. (ng/mL)	Exposure time (h)	Cell culture medium[a]
Human dermal fibroblast cells (17)	300	O.N.	RPMI-1640
Human lung fibroblast cell line (WI-38,MRC-5) (18)	100[b]	24	α-MEM
Human foreskin fibroblast cell line (BJ) (18)	100[b]	24	α-MEM
Human resting T cells (17)	300	O.N.	RPMI-1640
Human cervical cancer cell lines (SiHa,Hela,C33A) (17)	300	O.N.	DMEM
Human astrocyte cell line (NHA) (19) growth medium from Clonetics	500	48	Astrocyte
Human colorectal carcinoma cell line (SW-480) (20)	1000	24	IMEM
Human renal cortical epithelial cell line (HRCE) (21)	300	24	REGM™
Human osteosarcoma cell line (MG63) (22)	500	24	DMEM
Human osteosarcoma cell line (Saos-2) (17)	300	O.N.	DMEM
Human pro-B-cell lines (RS4,Nalm,16KM3,REH) (23)	300	24	IMDM
Human pre-B-cell line (OB5,697,Nalm 6) (23)	300	24	IMDM
Human intermediate B-cell line (1E8) (23)	300	24	IMDM
Human mature B-cell lines (Raji,Dakiki,IM9) (23)	300	24	IMDM
Human plasma B-cell (HS sultan, OPM2,U266) (23)	300	24	IMDM
Human breast carcinoma cell line (MCF/7) (23)	300	24	IMDM
Human embryonic kidney cell line (HEK) (18)	100[b]	24	α-MEM
Human lung adenocarcinoma cell line (LT23) (24)	50	16	1:1 mixture of DMEM and HAM's F12[c]
Human prostate cancer cell lines (LNCaP,PC3,DU145) (25)	100	24	RPMI-1640
Rat skin fibroblasts (26)	30	24	DMEM

(continued)

Table 1 *(continued)*

Cell line	TSA conc. (ng/mL)	Exposure time (h)	Cell culture medium[a]
Rat pulmonary arterial SMCs (PAC1) (27)	60	24	DMEM
Mouse primary embryonic fibroblast (EF1) (28)	100	6	DMEM
Mouse renal fibroblast cell line (NIH3T3) (29)	100	24	DMEM
Mouse peritoneal macrophages (30)	2.5	48	RPMI-1640
Mouse fibroblasts (10T1/2) (27)	60	24	DMEM

α-MEM, α-miminal essential medium; DMEM, Dulbecco's MEM; IMEM, improved MEM; REGM, renal epithelial cell medium (Clonefics).

[a]The cell culture medium should include appropriate antibiotics, fetal calf serum, and L-glutamine.

[b]Dissolved in Me_2SO.

[c]1:1 mixture of DMEM and HAM's F12, buffered with 22 mM $NaHCO_3$ and 15 mM HEPES, with addition of insulin (5 μg/mL), transferrin (5 μg/mL), epidermal growth factor (5 ng/mL), triiodthyronine (0.1 nM), Na-selenite (75 nM), and ethanolamine (8 μM).

4. ddH_2O autoclave twice.
5. Reagents for preparation of total cellular RNA or mRNA (e.g., ULTRASPEC-II RNA kit, Biotecx Laboratories, Houston TX).
6. Reagents for cDNA synthesis (e.g., murine Moloney leukemia virus [MMLV] reverse transcriptase, Gibco-BRL, and random priming [N6], Pharmacia, Uppsala, Sweden).
7. PCR reagents: *Taq* polymerase with 10X *Taq* DNA polymerase buffer, $MgCl_2$, deoxyribonucleoside triphosphates (dNTPs) (e.g., Pharmacia).
8. Competitive templates for competitive PCR (*see* **Note 5**).
9. Specific hTERT primers: forward 5'-CGG AAG AGT GTC TGG AGC AA 3' and reverse 5'-GGA TGA AGC GGA GTC TGG A 3'. Specific β$_2$-microglobulin (β$_2$M) primers: forward 5'-GAA TTG CTA TGT GTC TGG GT 3' and reverse 5'-CAT CTT CAA ACC TCC ATG ATG 3'.
10. Metaphor agarose gels (FMC, Rockland, ME).

2.2. Histone Isolation

1. Phosphate-buffered saline (PBS).
2. Lysis buffer for histone isolation: 10 mM Tris-HCl, pH 6.5, 50 mM sodium bisulfite, 10 mM $MgCl_2$, 10 mM sodium butyrate, 8.6% sucrose, 1% Triton X-100.
3. Dounce homogenizer.
4. Resuspension buffer: 10 mM Tris-HCl, pH 8.0, 13 mM EDTA.
5. Sulfuric acid, acetone (Sigma).

2.3. Western Blot Analysis of Acetylated Histone H4

1. 2X Sodium dodecyl sulfate-polyacrylamide gel electrophoresis (SDS-PAGE) loading buffer, 18% SDS-PAGE gels, gel running and protein transfer apparatus, and nitrocellulose membrane.
2. Rabbit antibody against acetylated histone H4, antirabbit secondary antibody (Upstate Biotechnology, Lake Placid, NY).
3. ECL kit (Pharmacia).

3. Methods

We describe a method to optimize TSA-mediated induction of hTERT mRNA in normal human resting T lymphocytes, and we examine the status of histone acetylation.

3.1. Optimal Incubation Time of Human T Cells With TSA

TSA inhibits HDAC activity and induces histone acetylation in a time-dependent manner. Shorter incubation is insufficient to induce maximal levels of hTERT mRNA, whereas longer exposure to TSA may be harmful to cells. Therefore, we first investigate the temporal profile of hTERT expression in resting T lymphocytes treated with TSA. As shown in **Fig. 1**, hTERT mRNA became detectable within 4 h of TSA exposure and a maximal level was reached by 16 h.

1. Prepare normal human T lymphocytes from peripheral blood of healthy individuals using standard techniques. Maintain cells in RPMI-1640 medium supplemented with 10% FCS, 100 U/mL penicillin, and 2 mM L-glutamine, and incubate at 37°C/5% CO_2 in a humidified atmosphere.
2. Dilute cells to 1×10^6/mL in culture flasks.
3. Aliquot cells in eight culture flasks of the same size. If adherent cells are used, check that the cells are approx 40–50% confluent (*see* **Note 6**).
4. Add TSA (dissolved in 100% ethanol) to culture medium at a concentration of 1 μM or vehicle (ethanol)-containing medium. Keep the final ethanol concentration <0.1% (v/v%) in the medium.
5. Incubate cells under the same conditions as described above in **Subheading 3.1.** and harvest them 1, 2, 4, 6, 10, 16, and 24 h post-TSA exposure, respectively.
6. Purify total cellular RNA from the harvested cells using an ULTRASPEC-II RNA kit, according to the manufacturer's instruction.
7. Synthesize first-strand cDNA from total RNA templates with random hexamers using a kit for reverse transcription (RT).
8. Perform a competitive polymerase chain reaction (PCR; 25 μL/each sample) using the following parameters: denaturation at 94°C for 3 min, followed by amplification with 34 PCR cycles (94°C for 45 s, 60°C for 45 s, 72°C for 90 s), and a final extension at 72°C for 10 min. Each reaction comprises 1 × PCR buffer, 2.5 mM $MgCl_2$, 0.2 mM each dNTP, 0.3 μM primers, first-strand cDNA (corresponding to 50 ng total RNA), 2000 competitive molecules, and 0.625 U/μL *Taq* poly-

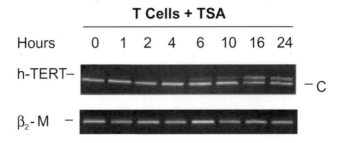

Fig. 1. Time-course study on induction of hTERT mRNA by trichostatin A (TSA) in normal human resting T lymphocytes. The levels of hTERT mRNA in the T cells treated with TSA for the indicated times were determined by using competitive RT-PCR *(17)*. C, competitive molecules; h-TERT, human telomerase reverse transcriptase; β_2-M, β_2-microglobulin. (Reproduced from **ref.** *17* with permission.)

merase. As a control for quantification, $\beta_2 M$ mRNA is amplified in parallel during 26 cycles using the same PCR parameters.

9. Run the products on 4% Metaphor agarose gels; the specific hTERT and its competitive amplicons are 145 and 166 bp in size, respectively.

3.2. Dose Course Study of T Cells Treated With TSA

The HDAC inhibitor TSA also upregulates hTERT expression in a dose-dependent manner. Within a certain range, the effect of TSA on gene activation is proportional to its concentrations in culture medium. Conceivably, however, too much TSA could be toxic to cells, thereby compromising or interfering with its gene *trans*-activating function. Because cells from different sources exhibit substantial variations in their sensitivity to TSA, it is necessary to test various concentrations of TSA to identify the best conditions for one's own experiments. In the case of human T cells, optimization of the experiment is performed as follows:

1. Prepare human T lymphocytes and culture them as described in **Subheading 3.1.**
2. Aliquot cells in five culture flasks of the same size.
3. Add TSA stock the culture medium with final concentrations of 100, 250, 500, and 1000 nM or to vehicle (ethanol)-containing medium.
4. Incubate cells as described above in **Subheading 3.1.**, and harvest them 16 h postincubation.
5. Isolate total cellular RNA and perform RT-PCR to determine the expression of hTERT mRNA as described in **Subheading 3.1.**

3.3. Identification of Histone Acetylation Status After TSA Treatment

A number of assays can be employed to examine the efficacy of TSA on HDAC inhibition. Chromatin immunoprecipitation (ChIP) is widely used to detect the in vivo association between acetylated histones and their target genes following treatment of cells with HDAC inhibitors (*see* **Chapters 2** and **3**). The abundance of acetylated histones is usually determined by using immunoblot of bulk histones separated on SDS-PAGE, Coomassie blue staining or Western blotting of bulk histones separated on acetic acid/urea/Triton X-100 (AUT) gels. Here we describe immunoblot analysis of acetylated histone H4 (*see* **Note 7**).

3.3.1. Histone Isolation

1. Wash cells (~5 × 10^6) with ice-cold PBS twice.
2. Resuspend cells in 1 mL lysis buffer.
3. Homogenize cells using a Dounce homogenizer according to the manufacturer's instruction.
4. Centrifuge the homogenates at 1000g for 5 min at 4°C.
5. Wash the pellets with 0.5 mL of suspension buffer.
6. Resuspend the pellets in 125 µL ice-cold sterile distilled water.
7. Add sulfuric acid to a final concentration of 0.4 N, and swirl to mix.
8. Incubate lysates on ice for 1 h.
9. Centrifuge lysates at 10,000g for 5 min at 4°C and discard the supernatant.
10. Add 10 vol of acetone to the pellet and place it at –20°C overnight.
11. Centrifuge at 10,000g for 5 min at 4°C, discard the supernatant, and use a vacuum to dry the pellet.
12. Resuspend the pellet with 50–200 µL ddH$_2$O.

3.3.2. Western Blot Analysis of Histone H4 Acetylation

1. Dilute equal amounts of histones in 2X SDS loading buffer, and boil them for 5 min.
2. Separate histones on 18% SDS-PAGE gels and blot them onto nitrocellulose membrane according to appropriate protocols.
3. Incubate the membrane in PBS with 3% dry milk for 20 min at room temperature.
4. Add the rabbit antibody against acetylated histone H4 at a dilution of 1:2000, and incubate the membrane with the diluted antibody overnight at 4°C.
5. Wash the membrane with PBS for 3 × 10 min.
6. Incubate the membrane with an antirabbit secondary antibody at a dilution of 1:3000 in PBS containing 3% dry milk at room temperature for 1.5 h.
7. Visualize the acetylated histone H4 with the ECL kit according to the manufacturer's protocol.

4. Notes

1. Although histones are associated with all eukaryotic chromatins, modification of histone acetylation status does not lead to a global change in gene expression. HDAC inhibitors act in a gene-selective manner, and differential display analysis demonstrates that only a small fraction of genes are transcriptionally affected by TSA treatment *(32)*. These histone-acetylation-sensitive genes are in general activated upon the increased histone acetylation resulting from HDAC inhibition.

However, a few genes such as *P57Kip2* have been shown to be repressed in some cell lines after treatment with the HDAC inhibitor *(33)*. It is unclear whether HDAC inhibitor-induced gene repression is a direct effect or caused by activation of a repressive element that in turn contributes to silencing of the specific gene(s).

2. It should be noted that a counteracting effect might occur when TSA and other compounds are added simultaneously. Rombouts et al. *(26)* showed that expression of the *procollagen* gene in skin fibroblasts was transcriptionally upregulated following transforming growth factor-β1 (TGF-β1) or TSA treatment alone, whereas the stimulatory effect of TGF-β1 on procollagen expression was significantly attenuated in the presence of TSA.

3. Human HDACs fall into three classes according to their similarity to yeast counterparts. Classes I (HDAC 1–3, 8, and possibly 11) and II (HDAC 4–7, 9–11) HDACs are all sensitive to inhibition by HDAC inhibitors such as TSA. The third class of HDACs (human sirtuins [SIRTs]) comprises NAD^+-dependent protein deacetylases. This family of HDACs is structurally and catalytically distinct from class I and II HDACs, and its enzymatic activity is not inhibited by TSA *(34)*. HDACs and their properties described in this chapter are limited to class I and II HDACs.

4. It has been suggested that histone hyper-/hypoacetylation is a common underlying feature of hTERT transcription regulation *(18,21)*, but the HDAC inhibitor TSA apparently inhibits hTERT expression in some prostate cell lines such as LNCaP and PC-3 *(35)*. There are no rational explanations for such a striking discrepancy at the moment.

5. The hTERT competitive template is made by inserting a 21-bp random sequence into the middle region of a wild-type (wt) hTERT PCR product. Therefore, both wt and competitive molecules can be amplified by using the same set of hTERT primers in the same reaction tubes. The resultant wt and competitive amplicons are separable in 4% Metaphor agarose gels. A ratio of wt *hTERT*/competitor signals represents relative abundance of hTERT mRNA. If there are no hTERT competitors available, or if one prefers, conventional or real-time RT-PCR may be used instead.

6. The efficacy of the HDAC inhibitor is cell density-dependent. Cells respond to TSA treatment only when they are cultured at an appropriate density and in an exponential growth phase. Cell density higher than a critical threshold may significantly compromise or even abolish *trans*-activating effects of TSA on acetylation-sensitive genes *(33)*.

7. The acetylation of histones H3 and H4 induced by HDAC inhibitors does not always occur at the same time and to the same degree *(36,37)*.

References

1. Bannister, A. J., and Miska, E. A. (2000) Regulation of gene expression by transcription factor acetylation. *Cell Mol Life Sci.* **57,** 1184–1192.
2. Struhl, K. (1998) Histone acetylation and transcriptional regulatory mechanisms. *Genes Dev.* **12,** 599–606.
3. Shankaranarayanan, P., Chaitidis, P., Kuhn, H., and Nigam, S. (2001) Acetylation by histone acetyltransferase CREB-binding protein/p300 of STAT6 is required for transcriptional activation of the 15-lipoxygenase-1 gene. *J Biol Chem.* **276,** 42,753–42,760.

4. Yoshida, M., Horinouchi, S., and Beppu, T. (1995) Trichostatin A and trapoxin: novel chemical probes for the role of histone acetylation in chromatin structure and function. *Bioessays* **17,** 423–430.

5. Nimmanapalli, R., Fuino, L., Stobaugh, C., Richon, V. M., and Bhalla, K. (2003) Co-treatment with the histone deacetylase inhibitor suberoylanilide hydroxamic acid (SAHA) enhances Gleevec-induced apoptosis of Bcr-Abl positive human acute leukemia cells. DOI 10.1182 *Blood* **101,** 3236–3239.

6. Colletti, S. L., Myers, R. W., Darkin-Rattray, S. J., et al. (2001) Broad spectrum antiprotozoal agents that inhibit histone deacetylase: structure-activity relationships of apicidin. *Bioorg. Med. Chem. Lett.* **11,** 107–117.

7. Lee, B. I., Park, S. H., Kim, J. W., et al. (2001) MS-275, a histone deacetylase inhibitor, selectively induces transforming growth factor beta type II receptor expression in human breast cancer cells. *Cancer Res.* **61,** 931–934.

8. Redner, R. L., Wang, J., and Liu, J. M. (1999) Chromatin remodeling and leukemia: new therapeutic paradigms. *Blood* **94,** 417–428.

9. Kamitani, H., Geller, M., and Eling, T. (1998) Expression of 15-lipoxygenase by human colorectal carcinoma Caco-2 cells during apoptosis and cell differentiation. *J. Biol. Chem.* **273,** 21,569–21,577.

10. Bernhard, D., Ausserlechner, M. J., Tonko, M., Loffler, M., Hartmann, B. L., Csordas, A., and Kofler, R. (1999) Apoptosis induced by the histone deacetylase inhibitor sodium butyrate in human leukemic lymphoblasts. *FASEB J.* **13,** 1991–2001.

11. Taplick, J., Kurtev, V., Lagger, G., and Seiser, C. (1998) Histone H4 acetylation during interleukin-2 stimulation of mouse T cells. *FEBS Lett.* **436,** 349–352.

12. Salminen, A., Tapiola, T., Korhonen, P., and Suuronen, T. (1998) Neuronal apoptosis induced by histone deacetylase inhibitors. *Brain Res. Mol. Brain Res.* **61,** 203–206.

13. Han, J. W., Ahn, S. H., Park, S. H., et al. (2000) Apicidin, a histone deacetylase inhibitor, inhibits proliferation of tumor cells via induction of p21WAF1/Cip1 and gelsolin. *Cancer Res.* **60,** 6068–6074.

14. Saito, A., Yamashita, T., Mariko, Y., et al. (1999) A synthetic inhibitor of histone deacetylase, MS-27-275, with marked in vivo antitumor activity against human tumors. *Proc. Natl. Acad. Sci. USA* **96,** 4592–4597.

15. Marks, P. A., Richon, V. M., and Rifkind, R. A. (2000) Histone deacetylase inhibitors: inducers of differentiation or apoptosis of transformed cells. *J. Natl. Cancer Inst.* **92,** 1210–1216.

16. Zhou, Q., Melkoumian, Z. K., Lucktong, A., Moniwa, M., Davie, J. R., and Strobl, J. S. (2000) Rapid induction of histone hyperacetylation and cellular differentiation in human breast tumor cell lines following degradation of histone deacetylase-1. *J. Biol. Chem.* **275,** 35,256–35,263.

17. Hou, M., Wang, X., Popov, N., et al. (2002) The histone deacetylase inhibitor trichostatin A derepresses the telomerase reverse transcriptase (hTERT) gene in human cells. *Exp. Cell Res.* **274,** 25–34.

18. Cong, Y. S. and Bacchetti, S. (2000) Histone deacetylation is involved in the transcriptional repression of hTERT in normal human cells. *J. Biol. Chem.* **275,** 35,665–35,668.

19. Taniura, S., Kamitani, H., Watanabe, T., and Eling, T. E. (2002) Transcriptional regulation of cyclooxygenase-1 by histone deacetylase inhibitors in normal human astrocyte cells. *J. Biol. Chem.* **277,** 16,823–16,830.

20. Kamitani, H., Taniura, S., Ikawa, H., Watanabe, T., Kelavkar, U. P., and Eling, T. E. (2001) Expression of 15-lipoxygenase-1 is regulated by histone acetylation in human colorectal carcinoma. *Carcinogenesis* **22,** 187–191.

21. Takakura, M., Kyo, S., Sowa, Y., et al. (2001) Telomerase activation by histone deacetylase inhibitor in normal cells. *Nucleic Acids Res.* **29,** 3006–3011.

22. Sowa, Y., Orita, T., Minamikawa-Hiranabe, S., Mizuno, T., Nomura, H., and Sakai, T. (1999) Sp3, but not Sp1, mediates the transcriptional activation of the p21/WAF1/Cip1 gene promoter by histone deacetylase inhibitor. *Cancer Res.* **59,** 4266–4270.

23. Schwab, J. and Illges, H. (2001) Regulation of CD21 expression by DNA methylation and histone deacetylation. *Int. Immunol.* **13,** 705–710.

24. Eickhoff, B., Germeroth, L., Stahl, C., et al. (2000) Trichostatin A-mediated regulation of gene expression and protein kinase activities: reprogramming tumor cells for ribotoxic stress-induced apoptosis. *Biol. Chem.* **381,** 1127–1132.

25. Nakayama, T., Watanabe, M., Yamanaka, M., et al. (2001) The role of epigenetic modifications in retinoic acid receptor beta2 gene expression in human prostate cancers. *Lab Invest.* **81,** 1049–1057.

26. Rombouts, K., Niki, T., Greenwel, P., et al. (2002) Trichostatin A, a histone deacetylase inhibitor, suppresses collagen synthesis and prevents TGF-beta(1)-induced fibrogenesis in skin fibroblasts. *Exp. Cell Res.* **278,** 184–197.

27. Qiu, P. and Li, L. (2002) Histone acetylation and recruitment of serum responsive factor and CREB-binding protein onto SM22 promoter during SM22 gene expression. *Circ. Res.* **90,** 858–865.

28. Gregory, R. I., O'Neill, L. P., Randall, T. E., et al. (2002) Inhibition of histone deacetylases alters allelic chromatin conformation at the imprinted U2af1-rs1 locus in mouse embryonic stem cells. *J. Biol. Chem.* **277,** 11,728–11,734.

29. Xiao, H., Hasegawa, T., and Isobe, K. (1999) Both Sp1 and Sp3 are responsible for p21waf1 promoter activity induced by histone deacetylase inhibitor in NIH3T3 cells. *J. Cell Biochem.* **73,** 291–302.

30. Wang, X. Q., Alfaro, M. L., Evans, G. F., and Zuckerman, S. H. (2002) Histone deacetylase inhibition results in decreased macrophage CD9 expression. *Biochem. Biophys. Res. Commun.* **294,** 660–666.

31. Xu, D., Popov, N., Hou, M., et al. (2001) Switch from Myc/Max to Mad1/Max binding and decrease in histone acetylation at the telomerase reverse transcriptase promoter during differentiation of HL60 cells. *Proc. Natl. Acad. Sci. USA* **98,** 3826–3831.

32. Van Lint, C., Emiliani, S., and Verdin, E. (1996) The expression of a small fraction of cellular genes is changed in response to histone hyperacetylation. *Gene. Expr.* **5,** 245–253.

33. Gray, S. G. and Ekstrom, T. J. (1998) Effects of cell density and trichostatin A on the expression of HDAC1 and p57Kip2 in Hep 3B cells. *Biochem. Biophys. Res. Commun.* **245,** 423–427.

34. Thiagalingam, S., Cheng, K. H., Lee, H. J., Mineva, N., Thiagalingam, A., and Ponte, J. F. (2003) Histone deacetylases: unique players in shaping the epigenetic histone code. *Ann. NY Acad. Sci.* **983,** 84-100.
35. Suenaga, M., Soda, H., Oka, M., et al. (2002) Histone deacetylase inhibitors suppress telomerase reverse transcriptase mRNA expression in prostate cancer cells. *Int. J. Cancer* **97,** 621–625.
36. Ito, K., Barnes, P. J., and Adcock, I. M. (2000) Glucocorticoid receptor recruitment of histone deacetylase 2 inhibits interleukin-1beta-induced histone H4 acetylation on lysines 8 and 12. *Mol. Cell. Biol.* **20,** 6891–6903.
37. Zhang, W., Bone, J. R., Edmondson, D. G., Turner, B. M., and Roth, S. Y. (1998) Essential and redundant functions of histone acetylation revealed by mutation of target lysines and loss of the Gcn5p acetyltransferase. *EMBO J.* **17,** 3155–3167.

9

Site-Specific Analysis of Histone Methylation and Acetylation

David Umlauf, Yuji Goto, and Robert Feil

Summary

Covalent modifications on the nucleosomal histones are essential in chromatin regulation and gene expression. Patterns of histone modifications may be somatically maintained and can thereby maintain locus-specific repression/activity in defined lineages or throughout development. During recent years, histone acetylation and methylation have emerged as key players in the repression or activation of genes and chromosomal domains. Histone methylation and acetylation patterns (and other histone modifications) can be analyzed by chromatin immunoprecipitation (ChIP). This chapter describes how ChIP can be performed on native chromatin prepared from cells and tissues, in order to analyze histone methylation and acetylation at specific sites in the genome. We also present different PCR-based assays that can be applied to analyze loci of interest in immunoprecipitated chromatin fractions.

Key Words: Chromatin immunoprecipitation; native chromatin; histone methylation; histone acetylation; quantitative PCR; allele-specific PCR.

1. Introduction

Covalent modifications on the nucleosomal histones are essential in chromatin regulation and gene expression. Patterns of histone modifications may be somatically maintained and can thereby maintain locus-specific repression/activity in defined lineages or throughout development. During recent years, histone acetylation and methylation have emerged as key players in the repression or activation of genes and chromosomal domains. Histone methylation and acetylation patterns (and other histone modifications) can be analyzed by chromatin immunoprecipitation (ChIP). This chapter describes how ChIP can be performed on native chromatin prepared from cells and tissues, in order to analyze histone methylation and acetylation at specific sites in the genome. We also present different PCR-based assays that can be applied to analyze loci of interest in immunoprecipitated chromatin fractions.

From: *Methods in Molecular Biology, vol. 287: Epigenetics Protocols*
Edited by: T. O. Tollefsbol © Humana Press Inc., Totowa, NJ

In cells and tissues, the histones that constitute the nucleosomes are subject to multiple posttranslational modifications *(1)*. These include lysine acetylation, lysine and arginine methylation, serine phosphorylation, and lysine ubiquitination. On their own, or in combination, these covalent modifications on the core histones are thought to play essential roles in chromatin organization and gene expression in eukaryotes *(2–6)*. In the last few years, many novel insights have emerged into the diverse roles of histone methylation and acetylation and its recognition by nuclear proteins *(5–7)*. For example, methylation *(7)* on different lysines of histone H3 can produce different, opposite outcomes. Methylation on lysine 4 (K4) of histone H3 is associated with heritable transcriptional activity in different eukaryotic model systems *(8–11)*, possibly because this modification somehow inhibits repressive chromatin remodeling complexes from binding to the chromatin *(12)*. Methylation at lysine residues K9 and K27, in contrast, seems to be involved in gene repression along chromosomal domains *(8,9,11,13,14)*. The heritable repressed/active states that these two methylated lysines can bring about may involve recognition by specific nuclear proteins. In particular, heterochromatin protein-1 (HP1) was found to be bound to methylated H3-K9 at pericentric heterochromatin *(15,16)*, and possibly at other heritably repressed chromosomal regions as well. H3-K27 methylation, on the other hand, is regulated and recognized by different polycomb group proteins *(17,18)*. Many insights into the roles of histone modifications have emerged from indirect immunofluorescence studies on cultured cells. These studies have been highly informative because they revealed the functions of specific histone modifications in, for instance, pericentric chromatin condensation *(13,19)* and X-chromosome inactivation *(20–22)* in mammals (H3 and H4 deacetylation, and H3-K9 methylation). However, particularly in mammalian model systems, little is known about how histone modifications are organized at specific chromosomal regions and genes. To address in detail what happens at specific sites in vivo, ChIP is the method of choice. Here we describe how ChIP can be performed on native chromatin from cells or tissues to analyze histone methylation and acetylation at specific sites. In addition, we present different polymerase chain reaction (PCR)-based methods that allow the analysis of a locus of interest in chromatin precipitated with antibodies to specific histone methylation marks.

1.1. Chromatin Immunoprecipitation

ChIP is performed by incubation of fractionated chromatin with an antiserum directed against the histone modification of interest. Broadly, there are two ways of preparing such *"input" chromatin*. Several groups in the field prepare *crosslinked chromatin*, for example, by photochemical crosslinking or by chemical crosslinking of proteins and DNA with specific substances such

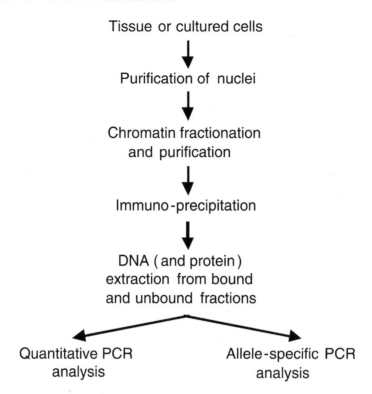

Fig. 1. Procedures used to investigate site-specific histone methylation and/or other covalent modifications on histones. Briefly, nuclei are purified from fresh/frozen tissues or cells. Chromatin is then fractionated with micrococcal nuclease and purified from the nuclei. The obtained input chromatin comprises fragments of up to five nucleosomes in length and is incubated with antiserum directed against the histone modification of interest. Subsequently, the antibody-bound fraction is separated from the unbound fraction. Genomic DNA is extracted from the bound and unbound fractions, and quantitative and qualitative PCR technologies are applied to investigate the gene or chromosomal region of interest.

as formaldehyde *(23)*. The latter method is particularly suitable for ChIP studies on histone modifications (see Chap. 2 for a detailed description). However, it has the slight handicap that usually only a small fraction of the chromatin is precipitated, and it relies on random shearing, which does not always produce small enough chromatin fragments at the regions of interest. Other methodologies, such as the one described in this chapter (**Fig. 1**), make use of *native chromatin (3,25)*. In these methods, usually the chromatin is fractionated by incubation of purified nuclei with micrococcal nuclease (MNase), an enzyme that preferentially cleaves the linker DNA between the nucleosomes *(26)*.

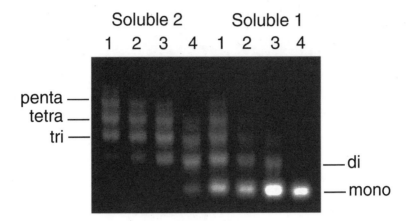

Fig. 2. Example of native chromatin preparation. Nuclei were purified from primary fibroblast cells and incubated for increasing lengths of time with MNase (6, 9, 12, 15 min, for lanes 1–4, respectively). The first soluble-1 (S1) fractions were obtained directly after MNase digestion, and the second soluble fraction (S2) was recovered from the nuclei by overnight dialysis. Electrophoresis of these fractions was through a 1.2% agarose gel. Bands corresponding to chromatin fragments of one nucleosome (mono) to five nucleosomes (penta) in length are indicated. In this example, our input chromatin for immunoprecipitation was obtained by combining S1 fractions 1 and 2 with S2 fractions 3 and 4. (Adapted from **ref. 27** with permission from S. Karger AG.)

Specifically, by performing partial digestions with MNase, it is possible to obtain native chromatin fragments of, on average, one to five nucleosomes in length. These mono- and oligonucleosome fragments are purified from the nuclei and are used to perform ChIP (**Fig. 2**). The advantage of using native, MNase-fractionated chromatin as the input material for ChIP is that epitopes recognized by the antibody remain intact during the chromatin preparation. As a consequence, native chromatin tends to give higher levels of precipitation for a specific histone modification than formaldehyde-crosslinked chromatin *(27)*. The ChIP protocol presented below describes in detail how to prepare and immunoprecipitate native chromatin. This protocol was adapted from a methodology originally described by O'Neill and Turner *(3)* and allows ChIP to be performed not only on chromatin from cultured cells, but also on freshly dissected and frozen tissues. It is adapted to the analysis of histone methylation and acetylation.

1.2. PCR-Based Analysis of Precipitated Chromatin

After ChIP, precipitated chromatin fractions are analyzed to assess the amount and the quality of the precipitated chromatin. DNA is then extracted to allow analysis of the chromosomal site(s) of interest. In several earlier studies on site-specific histone modifications, regions of interest were analyzed by Southern hybridization of slot blots *(3,24)*. During the last few years, however, with the availability of quantitative amplification techniques to many research laboratories, PCR has become the method of choice. To determine how much DNA is precipitated at a site of interest, one can choose between different PCR-based approaches. Apart from real-time PCR amplification to quantify the amounts of chromatin that are precipitated at specific loci, one possibility is to perform *duplex amplification*, which is coamplification of a fragment from the region of interest and a control fragment (e.g., the actin gene, or the tubulin gene). Duplex PCR amplification has been successful in studies on the *S. pombe* mating-type loci and for analysis of imprinted mammalian genes (**Fig. 3**) and allows one to determine relative levels of specific histone modifications along chromosomal domains *(9,25)*. Alternatively, in particular for allelic studies on dosage-compensation mechanisms, or on genomic imprinting in mammals, one can apply single-strand conformation polymorphism (SSCP; **Fig. 4**) *(28,29)*, or similar strategies such as *hot-stop PCR (30)*, to differentiate PCR products, which represent the silent allele, from those amplified from the active allele *(11,27)*. These different PCR-based approaches toward analysis of precipitated chromatin fractions are presented in this chapter.

2. Materials

2.1. Nuclei Preparation From Tissues and Cells

1. Appropriate medium for culturing cells, e.g., RPMI containing 10% (v/v) fetal calf serum.
2. Phosphate-buffered saline (PBS), pH 7.3.
3. 0.05% (w/v) Trypsin solution (Sigma).
4. Homogenizers. We use a tissue grinder/homogenizer (from BDH) that has a glass mortar (tube) and a pestle with a hard plastic head. The clearance between pestle and mortar is 0.15–0.25 mm.
5. 14-mL Polypropylene tubes (e.g., 17 × 100-mm Falcon tubes).
6. Muslin cheesecloth.
7. Buffer I: 0.3 *M* sucrose in 60 m*M* KCl, 15 m*M* NaCl, 5 m*M* MgCl$_2$, 0.1 m*M* ethyleneglycol-*bis N,N,N'*, or *N'*-tetraacetic acid EGTA, 15 m*M* Tris-HCl, pH 7.5, 0.5 m*M* dithiothreitol (DTT), 0.1 m*M* phenylmethylsulfonyl fluoride (PMSF), and 3.6 ng/mL aprotinin (Sigma) (*see* **Notes 1** and **2**).
8. Buffer II: 0.3 *M* sucrose in 60 m*M* KCl, 15 m*M* NaCl, 5 m*M* MgCl$_2$, 0.1 m*M* EGTA, 15 m*M* Tris-HCl, pH 7.5, 0.5 m*M* DTT, 0.1 m*M* PMSF, and 3.6 ng/mL aprotinin, 0.4% (v/v) IGEPAL CA-630® (formally called Nonidet®P40, from Sigma).
9. Buffer III: 1.2 *M* sucrose in 60 m*M* KCl, 15 m*M* NaCl, 5 m*M* MgCl$_2$, 0.1 m*M* EGTA, 15 m*M* Tris-HCl, pH 7.5, 0.5 m*M* DTT, 0.1 m*M* PMSF, and 3.6 ng/mL aprotinin.

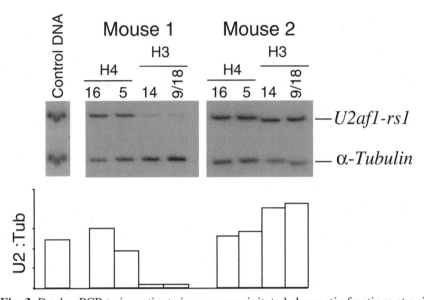

Fig. 3. Duplex PCR to investigate immunoprecipitated chromatin fractions at a site of interest relative to a control locus. In this example, from a study on the mouse by Gregory and co-workers *(25)*, histone modifications were investigated at the splice factor-encoding *U2af1-rs1* gene and were compared with those at the *a -Tubulin* gene. Two sets of PCR primers were designed, one for the splice factor-encoding gene *U2af1-rs1* and one for the *a -Tubulin* gene. When used in a single PCR reaction (duplex PCR), the two primer pairs amplified similar amounts of DNA from a control genomic DNA (left lane). The duplex PCR coamplification approach was then applied to analyze immunoprecipitated chromatin fractions obtained after ChIP on native liver chromatin. Two animals were compared: a normal control mouse (Mouse 2) and a mouse with genetically induced, aberrant DNA methylation at the *U2af1-rs1* gene (Mouse 1). ChIP was performed with antisera directed against acetylation at lysine residue 16 on histone H4, against acetylation on lysine 5 on H4, against acetylation on lysine 14 of H3, and against acetylation of lysines 9/18 on H3, respectively (for description of these affinity-purified polyclonal antisera (*see* **refs.** *3*,*25*). After duplex amplification from each of the antibody-bound fractions and electrophoresis through a gel the intensity of the *U2af1-rs1*-specific PCR product was compared to that of the Tubulin product. The calculated *U2af1-rs1*:Tubulin ratios are plotted underneath. It follows from this example that Mouse 1 has lower levels of H3 acetylation in comparison to Mouse 2. (Adapted from **ref.** *25*.)

10. Parafilm® (Sigma).
11. Equipment: a high-speed centrifuge with a swing-out bucket rotor that takes 14-mL polypropylene tubes.

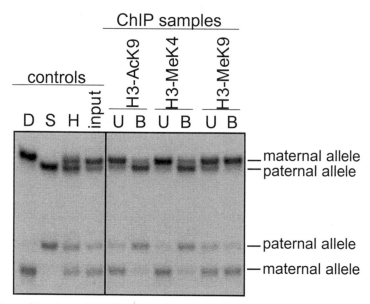

Fig. 4. Application of SSCP in combination with PCR to analyze allele-specific patterns of histone methylation. The example experiment concerns a regulatory CpG island (located in a gene called *Kvlqt1*) that controls the parental allele-specific gene expression across a cluster of imprinted genes on distal mouse chromosome 7. Lung tissue was dissected from a mouse that was an interspecific hybrid (H) between *Mus musculus domesticus* (D, paternal genome) and *Mus spretus* (S, maternal genome). After nuclei and native chromatin preparations, immunoprecipitation was performed with rabbit polyclonal antisera to acetylation at lysine 9 of H3 (H3-AcK9), to dimethylation at lysine 4 of H3 (H3-MeK4), and to dimethylation at lysine K9 of H3 (H3-MeK9). These antisera were commercially purchased (Upstate Ltd.) additional data are presented in **ref. *11***. Radioactive PCR was performed on bound (B) and unbound (U) fractions, with a pair of primers that amplified from a unique sequence at this imprinting-control center. After denaturing of the PCR products, electrophoresis was performed through a nondenaturing polyacrylamide gel (SSCP electrophoresis). The four lanes to the left show control amplifications from genomic DNAs (D, *Mus musculus domesticus* DNA; S, *Mus spretus* DNA; H, (*Mus musculus domesticus* × *Mus spretus*) F1 DNA. In the analysis of the antibody bound (B) and unbound (U) fractions (right panel), the bands representing the maternal and paternal alleles are indicated.

2.2. MNase Fractionation and Purification of Chromatin

1. MNase digestion buffer: 0.32 *M* sucrose, 50 m*M* Tris-HCl, pH 7.5, 4 m*M* MgCl$_2$, 1 m*M* CaCl$_2$, 0.1 m*M* PMSF.
2. MNase (Amersham Bioscience), at 10 U/mL in 50% (v/v) glycerol. Aliquots (10–20 µL) are frozen, and each aliquot should be used only once after thawing to ensure equal enzyme activity in different chromatin preparations.

3. Water bath set at 37°C.
4. Stop solution: 20 m*M* EDTA, pH 8.0.
5. Bench-top centrifuge for 1.5-mL Eppendorf tubes.
6. Dialysis tubing, 0.5 mm thick (VWR international).
7. Tubing preparation solution I: 2% (w/v) sodium bicarbonate, 1 m*M* EDTA, pH 8.0.
8. Tubing preparation solution II: 1 m*M* EDTA, pH 8.0.
9. Dialysis buffer: 1 m*M* Tris-HCl, pH 7.5, 0.2 m*M* EDTA, 0.2 m*M* PMSF.
10. 5-mm Universal tubing clamps (Spectrum Laboratories).

2.3. Assessment of Chromatin and Immunoprecipitation

1. Spectrophotometer.
2. Loading buffer, six times concentrated: 30% (v/v) glycerol in H_2O, 0.25% (w/v) bromophenol blue, 0.25% (w/v) xylene cyanol (store at 4°C).
3. 20% (w/v) Sodium dodecyl sulfate (SDS).
4. Horizontal gel electrophoresis tank for agarose gels.
5. 1X TBE electrophoresis buffer: 0.09 *M* Tris-borate, 2 m*M* EDTA, pH 8.0.
6. 100-bp DNA size-ladder (Promega).
7. ChIP incubation buffer: 50 m*M* NaCl, Tris-HCl, pH 7.5, 0.1 m*M* PMSF, 5 m*M* EDTA.
8. Affinity-purified antiserum raised against histone peptides with mono-, di-, or trimethylation at a specific lysine/arginine residue. We use approx 5–10 μg of antibody for ChIP on chromatin corresponding to approx 20 μg of genomic DNA.
9. Bench-top centrifuge for 1.5-mL Eppendorf tubes.
10. Protein A (e.g., CL-4B Sepharose from Amersham Bioscience), or G Sepharose, according to the characteristics of the antibody used for immunoprecipitation (*see* **Note 8**).
11. Washing buffer A: 50 m*M* Tris-HCl, pH 7.5, 10 m*M* EDTA, 75 m*M* NaCl. Store at 4°C.
12. Washing buffer B: 50 m*M* Tris-HCl, pH 7.5, 10 m*M* EDTA, 125 m*M* NaCl. Store at 4°C.
13. Washing buffer C: 50 m*M* Tris-HCl, pH 7.5, 10 m*M* EDTA, 175 m*M* NaCl. Store at 4°C.
14. 15-mL Tubes (e.g., 17 × 120-mm Falcon conical tubes).
15. Centrifuge with a swing-out bucket rotor that takes 15-mL polypropylene tubes.
16. Elution buffer: 50 m*M* NaCl, Tris-HCl, pH 7.5, 0.1 m*M* PMSF, 5 m*M* EDTA, 1% SDS (w/v).

2.4. DNA Extraction and Assessment of Precipitated Chromatin

1. Phenol/chloroform/isoamyl alcohol 25:24:1 (v/v/v). For extraction of genomic DNA, the phenol should be saturated beforehand with 100 m*M* Tris-HCl, pH 7.5, and stored at 4°C under 10 m*M* Tris-HCl, pH 7.5 *(32)*.
2. 5 *M* NaCl.
3. Glycogen solution at 20 mg/mL (Roche).

4. 2-Propanol.
5. 70% (v/v) Ethanol.
6. TE buffer: 10 mM Tris-HCl, pH 7.5, 1 mM EDTA.
7. Spectrophotometer.
8. Loading buffer, six times concentrated: 30% (v/v) glycerol in H_2O, 0.25% (w/v) bromophenol blue, 0.25% (w/v) xylene cyanol FF (store at 4°C).
9. 20% (v/v) SDS.
10. Horizontal electrophoresis tank for agarose gels.
11. 1X TBE electrophoresis buffer: 0.09 M Tris-borate, 2 mM EDTA, pH 8.0.
12. 100-bp DNA size-ladder (Promega).
13. 20 mg/mL Ethidium bromide solution in H_2O.

2.5. Quantitative PCR Analysis of Precipitated Chromatin

1. Template DNA: this is the genomic DNA extracted from the antibody-bound and antibody-unbound fractions. Control genomic DNAs should be used as well. For each PCR amplification, we use 50–100 ng of template DNA.
2. Quantitect SYBR Green PCR kit (QIAGEN).
3. LightCycler machine (Roche Diagnostics)

2.6. Allele-Specific PCR Analysis of Precipitated Chromatin

2.6.1. Hot-Stop Amplification Across Polymorphic Restriction Sites

1. Template DNA (50–100 ng of DNA).
2. Forward and reverse primers (stock solutions in H_2O at 100 μM).
3. dNTP mix: stock solutions at 25 mM for each dNTP.
4. [α^{32}P]dCTP (10 μC/μL, specific activity 3000 Ci/mmol).
5. 10X PCR amplification buffer (supplied with the *Taq* polymerase).
6. *Taq* polymerase (at 5 U/μL)
7. Thermal cycler.
8. 0.2-mL Thin-walled PCR tubes (e.g., from EUROGENTEC).
9. Restriction endonuclease that is specific for a polymorphic restriction site within the amplified DNA fragment.
10. 10X Digestion buffer (supplied with the restriction endonuclease).

2.6.2. Electrophoresis of Restriction Enzyme-Digested PCR Products

1. Acrylamide/*bis*-acrylamide 40% stock solution (29:1 ratio; Sigma).
2. 1X TBE buffer: 0.09 M Tris-borate, 2 mM EDTA.
3. N,N,N',N 9-tetramethyl-ethylene diamine (TEMED).
4. 10% (w/v) ammonium persulfate (APS), freshly prepared.
5. Vertical gel electrophoresis tank for polyacrylamide gels, with 21.7 × 16.5-cm glass plates, 0.4-mm spacers, and a shark-tooth comb.
6. PCR product.
7. Loading buffer, six times concentrated: 30% (v/v) glycerol in H_2O, 0.25% (w/v) bromophenol blue, 0.25% (w/v) xylene cyanol FF (store at 4°C).

8. Whatman 3-MM paper.
9. Thin transparent plastic wrap (e.g., Saran Wrap).
10. Gel dryer for acrylamide gels (e.g., Bio-Rad model 583).

2.6.3. SSCP-PCR Amplification and Electrophoresis of Amplification Products

1–8. Identical to **steps 1–8** of **Subheading 2.6.1.**
9. Acrylamide solution for SSCP gels: 2X MDE® solution (Sigma).
10. 0.6X TBE buffer: 0.054 M Tris-borate, 12 mM EDTA.
11. TEMED.
12. 10% (w/v) APS, freshly prepared.
13. A standard DNA sequencing gel apparatus with 31 × 38.5-cm glass plates, 0.4-mm spacers, and a shark tooth comb.
14. PCR product.
15. Loading dye: 95% (v/v) formamide, 10 mM NaOH, 0.25% (w/v) bromophenol blue, 0.25% (w/v) xylene cyanol.
16–18. Identical to **steps 8–10** of **Subheading 2.6.2.**

2.6.4. Gel Image Analysis

1. X-ray films and cassettes with scintillation screens for exposure of X-ray films.
2. Imaging equipment for densitometric measurements on exposed X-ray films (e.g., Geldoc-1000 system from Bio-Rad).
3. PhosphorImager (e.g., Molecular Imager FX system from Bio-Rad).

3. Methods

3.1. Nuclei Preparation From Tissues and Cells

3.1.1. Purification of Nuclei From Tissues

1. Dissect tissue, not more than 0.2 g in total, and rinse it in PBS (*see* **Notes 1** and **2**).
2. Homogenize tissue in a prechilled glass homogenizer with 5–10 mL of ice-cold buffer I, until no clumps of cells persist (about 10-20 strokes). Filter the cell suspension through four layers of muslin cheesecloth that have been moistened beforehand with 2 mL of buffer I.
3. Transfer the cell suspension to a 14-mL polypropylene tube, and spin cells down in a swing-out rotor (at 6000g for 10 min, at 4°C).
4. Pour off the supernatant and resuspend the cells in 2 mL of ice-cold buffer I. Then add 2 mL of ice-cold buffer II (*see* **Notes 3** and **4**), mix gently, and place on ice for 10 min.
5. Prepare two 14-mL tubes containing 8 mL of ice-cold buffer III each. Carefully layer 2 mL of each cell suspension (from **step 4**) on each 8-mL sucrose cushion. Cover the tube with a piece of parafilm.

6. Centrifuge in a prechilled swing-out rotor, at 10,000*g*, for 20 min at 4°C. During this centrifugation step, the nuclei will form a pellet on the bottom of the tube, whereas the cytoplasmic components will remain in the top layer (*see* **Note 5**).
7. Carefully take off the supernatant with a Pasteur pipet. This is a critical step; the top solution (which contains the detergent IGEPAL CA-630) *should not* come into contact with the nuclear pellet at the bottom of the tube. One way to achieve this is to remove the supernatant about three times, each time changing the Pasteur pipet (*see* **Note 6**).
8. Resuspend the nuclei pellet into 1 mL of MNase digestion buffer and put on ice. Nuclei can, at this point, be counted by using a microscope slide for counting cells. The number of nuclei obtained per gram of tissue varies between different tissue types. For liver, the above protocol yields approx 2×10^9 nuclei/g of tissue. Frozen tissues can be used for nuclei preparation as well; *see* **Note 7**.

3.1.2. Nuclei Preparation From Cultured Cells

1. Culture 5×10^7 to 5×10^8 cells in appropriate culture medium. Ensure that cells are not grown beyond semiconfluency.
2. Rinse cells in PBS, add 2 mL of trypsin solution (for adhering cells only), and incubate at 37°C. When trypsinization is complete, stop the reaction by adding 5 mL of culture medium to the cells.
3. Divide the cell suspension among two 14-mL tubes, and spin cells down in a swing-out rotor (4000*g*, 5 min at 4°C).
4–8. Identical to **steps 4–8** in **Subheading 3.1.1.**

3.2. MNase Fractionation and Purification of Chromatin

3.2.1. MNase Fractionation

1. Resuspend nuclei (purified as described in **Subheadings 3.1.1.** and **3.1.2.**) in 1 mL of ice-cold MNase digestion buffer and place on ice.
2. Aliquot two 1.5-mL Eppendorf tubes with 500 μL of re-suspended nuclei.
3. Add 1 μL of MNase enzyme to each tube and mix gently.
4. Put the two tubes in a 37°C water bath for 6 and 9 min, respectively.
5. Add 20 μL of stop solution.
6. Chill on ice. Continue from here with **step 1** of **Subheading 3.2.3.** after having prepared the dialysis tubing (*see* **Subheading 3.2.2.**).

3.2.2. Preparation of Dialysis Tubing

Dialysis tubing needs to be prepared before starting the purification of chromatin. This is done as follows:

1. Cut the tubing into pieces of convenient length (10–20 cm).
2. Boil the tubes for 10 min in 0.5 L of tubing preparation solution I.
3. Rinse the tubes twice in distilled water.

4. Boil the tubes for 10 min in 0.5 L of tubing preparation solution II.
5. Allow the tubes to cool, and store them in tubing preparation solution II at 4°C. Ensure that the tubes are entirely submerged.
6. Before use, wash the tubing twice inside and out with distilled water.

3.2.3. Recovery of Soluble Chromatin Fractions

1. Centrifuge the 1.5-mL tubes with the MNase-digested nuclei at 10,000 rpm (4°C) for 10 min to pellet the nuclei.
2. Transfer the supernatant into another 1.5-mL tube and store at 4°C. This supernatant contains the first soluble fraction of chromatin, S1, which comprises small fragments only. Do not discard the pellet.
3. Carefully resuspend the pellet in 500 μL of dialysis buffer.
4. Close one side of the dialysis tube with a universal closure clamp. Transfer the 500 μL of resuspended nuclei into the dialysis tube and close the other side with a second clamp.
5. Immerse the tube for 12–16 h in 1–2 L of dialysis buffer. Perform dialysis at 4°C in a beaker with constant mild stirring using a magnetic stirrer.
6. Transfer the dialyzed nuclei into a 1.5-mL Eppendorf tube.
7. Centrifuge for 10 min at 11,000g, at 4°C in a microcentrifuge.
8. Transfer the supernatant in a new 1.5-mL Eppendorf tube and store at 4°C. This is the second soluble chromatin fraction, S2, comprising larger fragments of chromatin that were removed from the nuclei during the dialysis.
9. Resuspend the pellet in 50 μL of lysis buffer and store at 4°C. This is the *pellet* chromatin fraction P.

3.3. Quality Control of Chromatin

1. Take the optical density (OD) of each fraction at 260 nm.
2. In separate 1.5-mL Eppendorf tubes, put 0.5 μg of chromatin for each of the fractions (S1, S2, and P) obtained as in **Subheadings 3.3.** and **3.4.**
3. Add 2 μL of loading buffer and 1 μL of 10% SDS. Adjust the volume to 10 μL and mix gently.
4. Load the samples onto a standard 1% (w/v) agarose gel (about 10–15 cm in length) in 1X TBE, with the 100-bp DNA ladder as a size control. Let the samples migrate at 2–3 V/cm until the fastest blue marker in the loading buffer has migrated until about halfway up the gel.
5. Stain the gel for 30 min in a tray with 500 mL of H_2O to which 10 μg of ethidium bromide is added.
6. Remove the background staining from the gel by rinsing for 15 min in H_2O.
7. Control the size of the chromatin fragments under an ultraviolet (UV) lamp and take a photograph (*see* **Fig. 2** for an example of typical S1 and S2 fractions). The pellet fraction, P, consists of chromatin fragments that are longer than five nucleosomes in length.

3.4. Chromatin Immunoprecipitation

3.4.1. Incubation of Chromatin With Antiserum

1. Mix 10–20 μg of the first (S1) and 10–20 μg of the second (S2) chromatin fractions (obtained as in **Subheadings 3.2.3.**) in a 1.5-mL Eppendorf tube (*see* also **Fig. 2**).
2. Complete the volume to 1 mL with ChIP incubation buffer.
3. Add 5–10 μg of the antibody of choice.
4. Close the tubes and seal the lids with parafilm. Rotate (20–30 rpm) the tubes in a rotating wheel for 12–16 h at 4°C. During this incubation, the antibodies will bind to their specific epitopes.
5. Proceed from here with **step 9** of **Subheading 3.4.2.** after having prepared the aliquots of protein A or G Sepharose (*see* **Subheading 3.4.2.**).

3.4.2. Incubation With Protein A Sepharose (or Protein G Sepharose; see **Notes 7** and **8**)

3.4.2.1. Preparation of Protein A Sepharose (Before Starting the Immunoprecipitation)

1. Weigh 0.25 g of protein A Sepharose beads into a 14-mL polypropylene tube.
2. Add 1 mL of water to moisten the beads.
3. Wash with 10 mL of water and mix.
4. Centrifuge for 3 min at 1500*g* in a swing-out rotor and discard the supernatant.
5. Repeat **steps 3** and **4** four times.
6. Add 1 mL of sterile water and resuspend the beads.
7. Distribute 100-μL aliquots in ten 1.5-mL Eppendorf tubes. Store these aliquots at 4°C. They can be used for the extraction of antibody-bound chromatin from multiple ChIP experiments.

3.4.2.2 Extraction of Immunoprecipitated Chromatin With Protein A Sepharose

1. Add 50 μL of protein A Sepharose to each tube after the immunoprecipitation (*see* **Note 8**).
2. Let the tubes rotate for 4 h at 4°C at 20–30 rpm.
3. Centrifuge the incubated chromatin at 1500*g* in a swing-out rotor for 3 min.
4. Transfer the supernatant to a 2-mL Eppendorf tube. This fraction contains the chromatin that did not link the antibody: the *unbound fraction*.
5. Resuspend the protein A Sepharose beads in 1 mL of buffer A.
6. Transfer the resuspended beads to a 15-mL Falcon tube.
7. Complete to 10 mL with buffer A. Mix briefly.
8. Centrifuge for 3 min at 1500*g* (4°C) in a swing-out rotor. Carefully discard the supernatant.

9. Resuspend beads in 10 mL of buffer B. Briefly mix.
10. Centrifuge for 3 min at 1500*g* (4°C) in a swing-out rotor. Carefully discard the supernatant.
11. Resuspend the Sepharose beads in 10 mL of buffer C.
12. Centrifuge for 3 min at 1500*g* (4°C) in a swing-out rotor. Carefully discard the supernatant.
13. To elute the chromatin from the washed beads, resuspend the Sepharose bead pellet in 500 µL of elution buffer and transfer to a 1.5-mL Eppendorf tube.
14. Incubate for approx 30 min at room temperature on a rotater machine (20–30 rpm). After this incubation, centrifuge for 3 min at 250*g* in a bench-top microcentrifuge.
15. Carefully transfer the supernatant into a 2-mL Eppendorf tube. The supernatant contains the chromatin eluted from the protein A Sepharose beads and is called the *bound fraction*.

3.5. DNA Extraction and Assessment of Precipitated Chromatin (see **Note 9**)

3.5.1. DNA Extraction From Precipitated Chromatin

1. Add 500 µL of phenol/chloroform/isoamyl alcohol 25:24:1 (v/v/v) to bound and unbound fractions.
2. Vortex for 30 s.
3. Centrifuge at 15,000*g* for 15 min in a bench-top microcentrifuge.
4. Carefully transfer the upper, aqueous, phase to another 2-mL Eppendorf tube.
5. Add NaCl to a final concentration of 250 m*M*.
6. Add 20–40 µg of glycogen and mix. Since the DNA concentration in the bound fraction is usually low, we recommended glycogen as a coprecipitator. This step is not necessary for the unbound fraction.
7. Add 1 vol of 2-propanol.
8. Mix and store at –80°C for at least 2 h.
9. Centrifuge at 18,000*g* in a microcentrifuge for 15 min. Carefully discard the supernatant.
10. Rinse the pellet with 1 mL of 70% (v/v) ethanol.
11. Centrifuge at 18,000*g* for 5 min in a microcentrifuge. Carefully discard the supernatant.
12. Dry the pellet for 5–10 min at room temperature. Resuspend the pellet in 10–50 µL of TE buffer.

3.5.2. Assessment of Precipitated Chromatin

Measure the OD_{260} of each of the samples to determine how much to take as template for the subsequent PCR amplification. The ratio between the bound fraction DNA vs total starting material (corresponding to the bound and unbound fractions together) indicates the efficiency of the ChIP assay and represents the percentage of immunoprecipitated chromatin. In a standard experiment on histone modifications, no more than 15% of the input native chromatin should be precipitated. However, the percentage of overall precipitation depends on the nature and abundance of the histone modification and on the characteristics and concentration of the antibody used (*see* **Note 10**).

3.6. Quantitative PCR Analysis of Precipitated Chromatin (*see* Note 11)

3.6.1. Real-Time PCR Amplification

For real-time PCR, each amplification is run in duplicate to control for PCR variation. The standard curve is constructed from the log-linear amplification phase using external DNA controls (we use four different concentrations of a control mouse genomic DNA). The amount of target DNA in the starting material is calculated from this standard curve. To be able to compare regions within the same ChIP, results are presented as the percentage of the input chromatin that is precipitated at the region of interest. The following steps are according to a standard protocol provided with the Quantitect SYBR Green PCR kit (Qiagen).

1. Put 20–50 ng of template DNA into a capillary that is specific for the real-time PCR machine.
2. Add forward and reverse primers to a final concentration each of 0.4 μ*M*.
3. Add 9 μL of QuantiTect SYBR Green, 2X PCR mixture.
4. Complete to 18 μL with sterile water.
5. Amplify for 40–50 cycles in a Light Cycler PCR machine (e.g., one from Roche Diagnostics), and follow the manufacturer's instructions precisely on how to calculate the site-specific amount of DNA in the template DNA from which the real-time amplification was performed.

3.6.2. Duplex PCR Amplification

A duplex PCR reaction consists of coamplification of a fragment from the region of interest and a control fragment (e.g., from the actin gene). Primers should be designed such that on control genomic DNA, there is more or less equal amplification of the specific fragment and the control fragment. Usually, there is no problem in saturating the reaction (30–35 cycles of amplification), provided that this does not change the ratio between the two PCR products. (This should be tested beforehand.) To determine the precise ratio between the two different PCR products, it is best to perform the PCR reaction by adding radioactive dCTP (*see* protocol for PCR-SSCP: **steps 1–8** of **Subheading 3.7.2.**). The radioactive PCR products should be run through a standard nondenaturing polyacrylamide gel, as described in **steps 1–6** of **Subheading 3.7.1.3.** An example of a typical duplex PCR assay, and its application to analysis of immunoprecipitated chromatin fractions, is presented in **Fig. 3**.

3.7. Allele-Specific PCR Analysis of Precipitated Chromatin (see **Note 11**)

3.7.1. Hot-Stop PCR Amplification
Across a Polymorphic Restriction Site

In many allele-specific PCR-based studies, one makes use of the presence of polymorphic restriction sites. During PCR amplification from DNA of mixed genetic background, heteroduplexes (e.g., association of the opposite single strands) can be formed. This will result in the polymorphic restriction site becoming nondigestible by the restriction enzyme and will lead to an estimation of the uncut material that is too high. Hot-stop PCR is based on a standard cold amplification of the DNA, followed by addition of radiolabeled [α^{32}] dCTP and fresh dNTPs for a last cycle of hot PCR amplification. Consequently, all radioactive products in the reaction are homoduplex species; digestion by the restriction enzyme allows the allelic ratio to be faithfully determined *(30)*.

3.7.1.1. Hot-Stop PCR Amplification in a Final Volume of 25 µL

1. Take 50–100 ng of template DNA, and put it in a 0.2-mL PCR tube.
2. Add forward and reverse primer mix to a final concentration of 0.4 µM each.
3. Add 2.5 µL of 10X buffer (supplied with *Taq* polymerase).
4. Add dNTP to a final concentration of 0.2 µM.
5. Add 18.4 µL of water.
6. Add 5 U of *Taq* polymerase (e.g., Hotstart-Taq enzyme, from Qiagen).
7. Amplify for 35–40 cycles in a thermal cycler.
8. Transfer 5 µL of the PCR product to another PCR tube.
9. Complete to 25 µL with a newly prepared PCR mix containing [α^{32}]dCTP (10 µCi, specific activity 3000Ci/mmol) and fresh dNTPs.
10. Amplify for one additional cycle only, in a thermal cycler.

3.7.1.2. Restriction Enzyme Digestion of PCR Products

1. Transfer 10 µL of the hot PCR product obtained as in **Subheading 3.7.1.** into a 1.5-mL Eppendorf tube.
2. Add 1.5 µL of 10X restriction enzyme buffer.
3. Add 10–20 U of restriction enzyme that cuts the polymorphic restriction site.
4. Let digest for 1–2 h (for most enzymes, this will be at 37°C).
5. Add 5 µL of loading dye.

3.7.1.3. Electrophoresis of Digested PCR Products

1. Prepare the solution for the polyacrylamide gel: mix 15 mL of acrylamide solution, 12 mL of 5X TBE buffer, and 32.5 mL of deionized water. Add 50 µL TEMED and 500 µL freshly prepared 10% APS.
2. Pour the gel immediately. Insert the shark-tooth comb, and clamp on all sides. Lay the gel flat, and let the matrix polymerize for at least 30 min.

3. After polymerization, place the glass plates into the gel apparatus, and add the TBE buffer.
4. Load samples into the gel and migrate at 120–200 V for 2–3 h.
5. After electrophoresis, transfer the gel to a sheet of Whatman 3MM paper and cover with plastic wrap. Dry for 45 min at 80°C in a gel dryer.
6. Expose the gel to an X-ray film at room temperature (for 4–16 h). In addition, a phosphorimager can be used to determine the relative intensities of the bands.

3.7.2. PCR Amplification to Generate SSCP Polymorphisms

For studies on genomic imprinting, and dosage compensation and for other analyses of allelic gene expression, one needs to distinguish the (parental) alleles of a gene faithfully. If there are single-nucleotide polymorphisms between the two alleles at the gene of interest, it is possible to discriminate (denatured) PCR products derived from the one or the other allele, because the secondary structure of each single strand will be directly dependent on the sequence itself. Hence, in nondenaturing gel conditions, there will be differential migration of each single strand (*see* **Fig. 4**). This is the SSCP technique *(28,29)* (*see* **Note 12**).

3.7.2.1. RADIOACTIVE PCR AMPLIFICATION FOR SSCP ANALYSIS

1–6. Identical to **steps 1–6** at **Subheading 3.7.1.**
7. Add 1 μL of [α^{32}]dCTP.
8. Amplify for 35–40 cycles in a thermal cycler.

3.7.2.2. SSCP ELECTROPHORESIS OF RADIOACTIVE PCR PRODUCTS

1. Prepare the solution for the nondenaturing MDE gel (a polyacrylamide-like matrix, specifically optimized for SSCP): mix 15 mL of 2X MDE solution, 7.2 mL of 5X TBE buffer, and 37.5 mL of deionized water. Add 40 μL TEMED and 400 μL freshly prepared 10% APS.
2. Pour the gel immediately. Insert the shark-tooth comb with teeth pointing upward to form a single well the width of the gel, and clamp on all sides. Lay the gel flat, and let the matrix polymerize for at least 30 min.
3. After polymerization, remove clamps, tape, and comb. Place the glass plates into the sequencing gel apparatus.
4. Take 2 μL of the PCR product and, add 8 μL of loading dye. Denature the sample at 95°C for 5 min, and then place on ice.
5. Load 5–7 μL of the sample into the gel. Run the gel at 400 V for 24 h (at room temperature *see* **Note 12**).
6–7. Identical to **steps 5** and **6**, at **Subheading 3.7.1.**

4. Notes

1. Wear gloves throughout all procedures, and respect other usual safety precautions, particularly when handling phenol, chloroform, and acrylamide solutions.

2. The described protocols work well on tissues, such as liver, brain, lung, and placenta, and also on early embryos. No more than approx 0.2 g of tissue should be used for the volumes and tube sizes indicated in the protocol. In case higher amounts of tissue are used, we recommend increasing the number of tubes accordingly. To analyze histone acetylation in the same cells/tissues used for assaying histone methylation, we recommend adding sodium butyrate (to a final conc. of 5 mM) to the solutions used for the purification of nuclei and the preparation of input chromatin. Sodium butyrate prevents loss of histone acetylation via the action of endogenous histone deacetylases. For the site-specific analysis of histone phosphorylation, different protocols are applied, which are described elsewhere *(34,35)*, with addition of specific inhibitors of phosphatases.

3. For many tissues (liver, kidney, placenta), a 0.2% concentration of the nonionic detergent IGEPAL CA-630 is sufficiently high to lyse the cellular membranes during the 10-min incubation. However, we recommend testing 0.4% IGEPAL for certain other tissues. For example, this higher concentration of detergent gives a slightly better yield of nuclei from brain and muscle tissue.

4. To prevent chromatin degradation by endogenous nucleases, and to keep the chromatin intact, all steps of the nuclei purification procedure should be performed on ice, or at 4°C (e.g., precool the centrifuge rotors). At **step 4** of this procedure (**Subheading 3.1.1.**), it is critical not to extend the incubation in the IGEPAL CA-630-containing buffer for more than 10 min (Start the subsequent centrifugation step at exactly 10 min after adding buffer II to the cells in buffer I).

5. At **step 6** of the nuclei purification procedure (**Subheading 3.1.1.**), the nuclei pellet should be white. For liver nuclei preparation, for instance, all the red color (owing to the presence of hemoglobin in the blood cells) should be in the layer on top of the sucrose cushion. At **step 7, Subheading 3.1.1.** keep any trace of the top layer (buffer I mixed with buffer II) from coming into contact with the nuclei pellet. Usually, we remove the top layer and the sucrose cushion from the tube by using Pasteur pipets. This is done by aspirating from the surface of the solution, while changing with a new Pasteur pipet two or three times. In case one suspects that the top layer has nevertheless come in contact with the nuclei pellet, the nuclei should be gently rinsed with 1 mL of buffer III in an additional step, before proceeding with **step 8, Subheading 3.1.1.**

6. In case frozen tissue is used for nuclei purification, one should proceed as follows. Grind the frozen tissue to powder in a mortar, while keeping it constantly under liquid nitrogen (prechill the mortar with liquid nitrogen). Transfer the finely ground tissue into 5–10 mL of ice-cold buffer I, and resuspend the cells. Filter this cell suspension through two layers of muslin cheesecloth that has been moistened beforehand with 2-mL of buffer I. Proceed from here with **step 3** of the nuclei purification procedure (**Subheading 3.1.1.**).

7. The immunoprecipitations and incubation with protein A Sepharose are performed in Eppendorf tubes. These tubes may be siliconized beforehand (e.g., with a 2% v/v dichloromethylsilane solution), to prevent a specific association of chromatin and antibodies to the interior wall of the tubes. In our laboratory

(11,27), however, we obtained comparable results with nonsiliconized and with siliconized tubes.

8. Proteins A and G are bacterial cell wall proteins that bind to the Fc region of antibodies. This interaction is strongest at neutral or slightly basic pH values. These proteins are covalently coupled to Sepharose. The choice between protein A or protein G Sepharose depends on the nature of the antibody used for ChIP. In general, protein A works best for polyclonal antisera from rabbit and for mouse monoclonal antibodies from the IgG2a,b and IgG3 subclasses. Protein G Sepharose should be used for mouse IgG1 monoclonal antibodies and for polyclonal antisera from mouse, rat, sheep, and goat. Chicken antisera do not bind well either to protein A or to protein G; thus, when using ChIP, we recommend adding 5 µg of a rabbit antichicken antiserum directly after **step 4** of **Subheading 3.4.1.**, for a second precipitation of 3–4 h, before proceeding with the extraction of the antibody-bound chromatin.

9. When an antiserum is used for the first time, it is important to verify that the histone modification it is directed against has become enriched in the antibody-bound fraction. This can be done by purifying the histone proteins from this fraction followed by electrophoresis through acid urea Triton gels *(3,31)*. After electrophoresis, proteins are Western blotted to nylon filters, and the Western blot is immunostained with the antiserum, following standard procedures *(32)*. An example of this procedure *(31)* is presented by Gregory et al. *(33)*, relative to a study on histone acetylation in ES cells and fibroblasts.

10. The percentage of input chromatin that is precipitated is not the same for different histone modifications. A histone modification that is abundantly present on the chromosomes will give more overall precipitation than one found only in a small proportion of the chromatin. In addition, the overall precipitation efficiency depends on the amount of antiserum used, and the "strength" of the antibodies (i.e., the affinity to their epitope). On the other hand, the efficiency of precipitation of modified histones at a locus of interest greatly depends on whether the modification is common or rare in the genome. For instance, a modification that is rare in the genome (e.g., H3-K4 methylation; *see* **Fig. 4**) usually gives good precipitation at the site at which it is present. This can be explained by the fact that in the ChIP the quantity of antibody added to the tube is high enough to precipitate all the chromatin that carries that specific modification. However, for a modification that is abundant in the genome, the indicated amount of antibody (5–10 µg) sometimes does not permit us to precipitate all the chromatin that has the modification.

11. Analysis of precipitated chromatin fractions by PCR requires extreme care. Depending on the amount of input chromatin and the abundance of the modification at the site of interest, sometimes only a little template DNA will be available for amplification. We recommend taking all the possible precautions *(32)* to prevent contamination from other DNA sources: amplification in a dedicated space (PCR hood), use of a set of pipets for PCR only, use of filter tips and so on. In addition, use one set of pipets solely for the preparation of nuclei, chromatin, and ChIP analysis.

12. In most cases, SSCP separates 150–300-bp single-stranded DNA molecules that have one or more nucleotide differences *(28)*. However, the migration of single-stranded fragments in the gel is strongly temperature-dependent. Ideally, therefore, the PCR samples to be compared should be run on the same gel. In addition, SSCP is more efficient for DNA, with a relatively high G+C content. SSCP analysis of fragments with a lower G+C content can be enhanced by electrophoresis at 4°C. Instead of adding radioactive [α^{32}P]dCTP to the PCR reactions for SSCP analysis, the PCR primers (forward and reverse) may be radioactively end-labeled by using T4 polynucleotide kinase and [γ^{32}P]dATP.

Acknowledgments

We thank Richard I. Gregory for his help with the design of methodologies and Bryan M. Turner and Laura P. O'Neill (Birmingham, UK) for introducing us to immunoprecipitation on native chromatin. The HFSP, the CNRS (ATIPE), and the Fondation pour la Recherche Médicale are acknowledged for their grant support.

References

1. Luger, K. and Richmond, T. J. (1998) Histone tails of the nucleosome. *Curr. Opin. Genet. Dev.* **8**, 140–146.
2. Hebbes, T. R., Clayton, A. L., Thorne, A. W., and Crane-Robinson, C. (1994) Core histone hyperacetylation co-maps with generalized DNase-I sensitivity in the chicken *a -Globin* chromosomal domain. *EMBO J.* **13**, 1823–1830.
3. O'Neill, L. P., and Turner, B. M. (1995) Histone H4 acetylation distinguishes coding regions of the human genome from heterochromatin in a differentiation-independent manner. *EMBO J.* **14**, 3946–3957.
4. Grunstein M. (1998). Inheritance by histones. *Cell* **93**, 325–328.
5. Turner, B. M. (2000) Histone acetylation and an epigenetic code. *Bioessays* **22**, 836–845.
6. Jenuwein, T. and Allis, C. D. (2001) Translating the histone code. *Science* **293**, 1074–1080.
7. Kouzarides. T. (2002) Histone methylation in transcriptional control. *Curr. Opin. Genet. Dev.* **12**, 198–209.
8. Litt, M. D., Simpson, M., Gaszner, M., Allis, C. D., and Felsenfeld, G. (2001) Correlation between histone lysine methylation and developmental changes at the chicken β-globin locus. *Science* **293**, 2453–2455.
9. Noma, K-I., Allis, C. D., and Grewal, S. I. S. (2001) Transitions in distinct histone H3 methylation patterns at the heterochromatin domain boundaries. *Science* **293**, 1150–1155.
10. Bernstein, B. E., Humphrey, E. L., Erlich, R. L., et al. (2002) Methylation of histone H3 Lys 4 in coding regions of active genes. *Proc. Natl Acad. Sci. USA* **99**, 8695–8700.
11. Fournier, C., Goto, Y., Ballestar, E., et al. (2002) Allele-specific histone lysine methylation marks regulatory regions at imprinted mouse genes. *EMBO J.* **23**, 6560–6570.

12. Zegerman, P., Canas, B., Pappin, D., and Kouzarides, T. (2001) Histone H3 lysine 4 methylation disrupts the binding of the nucleosome remodelling and deacetylase (NuRD) repressor complex. *J. Biol. Chem.* **277**, 11,624–11,624.

13. Peters, A.H., O'Carroll, D., Schertan, H., et al. (2001) Loss of the *Suv39h* histone methyltransferases impairs mammalian heterochromatin and genome stability. *Cell* **107**, 323–337.

14. Silva, J., Mak, W., Zvetkova, I., et al. (2003) Establishment of histone H3 methylation on the inactive chromosome requires recruitment of Eed-Enx1 polycomb-group complexes. *Dev. Cell* **4**, 481–495.

15. Jacobs, S. A., Taverna, S. D., Zhang, Y., et al. (2001) Specificity of the HP1 chromo domain for the methylated N-terminus of histone H3. *EMBO J.* **20**, 5232–5241.

16. Lachner, M., O'Carroll, D., Rea, S., Mechtler, K., and Jenuwein, T. (2001) Methylation of histone H3 lysine-9 creates a binding site for HP1 protein. *Nature* **410**, 116–120.

17. Cao, R., Wang, L., Wang, H., et al. (2002) Role of histone H3 lysine 27 methylation in polycomb-group silencing. *Science* **298**, 1039–1043.

18. Orlando, V. (2003) Polycomb, epigenomes, and control of cell identity. *Cell* **112**, 599–606.

19. Maison, C., Bailly, D., Peters, A. H. F. M., et al. (2002) Higher-order structure of pericentric heterochromatin involves a distinct pattern of histone modification and an RNA component. *Nat. Genet.* **30**, 329–334.

20. Heard, E., Rougeulle, C., Arnaud, D., Avner, P., Allis, C. D., and Spector, D. L. (2001) Methylation of histone H3 at lys-9 is an early mark on the X chromosome during X inactivation. *Cell* **107**, 727–738.

21. Boggs, B. A., Cheung, P., Heard, E., Spector, D. L., Chinault, A. C., and Allis, C. D. (2002) Differentially methylated forms of histone H3 show unique association with inactive human X chromosomes. *Nat. Genet.* **30**, 73–76.

22. Peters, A. H., Mermoud, J. E., O'Carroll, D., et al. (2002) Histone H3 methylation is an epigenetic imprint of facultative heterochromatin. *Nat. Genet.* **30**, 77–80.

23. Orlando, V. (2000) Mapping chromosomal proteins *in vivo* by formaldehyde-crosslinked-chromatin-immunoprecipitation. *Trends Biochem. Sci.* **25**, 99–104.

24. Hebbes, T. R., Thorne, A. W., and Crane-Robinson, C. (1988) A direct link between core histone acetylation and transcriptionally active chromatin. *EMBO J.* **7**, 1395–1403.

25. Gregory, R. I., Randall, T. E., Johnson, C. A., et al. (2001) DNA methylation is linked to deacetylation of histone H3, but not H4, on the imprinted genes *Snrpn* and *U2af1-rs1*. *Mol. Cell. Biol.* **21**, 5426–5436.

26. Drew, H. J. (1984) Structural specificities of five commonly used DNA nucleases. *J. Mol. Biol.* **176**, 535–557.

27. Goto, Y., Gomez, M., Brockdorff, N., and Feil, R. (2003) Differential patterns of histone lysine methylation and acetylation distinguish active and repressed alleles at X-linked genes. *Cytogenet. Genome Res.* **99**, 66–74.

28. Orita, M., Iwahana, H., Kanazawa, K., and Sekiya, T. (1989) Detection of polymorphisms of human DNA by gel electrophoresis as single-strand conformation polymorphisms. *Proc. Natl. Acad. Sci. USA* **86**, 2766–2770.

29. Gregory, R. I. and Feil, R. (1999) Analysis of chromatin in limited numbers of cells: a PCR-SSCP based assay of allele-specific nuclease sensitivity. *Nucleic Acids Res.* **27,** e32i–iv.

30. Uejima, H., Lee, M. P., Cui, H., and Feinberg, A. P. (2000) Hot-stop PCR: a simple and general assay for linear quantitation of allele ratios. *Nat. Genet.* **25,** 375–376.

31. Bonner, W. M., West, M. H., and Stedman, J. D. (1980) Two dimensional gel analysis of histones in acid extracts of nuclei, cells, and tissues. *Eur. J. Biochem.* **109,** 17–23.

32. Sambrook, J. and Russell, D.W. (2001). *Molecular Cloning. A Laboratory Manual.* Cold Spring Harbor Laboratory Press, Cold Spring Harbor, NY.

33. Gregory, R. I., O'Neill, L. P., Randall, T. E., et al. (2002) Inhibition of histone deacetylases alters chromatin conformation at the imprinted mouse *U2af1-rs1* locus in mouse embryonic stem cells. *J. Biol. Chem.* **277,** 11,728–11,734.

34. Clayton, A.L., Rose, S., Barratt, M.J., and Mahadevan, L.C. (2000) Phosphoacetylation of histone H3 on c-fos and c-jun associated nucleosomes upon gene activation. *EMBO J.* **19,** 3714–3726.

35. Thomson, S., Clayton, A. L., and Mahadevan, L. C. (2001) Independent dynamic regulation of histone phosphorylation and acetylation during immediate-early gene induction. *Mol. Cell* **8,** 1231–1241.

10

Analysis of Mammalian Telomere Position Effect

Joseph A. Baur, Woodring E. Wright, and Jerry W. Shay

Summary

Methods relating to the positioning of a transgene next to a newly formed telomere in human (HeLa) cells and the subsequent analysis of the resulting clones are described. These include vector design, analysis of integration sites by Southern blotting, pharmacological relief of silencing, and enhancement of silencing by telomere elongation. Several potential pitfalls of applying these techniques to other cell lines are discussed. In addition, detailed instructions are provided for several more general methods related to human telomeres including terminal restriction fragment analysis and purification of telomeres from digested genomic DNA. This chapter summarizes the techniques currently in use that relate to human telomere position effect.

Key Words: Chromosome; healing; position effect; repression; seeding; silencing; subtelomeric; telomerase; telomere; truncation; variegation.

1. Introduction

Reversible silencing of genes near telomeres, termed telomere position effect (TPE), has been studied in lower organisms for over a decade *(1,2)*. Although the mechanism of silencing, particularly in *Streptomyces cerevisiae*, is becoming clearer, its biological significance remains a mystery *(3)*. This phenomenon has recently been described in human cells *(4,5)*. Since the strength of silencing is proportional to telomere length and human telomeres shorten with each cell division *(6)*, loss of TPE has the potential to play a role in human aging. Positioning a reporter gene next to a human telomere and subsequent analysis of the resulting clones require utilization of several nonstandard molecular techniques. The generation and analysis of clones of human (HeLa) cells bearing a subtelomeric reporter gene (**Fig. 1**) is described here to illustrate these methods.

From: *Methods in Molecular Biology, vol. 287: Epigenetics Protocols*
Edited by: T. O. Tollefsbol © Humana Press Inc., Totowa, NJ

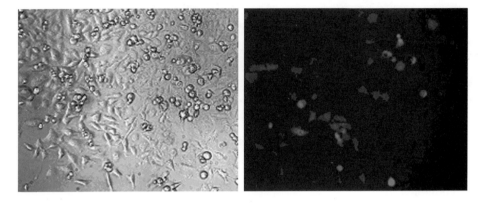

Fig. 1. Expression of a telomeric DsRed2 reporter in HeLa cells. A HeLa clone bearing the DsRed2 reporter at a telomeric site was examined (unfixed) on a Zeiss Axiovert 100M inverted fluorescent microscope. The mosaic pattern of expression is characteristic of transgenes in mammalian cells *(20–24)* and is particularly prominent for those at telomeric locations *(5)*.

2. Materials

1. Plasmid containing 1.6-kb human telomere repeats $(T_2AG_3)_n$ *(7)*.
2. Expression cassette for the reporter gene of interest (DsRed2-N1, Clontech, Palo Alto, CA, in this example).
3. Appropriate drugs for selection based on the final plasmids and retroviruses used.
4. Restriction enzymes, T4 polymerase (for blunting ends if necessary), T4 ligase.
5. Bacteria and related materials for plasmid transformation and amplification.
6. HeLa cells and a culture facility.
7. Materials for Southern blotting.
8. Random-primer labeling kit.
9. Phosphate-buffered saline (PBS).
10. Digestion buffer: 100 mM NaCl, 10 mM Tris-HCl, pH 8.0, 25 mM EDTA, pH 8.0, 0.5% sodium dodecyl sulfate (SDS), and 0.1 mg/mL proteinase K.
11. Phenol/chloroform/isoamyl alcohol.
12. Large volume of TE, membrane, and equipment for dialysis.
13. Trichostatin A (TSA) and/or 5-bromodeoxyuridine (BrdU), stored at –20°C at stock concentrations of 1 mg/mL in dimethyl sulfoxide (DMSO) and 1 M in H_2O, respectively.
14. Retroviral vector encoding hTERT and empty vector control.
15. Ecotrophic retroviral packaging cell line such as PE501 *(8)*.
16. Amphotrophic retroviral packaging cell line such as PA317 *(8)*.
17. Resuspension buffer: 100 mM NaCl, 100 mM EDTA, and 10 mM Tris-HCl, pH 8.0.
18. Proteinase K.
19. Triton X-100.
20. Denaturing solution: 0.5 M NaOH and 1.5 M NaCl.

21. Neutralization buffer: 1.5 M NaCl and 0.5 M Tris-HCl, pH 8.0.
22. ^{32}P-labeled (T$_2$AG$_3$)$_4$ oligonucleotide.
23. SDS.
24. Sodium chloride/sodium citrate buffer (SSC).
25. Phosphor screen or film and apparatus for detection/quantification (Amersham, Piscataway, NJ).
26. Fluorescence microscope, fluorescence-activated cell sorter, or other appropriate apparatus for detection of the chosen reporter gene.

For optional telomere purification (*see* **Subheading 3.2.4.**):

27. Biotinylated (CCCTAA)$_6$ oligonucleotide.
28. Streptavidin-coated magnetic beads such as Dynabeads (Dynal, Oslo, Norway).
29. 5X Denhardt's solution.
30. Samarium-cobalt or other strong magnet (Edmund Scientifics, Tonawanda, NY).

3. Methods

The methods described below outline (1) construction of the chromosome truncation vector, (2) analysis of the resulting clones by telomere purification and Southern blotting, (3) relief of silencing by TSA or BrdU, (4) elongation of telomeres by hTERT overexpression, and (5) representative results.

3.1. Truncation Vector

The construction of a vector designed to place a gene of interest next to a newly formed telomere by chromosome truncation is described here. A tract of telomere repeats contained within the vector "seeds" the formation of a new telomere at the site of integration when this construct is transfected into cells *(7,9–11)*, resulting in the truncation of a chromosome (*see* **Note 1**).

3.1.1. T$_2$AG$_3$-Containing Plasmid

A plasmid (pSXneo-1.6-T$_2$AG$_3$) containing a 1.6-kb tract of telomere repeats *(7)* was kindly provided by the laboratory of T. de Lange (*see* **Note 2**). The backbone containing telomere repeats, the origin of replication, and the β-lactamase (ampicillin resistance) gene was obtained by digestion with *Sma*I and *Hpa*I using standard molecular biology techniques *(12)*.

3.1.2. Expression Vector

The plasmid DsRed2-N1 (Clontech, Palo Alto, CA) contains a mammalian expression cassette for the fluorescent protein DsRed2 consisting of the cytomegalovirus (CMV) promoter, the coding region, and the SV40 poly-adenylation signal. A fragment containing an internal ribosome entry site (IRES) in front of the blasticidin-resistance gene was excised from the vector pWZL-Blast (gift of J. Morgenstern, Millennium Pharmaceuticals, Cambridge,

MA) and inserted into the *Hpa*I site between the DsRed2 coding region and the SV40 polyadenylation signal by standard molecular biology techniques *(12)*, to allow translation of two proteins from only one mRNA *(13)*, thus ensuring that blasticidin-resistant cells also expressed mRNA for DsRed2 (*see* **Note 3**).

3.1.3. Cloning

DNA manipulations were performed by standard methods and are described here briefly *(12)*.

1. The DsRed2/IRES-Blast expression cassette was removed from the modified DsRed2-N1 by digestion with *Afl*III and *Bfr*I, and the ends were blunted with T4 DNA polymerase.
2. This fragment was ligated into the backbone derived from pSXneo-1.6-T_2AG_3 such that the CMV promoter was placed adjacent to the base of the T_2AG_3 repeats (**Fig. 2**).
3. A control vector lacking telomere repeats was generated by excision of the telomere tract using *Cla*I and *Sac*II, followed by blunting with T4 DNA polymerase and religation (*see* **Note 4**).
4. After ligation, the DNA was transformed into DH5α (Invitrogen, Carlsbad, CA) by standard methods, plated on media containing 75 mg/mL ampicillin, and grown overnight at 37°C.
5. Single colonies were then isolated and grown overnight in liquid media containing 75 µg/mL ampicillin.
6. Plasmid DNA was isolated and checked for the presence and correct orientation of the insert by restriction enzyme digest.

3.2. Generation and Analysis of Clones

3.2.1. Generation of Clones

1. The vectors were linearized with *Cla*I and *Pvu*I (truncation vector) or *Pvu*I alone (control vector) as shown (**Fig. 2**) and gel-purified.
2. HeLa cells at 30-50% confluence on 10-cm dishes were transfected with 10 µg of plasmid using the FuGENE 6 transfection reagent (Roche, Basel, Switzerland) according to the manufacturer's instructions.
3. Cells were grown in 4:1 Dulbecco's modified Eagle's medium (DMEM)/Medium 199 (Invitrogen, Carlsbad, CA; *see* **Note 5**) containing 10% calf serum and 1 µg/mL blasticidin until individual clones could be easily distinguished (approx 2 wk).
4. Clones were then transferred to separate dishes by ring-cloning (*see* **Note 6**). A glass ring, sealed with sterile silicone vacuum grease, was placed over each clone, and the cells were then released by standard trypsinization methods.
5. Clones were then cultured until a sufficient number of cells were obtained from which to extract genomic DNA (10–20 million).
6. DNA was extracted by standard methods and used in the subsequent analysis.

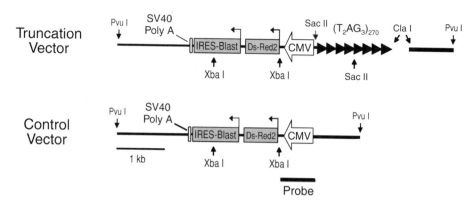

Fig. 2. Structure of the truncation and control vectors. Expression of a single transcript encoding both the DsRed2 and the blasticidin-resistance proteins is driven by the cytomegalovirus (CMV) promoter. The linearized forms (as transfected) are shown. Gel purification was used to remove the smaller *Cla*I/*Pvu*I fragment from the truncation vector prior to transfection. The restriction sites (*Xba*I) and probe region used during Southern blotting are indicated below.

3.2.2. Extraction of Genomic DNA

DNA was extracted using a standard dialysis procedure *(14)* instead of precipitation both to preserve the integrity of large DNA fragments and because genomic DNA from our HeLa cells was extremely difficult to redissolve after pelleting.

1. Trypsinize cells, wash in PBS, and pellet.
2. Resuspend cells at 10^8/mL in digestion buffer (100 mM NaCl, 10 mM Tris-HCl, pH 8.0, 25 mM EDTA, pH 8.0, 0.5% SDS, and 0.1 mg/mL proteinase K).
3. Incubate at least 12 h at 50°C with shaking.
4. Extract with phenol/chloroform/isoamyl alcohol, sacrificing volume if necessary to avoid any white precipitate when transferring the aqueous layer to a new tube. Repeat if necessary.
5. Dialyze the aqueous layer twice against 100 vol of Tris-HCl/EDTA (TE) buffer for a total of at least 24 h.

3.2.3. Digestion of DNA

Genomic DNA (60–80 μg if performing telomere purification, 15–20 μg if not) was digested with an enzyme (*Xba*I) that cut within the vector sequence, leaving a region corresponding to the Southern blot probe attached to the telomere repeats (**Fig. 2**). If the vector had integrated at an internal site, this digest produced a discreet band on a Southern blot since a second restriction site was present in the genomic DNA. If the vector sequences had seeded the

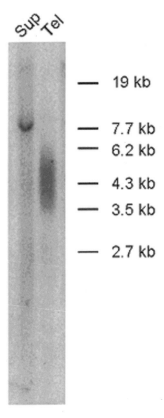

Fig. 3. Southern blot showing telomeric and internal integration sites. Genomic DNA was extracted from a clone in which both a telomeric and an internal integration have taken place. After digestion with *Xba*I, telomeres were purified by the optional procedure described in **Subheading 3.2.4.** Both the supernatant (Sup; containing bulk genomic DNA) and the purified telomeres (Tel) were analyzed by Southern blot using the CMV promoter region as a probe. Because the heterogeneous telomere fragments remain attached to the CMV promoter after digestion, the telomeric integration site is indicated by a smear in the telomere fraction, whereas the internal integration site is indicated by a single band in the supernatant fraction. Size markers (λ *Sty*I) are indicated in kilobases.

formation of a new telomere, however, this digest produced a smear on a Southern blot because the heterogeneous repetitive telomere fragments (which do not contain an *Xba*I site) remained attached to the probed vector sequences (**Fig. 3**).

3.2.4. (Optional) Telomere Purification

This protocol allows purification of telomere-containing DNA fragments after digestion based on the 3' overhang that is present at each chromosome end. This eliminates most of the background signal on a Southern blot, allowing a smear indicating a telomeric integration site (*see* **Subheading 3.2.5.**) to be more clearly distinguished. This method also provides an additional confirmation of a telomeric or internal integration site since telomeric fragments will be present in the telomere fraction whereas internal fragments will be present only in the supernatant.

1. To the digested DNA (it is not necessary to remove the digestion buffer), add 12.5 µL 20X SSC, 1.5 µL 25% Triton X-100, 4.5 pmol biotinylated (CCCTAA)$_6$ oligonucleotide, and water up to 250 µL.
2. Anneal the biotinylated oligonucleotide to the telomeric 3' overhangs by heating to 80°C for 20 min, 65°C for 30 min, 55°C for 20 min, 45°C for 15 min, and 35°C for 15 min.
3. Add 20 µL of a 10 mg/mL stock of streptavidin-coated magnetic beads (Dynabeads) that have been washed in 1X SSC, coated with 5X Denhardt's solution for 30 min, and resuspended in 1X SSC.
4. Incubate at 4°C overnight, rotating the sample end over end at approx 3 rpm to keep the beads suspended.
5. On d 2, prechill (on ice) a magnet (Edmund Scientifics, Tonawanda, NY), 1X SSC with 1% Triton X-100, 0.2X SSC with 1% Triton X-100, and TE, pH 8.0. Perform the remaining steps keeping all materials (including samples) on ice.
6. Spin tubes briefly to collect samples at the bottom, and then "pellet" beads by holding the samples against the magnet. While holding the sample tube against the magnet, carefully remove the supernatant with a pipetor and save. (This contains genomic DNA excluding telomere fragments.)
7. Resuspend using a wide-bore pipet tip in 150 µL of the1X SSC buffer, "pellet" the beads with the magnet, and discard the supernatant. (Remove either by pipeting or with a vacuum.)
8. Resuspend in 150 µL 1X SSC, this time transferring the slurry to a new tube to avoid recovering DNA nonspecifically bound to the walls of the tube. "Pellet" beads and discard supernatant as in the previous step.
9. Resuspend in 150 µL 0.2X SSC, "pellet" beads, and discard supernatant.
10. Without disturbing the pellet, hold tube against the magnet and gently add and remove 50 mL of TE with a pipetor. (This step is to remove residual SSC that could interfere with elution in the next step.)
11. Resuspend in 20 µL of TE and elute beads by heating to 65°C for 10 min.
12. Spin tubes briefly, "pellet" beads on a warmed magnet, and this time recover the supernatant containing telomere fragments.

3.2.5. Southern Blotting

Southern blotting was performed by standard methods according to the instructions provided with the Zeta Probe GT (Bio-Rad, Hercules, CA) nylon membrane.

1. Samples were run on a 0.7% agarose gel and capillary-transferred for at least 12 h in 10X SSX.
2. The membrane was then crosslinked twice in a Stratalinker ultraviolet (UV) crosslinker (Stratagene, La Jolla, CA) at the "autocrosslink" setting.
3. An $[\alpha\text{-P}^{32}]$-dCTP labeled probe was generated from a 600-bp fragment of the truncation vector containing primarily the CMV promoter by random priming.
4. Blocking and hybridization were performed in 0.25 M PBS, pH 7.2, 7% SDS at 65°C.
5. Washing steps were performed according to the membrane manufacturer's instructions and the blot was exposed to a Phosphor screen and visualized using a STORM 860 Phosphorimager (Amersham, Piscataway, NJ).
6. Telomeric insertions were indicated by a smear, and internal insertions gave discreet bands (of characteristic size; **Fig. 3**).
7. If telomeres were purified in the previous step, then telomeric clones also gave a positive signal in the telomere fraction and internal clones did not.

3.3. Relief of Silencing

Silencing can be relieved in telomeric clones (and internal controls) by treatment with either TSA *(4)* or BrdU *(15)*. TSA has the advantage that the mechanism is understood, since it is a known histone deacetylase inhibitor; however, this drug is highly toxic to HeLa cells, killing more than 50% during the treatment required for the assay. BrdU, on the other hand, is less toxic, but its mechanism of action is unknown.

3.3.1. TSA

Cells were treated with 200 ng/mL trichostatin A in regular medium for 24 h. The TSA-containing medium was then replaced with fresh medium, and the cells were incubated an additional 24 h before assaying (*see* **Note 7**).

3.3.2. BrdU

Cells were treated for 72 h with 50 μM BrdU in regular medium. Effects were visible by about 48 h and persisted for several days.

3.4. Enhancement of Silencing by Telomere Elongation

Telomerase is the enzyme that maintains telomeres in germline and most tumor cells. It consists of an integral RNA component and a catalytic protein component. Although HeLa cells are telomerase-positive, additional exogenous telomerase protein (hTERT) can dramatically increase telomere length (*see* **Note 8**).

3.4.1. Retroviral Vectors

The telomerase catalytic component, kindly provided by the Geron Corporation (Menlo Park, CA), was subcloned into the *Eco*RI site of the retroviral vector pBabe-puro *(16)*. Retroviral supernatant was obtained from this and a control (empty) vector by standard methods *(16)*. The vector was transiently transfected into the ecotropic packaging cell line PE501 *(8)*, and supernatant from these cells was used to infect stably the amphotrophic cell line PA317 *(8)*. Supernatant from PA317 was then used to infect HeLa cells.

3.4.2. Changes in Telomere Length

Telomere length in HeLa cells increased from approx 5 kb to approx 15 kb within 1 mo after hTERT infection. Changes in telomere length were monitored by Southern blot (as described above) for telomeric clones, since the size of the plasmid sequences attached to the telomeric smear was known and could be subtracted, or alternatively by terminal restriction fragment (TRF) analysis as described in the next section.

3.4.3. Terminal Restriction Fragment Analysis

TRF is a generally applicable method for determining telomere length, first described in **ref. *17*** and further developed in **ref. *18***. This method saves a few steps relative to the Southern blotting technique described previously and can be used to determine telomere length in both telomeric and internal clones. Genomic DNA is digested with a mixture of restriction enzymes so that only repetitive sequences (such as telomeres) that contain no restriction sites remain intact. Samples are run on an agarose gel, which is then probed for telomere sequences (**Fig. 4**). A more detailed description of the TRF procedure is provided in **ref. *19***.

1. Resuspend cells in 100 m*M* NaCl, 100 m*M* EDTA, and 10 m*M* Tris-HCl, pH 8.0, at 20,000 cells/µL.
2. Extract genomic DNA by bringing the final concentrations of Triton X-100 and proteinase K up to 1% and 2 mg/mL, respectively, and incubate for 2–16 hours at 55°C.
3. Inactivate proteinase K at 70°C for 30 min.
4. (Optional) Extract with an equal volume of phenol/chloroform/isoamyl alcohol. This step is not necessary when using the restriction enzymes specified in **step 6**; however, some enzymes may cut less efficiently if this extraction has not been carried out.
5. Dialyze samples overnight against TE, pH 8.0.

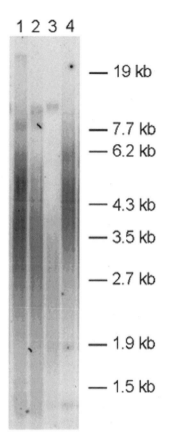

Fig. 4. Terminal restriction fragments from human cells. Genomic DNA from four human cell lines was digested with a mixture of restriction enzymes with four-base recognition sites in order to degrade nonrepetitive DNA. Samples were then run on an agarose gel, which was subsequently dried and probed with a $(T_2AG_3)_4$ oligonucleotide (corresponding to the telomere repeat sequence). Care must be taken when determining average size (*see* **Note 9**) owing to the extensive heterogeneity. Lane 2, in particular, is a good example of this. Size markers (λ *Sty*I) are indicated in kilobases.

6. After dialysis, digest 1 µg DNA with a mixture of six restriction enzymes (1–2 U each of *Alu*I, *Cfo*I, *Hae*I, *Hinf*I, *Msp*I, and *Rsa*I) with 4-bp target sites.
7. Run on a 0.7% agarose gel overnight at approx 2.5 V/cm.
8. Denature the gel for 20 min in 0.5 *M* NaOH and 1.5 *M* NaCl.
9. Rinse for 10 min in water.
10. Dry for 1 h at 55°C. The gel is delicate at this stage and can be transported by rolling loosely around a 10- or 25-mL pipet.
11. Neutralize for 15 min in 1.5 *M* NaCl and 0.5 *M* Tris-HCl, pH 8.0.

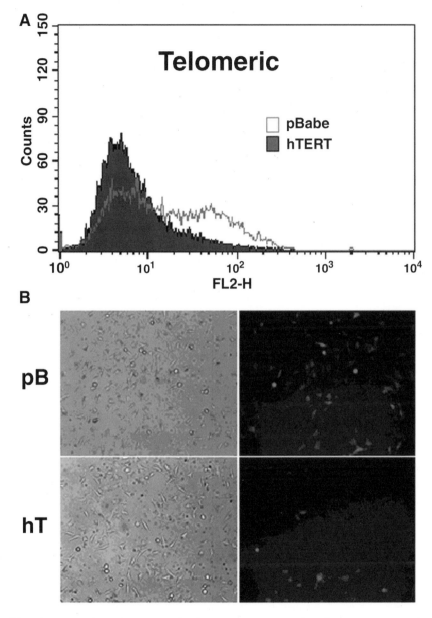

Fig. 5. Elongation of telomeres by hTERT overexpression decreases expression of DsRed2 in telomeric clones. Clones were infected with an empty vector (pBabe) or a retrovirus encoding the telomerase catalytic component (hTERT). (**A**) FACS analysis of a clone bearing a telomeric DsRed2 reporter with short telomeres (red outline) or long telomeres (solid blue histogram). (**B**) Brightfield and fluorescent images for the cells analyzed in A.

12. Probe with ^{32}P-labeled $(T_2AG_3)_4$ oligonucleotide (end-labeled using T4 poly-nucleotide kinase).

13. Wash in 2X SSC for 15 min and 0.1X SSC with 0.1% SDS twice for 10 min.

14. Expose the gel to a phosphor screen or film and analyze, keeping in mind that signal strength will be proportional to both the number of telomeres and the length of each telomere (*see* **Note 9**).

3.5. Detection of Reporter Expression

DsRed2 expression was detected by a combination of fluorescence micros-copy and fluorescence-activated cell sorting. Expression was highly variable in internal clones, in terms of both the fraction of cells positive and the inten-sity within each positive cell. Expression in telomeric clones was always lim-ited to a few percent of the cells (**Fig. 5**; *see* **Note 10**).

4. Notes

1. This procedure was originally used in mammalian cells that were telomerase-positive and aneuploid *(7,9–11)*, such as the HeLa cells described here. Telomerase was thought to be necessary for the "healing" of a new telomere by extension of the plasmid-based telomere repeats, and aneuploidy was thought to indicate that cells might tolerate the loss of a chromosome arm after a truncation event. More recently, it was shown that telomere-healing events can be detected in some normal (telomerase-negative) human fibroblast strains using a 2-kb tract of telomere repeats and that overexpression of TRF1 can enhance this process in telomerase-positive cells *(25)*. In another report, telomere-healing was demon-strated in SV40-transformed human embryonic kidney (HEK) cells in the pres-ence of wild-type or catalytically inactive telomerase, but not in the absence of telomerase *(26)*. In this report, no telomere-healing events were detected in human diploid fibroblasts transfected with a 1.6-kb tract of telomere repeats or in HEK cells transfected with a 3.2-kb tract of telomere repeats (both telomerase-negative), even in the presence of SV40 T antigen. It is therefore necessary to consider carefully the cell type that will be used (*also see* **Note 8**) and the strat-egy for generating telomere-healing events.

2. Telomere (T_2AG_3) repeats are unstable in certain positions and/or orientations within a plasmid for reasons that are not well understood *(27)*. Rearrangements can be minimized by harvesting bacteria containing the plasmid before the end of log phase growth (usually 10–12 h for a 250-mL culture). It is necessary to check the integrity of the telomere repeat array by restriction digest at each step in the cloning process. Smaller, substoichiometric bands below the band containing telomere re-peats are indicative of deletion products. In some cases, it may be necessary to adopt an alternative strategy if the desired product cannot be obtained intact.

3. An important caveat to keep in mind is that, regardless of the way the vector is organized, this type of strategy will produce only clones in which there is suffi-cient expression of the marker gene to get drug resistance. It is possible that

many telomeric clones exhibiting complete silencing are lost during the selection process. Linking the reporter to the resistance marker, as is done here, simply ensures that the reporter will be intact in the isolated clones (i.e., prevents the isolation of clones in which the reporter gene has become damaged or lost during integration but that still contain the resistance marker).

4. A linearized control vector could be generated simply by cutting the truncation vector on both sides of the telomere repeats. However, inclusion of extraneous sequences at the end of the linearized control vector (as shown in **Fig. 1**) increases the number of expressing clones that are obtained in some systems *(27)*. It is not clear whether this is owing to degradation of the transfected material, loss of some sequences during integration, or some other mechanism.

5. Our lab uses this particular mix of cell culture media for historical reasons. It is not expected to differ significantly from 100% DMEM.

6. Transfection of a repeat-containing vector typically produces one to three times as many clones as the corresponding vector lacking repeats *(27)*. Within these clones, it is not unusual for >50% to be telomeric integration events *(7)*, although as few as 10% may be obtained, depending on the construct and/or cell line *(27)*.

7. TSA induces either apoptosis, differentiation, or senescence, depending on the cell line *(28)*. HeLa cells treated with TSA undergo apoptosis, and the effective doses for killing cells and relieving transgene silencing are very similar. The procedure described here results in the apoptosis of over half of the treated cells; however, lower doses are much less effective at relieving silencing. The effects of TSA (and BrdU) are not specific to telomeric clones *(4)*. Both of these agents appear to relieve silencing of transgenes generally but have more dramatic effects on telomeric clones owing to the stronger initial repression.

8. The behavior of telomeres in the presence of exogenous telomerase is characteristic of each cell line *(29)*. Some, like the HeLa cells described here, will elongate their telomeres rapidly and almost indefinitely in the presence of excess hTERT, whereas others elongate their telomeres more slowly and can reach a stable length that may be very close to the starting length. This should be determined beforehand for the cell line in question if telomere elongation will form an important part of the experiment.

9. Since the probe can bind along the length of the entire telomere, long telomeres will not only run at a higher molecular weight, they will also give a more intense signal per end. This becomes important when attempting to determine the average telomere length. Mean size can be estimated by subdividing the telomere smear into discreet regions and then dividing the sum of volume (PhosphorImager) or optical density (film) minus backgound for all regions by the sum of volume minus background divided by length (of the fragments in that region) for all regions *(6)*. The formula for estimating average telomere length by this method is this method is $\Sigma(\text{volume}i - \text{background})/\Sigma[(\text{volume}i - \text{background})/Li]$, where volume$i$ is the signal intensity and Li is the length of telomere

fragments in region *i*. The program Telorun for this analysis is available at URL: http://www.swmed.edu/home_pages/cellbio/shay-wright/research/ sw_lab_methods.htm.

10. In contrast to the stable expression typically observed for transgenes in yeast and other model systems, transgenes in mammalian cells are typically repressed to some degree and are frequently expressed in a mosaic pattern even within clones *(20–24)*. Repression at telomeres appears to be particularly strong since there are no reported cases of telomeric transgenes being expressed in a high fraction of cells and the average expression at telomeres is 10-fold lower than at internal loci *(4)*. However, any experiment involving telomere position effect in human cells should take into account the variability inherent in the expression of mammalian transgenes.

Acknowledgments

The authors thank T. de Lange for providing the plasmid-containing telomere repeats. This work was supported by the Department of Defense grant BC000422 (to Joseph A. Baur) and NIH grant AG07792 (to Woodring E. Wright and Jerry W. Shay).

References

1. Hazelrigg, T., Levis, R., and Rubin, G. M. (1984) Transformation of white locus DNA in drosophila: dosage compensation, zeste interaction, and position effects. *Cell* **36**, 469–481.
2. Gottschling, D. E., Aparicio, O. M., Billington, B. L., and Zakian, V. A. (1990) Position effect at S. cerevisiae telomeres: reversible repression of Pol II transcription. *Cell* **63**, 751–762.
3. Tham, W. H. and Zakian, V. A. (2002) Transcriptional silencing at Saccharomyces telomeres: implications for other organisms. *Oncogene* **21**, 512–521.
4. Baur, J. A., Zou, Y., Shay, J. W., and Wright, W. E. (2001) Telomere position effect in human cells. *Science* **292**, 2075–2077.
5. Koering, C. E., Pollice, A., Zibella, M. P., et al. (2002) Human telomeric position effect is determined by chromosomal context and telomeric chromatin integrity. *EMBO Rep.* **3**, 1055–1061.
6. Harley, C. B., Futcher, A. B., and Greider, C. W. (1990) Telomeres shorten during ageing of human fibroblasts. *Nature* **345**, 458–460.
7. Hanish, J. P., Yanowitz, J. L., and de Lange, T. (1994) Stringent sequence requirements for the formation of human telomeres. *Proc. Natl. Acad. Sci. US,* **91**, 8861–8865.
8. Miller, A. D. and Rosman, G. J. (1989) Improved retroviral vectors for gene transfer and expression. *Biotechniques* **7**, 980–982, 984–986, 989,990.
9. Farr, C., Fantes, J., Goodfellow, P., and Cooke, H. (1991) Functional reintroduction of human telomeres into mammalian cells. *Proc. Natl. Acad. Sci. USA* **88**, 7006–7010.

10. Farr, C. J., Stevanovic, M., Thomson, E. J., Goodfellow, P. N., and Cooke, H. J. (1992) Telomere-associated chromosome fragmentation: applications in genome manipulation and analysis. *Nat. Genet.* **2,** 275–282.

11. Barnett, M. A., Buckle, V. J., Evans, E. P., Porter, A. C., Rout, D., Smith, A. G., and Brown, W. R. (1993) Telomere directed fragmentation of mammalian chromosomes. *Nucleic Acids Res.* **21,** 27–36.

12. Sambrook, J., Fritsch, E. F., and Maniatis, T. (1989) *Molecular Cloning: A Laboratory Manual*, 2nd ed. Cold Spring Harbor Laboratory Press, Cold Spring Harbor, NY.

13. Jang, S. K., Pestova, T. V., Hellen, C. U., Witherell, G. W., and Wimmer, E. (1990) Cap-independent translation of picornavirus RNAs: structure and function of the internal ribosomal entry site. *Enzyme* **44,** 292–309.

14. Ausubel, F. M. (1993) *Current Protocols in Molecular Biology*. Greene and Wiley-Interscience, New York.

15. Suzuki, T., Yaginuma, M., Oishi, T., Michishita, E., Ogino, H., Fujii, M., and Ayusawa, D. (2001) 5-Bromodeoxyuridine suppresses position effect variegation of transgenes in HeLa cells. *Exp. Cell Res.* **266,** 53–63.

16. Morgenstern, J. P. and Land, H. (1990) Advanced mammalian gene transfer: high titre retroviral vectors with multiple drug selection markers and a complementary helper-free packaging cell line. *Nucleic Acids Res.* **18,** 3587–3596.

17. de Lange, T., Shiue, L., Myers, R. M., Cox, D. R., Naylor, S. L., Killery, A. M., and Varmus, H. E. (1990) Structure and variability of human chromosome ends. *Mol. Cell Biol.* **10,** 518–527.

18. Allsopp, R. C., Vaziri, H., Patterson, C., et al. (1992) Telomere length predicts replicative capacity of human fibroblasts. *Proc. Natl. Acad. Sci. USA* **89,** 10114–10118.

19. Herbert, B.-S., Shay, J. W., and Wright, W. E. (2003) in *Current Protocols in Cell Biology* (Dasso, M., and Morgan, K., eds.), in press.

20. Kalos, M. and Fournier, R. E. (1995) Free in PMC Position-independent transgene expression mediated by boundary elements from the apolipoprotein B chromatin domain. *Mol. Cell Biol.* **15,** 198–207.

21. Walters, M. C., Fiering, S., Eidemiller, J., Magis, W., Groudine, M., and Martin, D. I. (1995) Enhancers increase the probability but not the level of gene expression. *Proc. Natl. Acad. Sci. USA* **92,** 7125–7129.

22. Walters, M. C., Magis, W., Fiering, S., Eidemiller, J., Scalzo, D., Groudine, M., and Martin, D. I. (1996) Transcriptional enhancers act in cis to suppress position-effect variegation. *Genes Dev.* **10,** 185–195.

23. Martin, D. I. and Whitelaw, E. (1996) The vagaries of variegating transgenes. *Bioessays* **18,** 919–923.

24. Dorer, D. R. (1997) Do transgene arrays form heterochromatin in vertebrates? *Transgenic Res.* **6,** 3–10.

25. Okabe, J., Eguchi, A., Masago, A., Hayakawa, T., and Nakanishi, M. (2000) TRF1 is a critical trans-acting factor required for de novo telomere formation in human cells. *Human Mol. Genet.* **9,** 2639–2650.

26. Guiducci, C., Anglana, M., Wang, A., and Bacchetti, S. (2001) Transient expression of wild-type or biologically inactive telomerase allows the formation of artificial telomeres in mortal human cells. *Exp. Cell Res.* **265,** 304–311.
27. Baur, J. A., Shay, J. W., and Wright, W. E., unpublished results.
28. Marks, P. A., Richon, V. M., and Rifkind, R. A. (2000) Histone deacetylase inhibitors: inducers of differentiation or apoptosis of transformed cells. *J. Natl. Cancer Inst.* **92,** 1210–1216.
29. McChesney, P. A., Aisner, D. L., Frank, B. C., Wright, W. E., and Shay, J. W. (2000) Telomere dynamics in cells with introduced telomerase: a rapid assay for telomerase activity on telomeres. *Mol. Cell Biol. Res. Commun.* **3,** 312–318.

11

Activity Assays for Poly-ADP Ribose Polymerase

Eva Kirsten, Ernest Kun, Jerome Mendeleyev, and Charles P. Ordahl

Summary

Poly(ADP-ribose) polymerase (PARP-1) is a nuclear enzyme that has traditionally been thought to require discontinuous or "damaged" DNA (dcDNA) as a coenzyme, a preconception that has limited research mainly to its role in cell pathology, i.e., DNA repair and apoptosis. Recent evidence has shown that this enzyme is broadly involved in normal cell physiological functions including chromatin modeling and gene regulation when DNA strand breaks are absent. We have recently shown that double-stranded DNA (dsDNA) serves as a more efficient coenzyme for PARP-1 than dcDNA (Kun, Kirsten, and Ordahl [2002] *J. Biol. Chem.* **277**, 39,066–39,069), providing a mechanistic basis for PARP-1 function in normal cell physiology. Here we provide a detailed outline of methods for analyzing PARP-1 enzymatic activity using dsDNA as a coenzyme compared with broken or damaged DNA. Two procedures are described, one for analysis of auto-, and the other for trans-ADP-ribosylation. These assays provide a means of investigating the physiological role(s) of PARP-1 in normal cells.

Key Words: NAD; nuclear enzyme; coenzymic DNA; histone modification; chromatin remodeling; polypeptide posttranslational modification.

1. Introduction

Poly(ADP-ribose) polymerase (PARP-1; E.C. 2.4.2.30) is a chromatin-associated enzyme thought to be present in all cell types. The PARP-1 primary structure (**Fig. 1A**) consists of three major domains: (1) an N-terminal DNA binding domain containing two zinc fingers, (2) a C-terminal catalytic domain containing an NAD binding site, and (3) an "auto-modification" domain between these with multiple glutamic acid residues to which poly(ADP-ribose) chains (ADPR)n attach. At approx 0.5×10^6 molecules per nucleus, PARP-1 is the second most abundant nonhistone nuclear protein *(1)*. PARP-1 uses nicotine adenine dinucleotide (NAD) as a substrate to catalyze the addition of (ADPR)n to acceptor proteins (**Fig. 1B** and **C**, respectively). *Auto-modification* refers to addition of (ADPR)n to one PARP-1 molecule within a homodimer. *Hetero-* or

From: *Methods in Molecular Biology, vol. 287: Epigenetics Protocols*
Edited by: T. O. Tollefsbol © Humana Press Inc., Totowa, NJ

A   PARP I primary structure

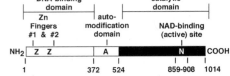

B   NAD structure   **C   ADPRn structure**

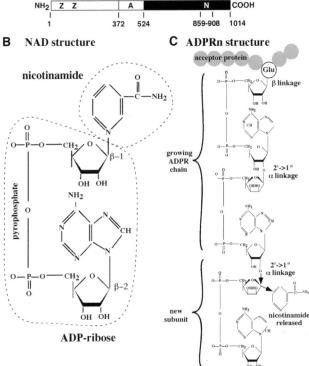

Fig. 1. Schematic diagrams of PARP-1 (A), NAD (B), and poly(ADP-ribose) polymer formation (C). (**A**) PARP-1 enzyme primary structure and functional domains. The three-domain structure of PARP-1 (DNA binding, auto-modification, and catalytic) first proposed *(36)* has been both confirmed and refined by gene and cDNA nucleotide sequence determination *(37)*. (**B**) NAD structure. Dashed lines encircle the nicotinamide and ADP-ribose moieties, which are joined at the β C-1″ position of the ribose moiety (indicated as β-1). The linkage marked β-2 is not affected during ADP-ribose polymerization. (**C**) Subunit addition. The ADP-ribose polymer is stably attached to a glutamate (Glu) reside of the modified protein via a β-1 linkage. The addition of a new subunit is shown at the bottom of the chain, where a ribose-ribose is formed between the incoming ADP ribose and the 2′ ribose at the terminus of the growing chain *(38,39)*. Specifically, the α-linkage occurs by an inversion process at the anomeric 1″-carbon atom of the ribose of substrate NAD. Thus, the configuration at the detectable stable 1″-carbon in the resultant 2′->1″ linkage is α, as determined by NMR *(40–42)*. This diagram is intended for schematic purposes only and does not attempt to portray accurately either molecular conformations or mechanisms.

trans-modification occurs when PARP-1 adds (ADPR)n to a second acceptor protein. Histone H_1 is the most frequent acceptor, followed by octameric histones (histones within nucleosomes, but not free histones) and a variety of other nonhistone proteins including a growing list of transcription factors. The secondary structure of (ADPR)n chains predicts that proteins so modified will be altered in their binding to other proteins or DNA *(2,3)*. Maximal PARP-1 catalytic activity requires DNA, and PARP-1 has two zinc-finger DNA binding domains located near the NH_2 terminus (**Fig. 1A**). The PARP-1 substrate is NAD, a nucleotide that is intimately connected to cellular redox systems, which regulate NAD/NADH ratios. Because NAD is the *only* ADPR donor for PARP-1 activity, the redox state of the cell exerts control over the active vs inhibited status of PARP-1, thereby linking its epigenetic gene regulatory properties to cellular metabolism.

1.1. Pathophysiology of PARP-1

Under some circumstances PARP-1 can become *superactivated*, a condition that can lead to diminution of NAD to levels incompatible with cell survival. For example, in cells with extensive DNA breakage, owing to ionizing radiation or other emergency, binding of PARP-1 to the broken ends of "damaged" DNA leads to an increase in auto-(ADPR)n and ultimately becomes a component of the cell death pathway. The role of PARP-1 in these aspects of DNA damage and apoptosis has been extensively studied and is reviewed in **ref. 4**.

1.2. Evidence for a Normal, Physiologic Role for PARP-1 in the Transcription and Replication of DNA

DNA breaks are absent in normal cellular chromatin and a requirement for such breaks to activate PARP-1 is not consistent with a normal, physiologic function. Nonetheless, (ADPR)n is known to be abundant in the nuclei of normal cells, and PARP-1 activity changes in concert with the cell cycle *(4)*. There is substantial evidence indicating an association of PARP-1 with a number of transcriptional factors, exerting both positive and negative regulation *(5–26)*. PARP-1 has recently been shown to serve a coenzymic function to Topo I *(27)*. PARP-1 has also been implicated as playing a role in DNA replication, a function supported by its colocalization with DNA polymerase *(28)* and localization at DNA replication sites *(29)*. A major limitation in this field has been the persistent postulate that discontinuous DNA (dcDNA) is the exclusive coenzyme of PARP-1 and that "DNA strand breaks" are the sole sites in DNA to which PARP-1 molecules bind. That widespread preconception has limited model building even as data increasingly accumulate that implicate this enzyme in chromatin modification and gene regulation (for a recent example, see **refs. 22** and **23**).

1.3. PARP-1 Prefers Linear, Double-Stranded DNA as Coenzyme for the Auto- and Trans-(ADPR)n Reactions

The notion that "broken DNA" is the exclusive coenzyme for PARP-1 enzymatic activity was recently disproven by showing that intact double strand DNAs (dsDNAs) serve as efficient coenzymes even when end-protected *(30)*. More importantly, from a DNA binding perspective, the K_a for PARP-1–DNA binding to dsDNA was found to be at least 100 times lower than that for "broken DNA." These results provide a mechanism whereby PARP-1 can be directly associated with, and activated by, the unbroken dsDNA found in the chromatin of normal cells. As noted above, PARP-1 and PARP-1 activity have been implicated in many cell functions including DNA replication and gene transcription. This avid association between PARP-1 and dsDNA may provide a crucial link in understanding the role of this chromatin-associated enzyme in these fundamental activities of eukaryotic cells.

2. Materials

1. 10X Buffer (stock solution 1): 500 mM Tris-HCl, pH 8.0, (for all reactions).
2. 10X DNA (stock solution 2): either end-protected, 23-nucleotide pair dsDNA (100 nM), or, alternatively, the weight equivalent of dcDNA. Both are dissolved in annealing buffer; 20 mM Tris-HCl, pH 7.0, 50 mM KCl (*see* **Note 1**).
3. Divalent cation-stimulated auto-poly-ADP-ribosylation assays: 10X cation salts.
   a. 250 mM MgCl$_2$.
   b. 120 mM CaCl$_2$.
   c. 30 mM Spermine.
4. Histone-stimulated poly-ADP-ribosylation assays (stock solution 4): cation salts are omitted and replaced with histone (Roche Applied Sciences, stored at –20°C in Ca^{2+}/Mg^{2+}-free phosphate-buffered saline).
   a. 1 mg/mL Histone H$_1$ (optimum concentration 2.5 µg/50 µL assay).
   b. 1 mg/mL Histone H$_3$ (optimum concentration 2.5 µg/50 µL assay).
5. Two 10X PARP-1 enzyme solutions (stock solution 5): 320 nM and 80 nM. PARP-1 enzyme (human) comes at a concentration of 0.1 mg/ml (~830 nM) from the manufacturer (Trevigen, high activity grade) and is stored at –80°C.
6. Hot NAD cocktail (concentrated stock solution 6): Mix cold and ^{32}P-labeled NAD to a final concentration of 1 mM in H$_2$O. Radiolabeled (^{32}P) NAD solution (Amersham) is stored at –20°C. As needed, it is diluted with a 1 mM NAD solution to obtain a "hot cocktail" containing approx 1×10^6 dpm in 20 µL. This diluted solution can be stored at –20°C.
7. Biotinylated NAD cocktail (Trevigen), stored at –20°C.
8. 20% Trichloroacetic acid (TCA), kept ice cold.
9. 10 mg/mL Bovine serum albumin (BSA).
10. 96-Well flat-bottomed tissue culture plates (preferably Nunc Maxi-sorp; Trenigen).

11. 1 mg/mL Streptavidin-horseradish peroxidase and the peroxidase substrate TACS-Sapphire (both from Trevigen), stored at 4°C.
12. Other reagents such as spermine, magnesium chloride, NAD, Tris-base, and others were obtained as ultrapure-grade reagents from Sigma-Aldrich.

3. Methods

3.1. Soluble Assay Systems

Auto-(ADPR)n involves one member of a PARP-1 dimer acting as target for modification by the other member. In this case, the only protein present is both enzyme and target, making simple acid precipitation suitable to measure the amount of label incorporated into auto-(ADPR)n. Because solution conditions permit an infinite range of reagent concentration they are ideal for analysis of enzyme kinetics by classical methods. The auto-(ADPR)n assay outlined below (6 time/concentration points) can be considered as a module that can be replicated in parallel to simultaneously analyze multiple reaction components/conditions, including the effects of activators and inhibitors.

3.1.1. Divalent Cation-Stimulated Auto-ADP-Ribosylation

Each reaction is conducted in microcentrifuge tubes containing 50 µL final volume and the incorporation of ^{32}P-NAD into acid-precipitable material is assayed.

1. Assay buffer solution components: 50 mM Tris-HCl, pH 8.0; plus divalent cation (25 mM MgCl$_2$) or 12 mM CaCl$_2$; or, 3 mM spermine, a polymeric cation (these concentrations reflect maximal activity); plus 10 or 20 nM dsDNA (synthetic end-protected 23-mer) or weight equivalent of dcDNA (*see* **Note 1**); and either 8 or 32 nM PARP-1 enzyme. (Concentrations for all reagents represent that of final reaction conditions.)
2. To assemble a reaction with six time-points, each of six microcentrifuge tubes is charged with: 5 µL H$_2$O, 5 µL 10X buffer (concentrated stock solution 1), 10 µL DNA solution (concentrated stock solution 2); or 5 µL DNA + 5 µL H$_2$O, 5 µL cation salts (concentrated stock solution 4), and 5 µL PARP-1 cocktail (from 320 or 80 nM concentrated stock solution 5); total reaction volume, 30 µL.
3. Initiate reactions by adding 20 µL hot NAD cocktail (concentrated stock solution 6), mix, and incubate at room temperature for up to 20 min.
4. At convenient points during the 20 min incubation period, individual microcentrifuge tubes are mixed with 950 µL ice cold 25% TCA, which stops the reaction. This is followed by addition of 30 µL 10 mg/mL BSA (concentrated stock solution) mixed by vortexing. Collected samples are kept on ice until the end of the 20-min incubation and, after brief vortexing, the samples are centrifuged at 14,000g at 4°C for 10 min. After carefully removing the supernatant (*see* **Note 2**), the sediments are washed three times with 20% ice cold TCA, vortexed, centrifuged and TCA removed.

5. Quantification of incorporated ^{32}P-NAD is made by adding scintillation fluid to the final sediments and, after vigorous vortexing, placing the tube in a scintillation vial filled with scintillation cocktail. Radioactivity is then determined in a scintillation counter.

3.1.2. Histone-Stimulated ADP-Ribosylation in Solution

This procedure is identical to that described in **Subheading 3.1.1.**, except for the following variations:

1. Omit the cation stimulators and replace with histone H_1 or H_3 to give a final concentration of 20–100 µg/mL (i.e., 1–5 µg per 50-µL assay; maximal activation is obtained ~2.5 µg/50 µL).
2. If necessary for detailed analysis, lower the PARP-1 concentration to 8 nM final concentration. PARP-1 at a concentration of 32 nM was used here (**Fig. 2A**).

3.2. Solid-State Poly-ADP-Ribosylation Assay

Because trans-(ADPR)n involves the modification of a second protein by PARP-1, a simple solution assay, such as that employed for auto-(ADPR)n in **Subheading 3.1.**, is not suitable. To selectively measure trans-(ADPR)n, therefore, the target protein is fixed to plastic prior to addition of the soluble reaction components. This allows enzyme and unincorporated substrate to be washed away leaving trans-(ADPR)n label attached to the protein target on the plastic surface.

A second, less obvious, advantage for using a solid state assay for trans-(ADPR)n is that potential direct effects of the target protein on PARP-1 activity can be eliminated or minimized. In the case of histones this effect can be profound because histone proteins act as polyanions that affect PARP-1 activity (*see* **Subheading 3.1.2.2.**) but it is minimized in the solid state system. These attributes make the solid state system adaptable for testing a variety of protein targets.

3.2.1. Trans-ADP-Ribosylation to "Fixed" Histone H_1

This is a modification of the assay described by Trevigen, Inc. Histone H_1 is coated to the well bottoms in 96-well plates by adding 50 µL per well of a 100 µg/mL solution of histone H_1 in PBS and allowing it to stand at 4°C for 20 h. Then the solutions were removed by aspiration and the wells washed five times by adding 100 µL /well of PBS (*see* **Note 3**) and removing each wash by tapping the inverted plate onto a paper towel, the final tapping being vigorous so as to achieve virtually dry wells.

3.2.2. Reaction Components

For enzymatic trans-poly-ADP-ribosylation system (50 µL final vol per well) all concentrations final:

1. 50 mM Tris-HCl, pH 8.0.
2. 400 µM NAD.

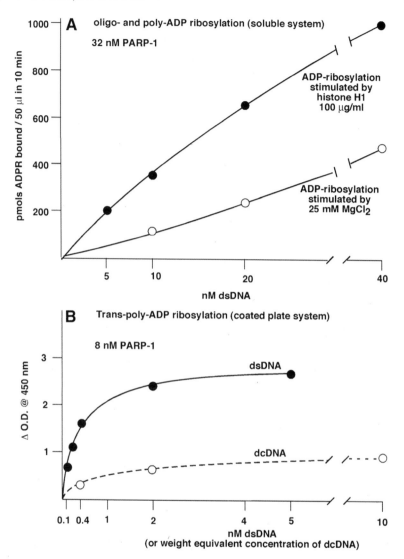

Fig. 2. PARP-1 activity in soluble and solid-state systems. (**A**) Soluble system assay of poly-ADP-ribosylation stimulated by divalent cation and histone and PARP-1 at a concentration of 32 n*M*. (**B**) Solid-state system assay of trans-poly-ADP-ribosylation (of histone H1) using dsDNA and dcDNA as coenzyme with PARP-1 at a concentration of 8 n*M*.

3. 25 μ*M* Biotinylated NAD (Trevigen).
4. 0.4–10 n*M* dsDNA or weight equivalent of randomly broken dcDNA (*see* **Note 1**).
5. 8 n*M* PARP-1 (Trevigen).

3.2.3. Reaction

Mix these components (from 10X stock solutions, from 2X stocks for NAD + biotinylated NAD) in a total volume of 40 μL/well, and start the reaction by adding 10 μL/well of diluted PARP-1 (50 ng/well; *see* **Note 3**), mixing, and allowing the reaction to proceed at room temperature for 10 min.

3.2.4. Stopping the Reaction

1. Stop the reaction by rapid decanting followed by 5 washes with 100 μL/well of PBS.
2. Quantify the biotinylated poly-ADP-ribose attached to the histone H_1-coated wells by reacting it with streptavidin-horseradish peroxidase (Trevigen; 50 μL of a 1:500 dilution of the 1 mg/mL original solution per well) for 30 min at 37°C followed by decanting and washing five times with 100 μL PBS/well as before.
3. After tap-drying the wells, add 50 μL per well of peroxidase substrate in the dark and allow to stand for 10 min at room temperature (*see* **Note 4**).
4. After addition of 50 μL/well of 0.2 *N* HCl, record the absorbance at 450 nm with a plate reader.

3.2.5. Assay Modification

A modification of the above assay which allows assessment of both auto- and trans-ADP-ribosylation and using ^{32}P-labeled NAD is outlined in **ref. 43**.

3.3. Discussion: Mechanistic Outline of Auto- and Trans-poly-ADP-Ribosylation Reactions

A complete, detailed picture of the mechanism of PARP-1 enzymatic activity has not yet been composed, but it is potentially useful to build reasonable models based on available information. Available evidence indicates that PARP-1 forms homodimers as a prerequisite for enzymatic activity *(31)*, and this has recently been confirmed by fluorescence methods *(32)*.

The following reaction equations outline the enzymatic steps in auto- and trans-modification that are schematically illustrated in **Fig. 3**.

3.3.1. Auto-ADP-Ribosylation Modification

1. NAD$^+$ + PARP-1 (a + b) $\longleftrightarrow$ {NAD-Trp$_{1014}$-Pa} $\longleftrightarrow$ [Pa-His~ADPr].
2. [Pa-His ~ ADPR] + [Pb-Glu] $\xrightarrow{coDNA}$ [Pb-Glu-ADPR] <initiation complex>.
3. <Repeating reaction 1> [Pa-His ~ ADPR] + [Pb-Glu-ADPR] $\xrightarrow{coDNA + Mg^{2+}}$ [Pb-Glu-ADPRn]

3.3.2. Trans-ADP-Ribosylation Modification

1. NAD$^+$ + PARP-1 (a + b) $\longleftrightarrow$ {NAD-Trp$_{1014}$-Pa} $\longleftrightarrow$ [Pa-His ~ ADPR].
2. [Pa-His~ADPr] + [histone H_1-Glu] $\xrightarrow{coDNA}$ [histone H_1-Glu-ADPR] <initiation complex>.
3. <Repeating reaction 1> [Pa-His ~ ADPR] + [histone H_1-Glu-ADPR] $\xrightarrow{coDNA}$ [histone H_1-Glu-ADPRn].

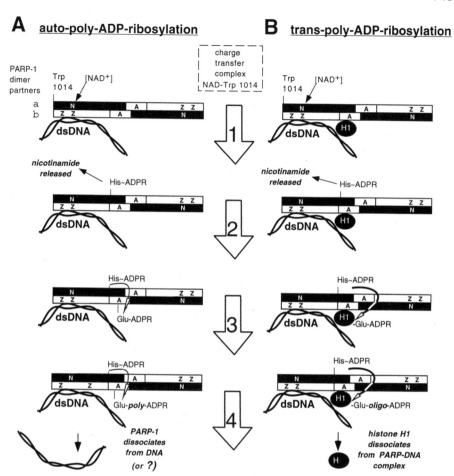

Fig. 3. Schematic of PARP-1 enzymatic activity. The key to the domain structure of PARP-1 is shown in **Fig. 1A**. The suggested antiparallel arrangement of PARP-1 dimer subunits permits the catalytic and the DNA binding domains to be in close association. Details regarding this schematic are given in **reactions 1** and **2**, **Subheading 3.3.** and the accompanying text.

The first step is essentially identical in both reactions; after binding to the NAD binding site of one dimer partner (*a*), NAD forms a transient charge transfer complex intramolecularly with Trp_{1014} *(33,34)* followed by cleavage of the NAD to release nicotinamide and transfer ADP-ribose, once again intramolecularly, to a His residue *(35)*. During the second step, the His-bound ADP-ribose is transferred to a Glu residue, either to one of the dimer partners in the case of auto-modification, or to histone H_1 in the case of trans-modification (**Fig. 1C**), forming an initiation complex. The displacement of nicotinamide by His to form [Pa-His–ADPR], is probably by way of an inversion at ribose C-1″

of substrate NAD (**Fig. 1B**). Thus, the His would be oriented at the α-side of the ribose. Subsequent displacement of His by Glu, to form [Pb-Glu-ADPR], is also likely to proceed by way of an inversion, leaving the Glu residue oriented at the β-side of the ribose, as depicted in **Fig. 1C**. The β-configuration is probably enzymatically reversible with the α-configuration.

Step 3 involves repetition of reaction **steps 1** and **2** to elongate the poly(ADP-ribose) chain. A fourth step would constitute the possible consequence(s) of poly(ADP-ribose) modification. In the case of auto-modification it has been proposed that dissociation between the modified PARP-1 dimer and the coenzymic DNA molecule is a likely outcome. In the case of trans-modification, dissociation of histone H1 from the DNA-PARP-1 complex is one possible consequence. Neither outcome exhausts the full range of potential outcomes, such as, for example, the possibility that poly-ADP-ribosylation acts to stabilize protein–protein and/or DNA–protein interactions in some cases.

4. Notes

1. End-protected, 23-nucleotide complementary oligodeoxynucleotides (synthesized by QIAGEN) are dissolved at 1 mg/mL (72 µM) in annealing buffer. These original solutions of each strand are stored at –80°C. To anneal the complementary strands, 10-µL aliquots of each original strand solution are mixed together (in a microcentrifuge tube) and after adding 10 µL of annealing buffer, the mixture (30 µL total volume) is heated for 10 min in a boiling water bath and, then cooled down slowly for annealing. Annealed oligodeoxynucleotides are diluted in annealing buffer to 2 µM to serve as stock solutions (store at 4°C) and aliquots are taken and subdiluted as needed. The weight-equivalent of dcDNA (DNAase-treated salmon sperm DNA referred to elsewhere as "damaged" or "broken" DNA) can also be used as an coenzymic DNA alternative but with lower efficiency than dsDNA (**Fig. 2B**).
2. Tubes should be oriented in the rotor so as to know on which side the pellet is located; this side should be avoided when the supernatant is aspirated with a micropipet.
3. It is preferable to use multichannel pipetors for the starting and washing of these solid-state reactions.
4. The plate should be covered with aluminum foil to protect it from light.

Acknowledgments

This work was supported by research grants to C.P.O. from the NIH (RO1-AR44483, RO1-HL35561, and RO1-HL59693) and from the Muscular Dystrophy Association of America.

References

1. Althaus, F. R. and Richter, C. (1987) ADP-ribosylation of proteins. Enzymology and biological significance. *Mol. Biol. Biochem. Biophys.* **37,** 1–237.

2. Alvarez-Gonzalez, R., Watkins, T. A., Gill, P. K., Reed, J. L., and Mendoza-Alvarez, H. (1999) Regulatory mechanisms of poly(ADP-ribose) polymerase. *Mol. Cell. Biol.* **193**, 19–22.

3. Minaga, T., Romaschin, A. D., Kirsten, E., and Kun, E. (1979) The in vivo distribution of immunoreactive larger than tetrameric polyadenosine diphosphoribose in histone and non-histone protein fractions of rat liver. *J. Biol. Chem.* **254**, 9663–9668.

4. deMurcia, G. and Shall, S. (2000) From DNA-Damage and Stress Signaling to Cell Death: Poly ADP-Ribosylation Reactions. Oxford University Press, New York.

5. Akiyama, T., Takasawa, S. Nata, K., et al. (2001) Activation of Reg gene, a gene for insulin-producing beta-cell regeneration: poly(ADP-ribose) polymerase binds Reg promoter and regulates the transcription by autopoly(ADP-ribosyl)ation. *Proc. Natl. Acad. Sci. USA* **98**, 48–53.

6. Anderson, M. G., Scoggin, K. E., Simbulan-Rosenthal, C. M., and Steadman, J. A. (2000) Identification of poly(ADP-ribose) polymerase as a transcriptional coactivator of the human T-cell leukemia virus type 1 *Tax protein. J. Virol.* **74**, 2169–2177.

7. Butler, A. J. and Ordahl, C. P. (1999) Poly(ADP-ribose) polymerase binds with transcription enhancer factor 1 to MCAT1 elements to regulate muscle-specific transcription. *Mol. Cell. Biol.* **19**, 296–306.

8. Cervellera, M. N. and Sala, A. (2000) Poly(ADP-ribose) polymerase is a B-MYB coactivator. *J. Biol. Chem.* **275**, 10,692–10,696.

9. Chang, W. J. and Alvarez-Gonzalez, R. (2001) The sequence-specific DNA binding of NF-kappa B is reversibly regulated by the automodification reaction of poly (ADP-ribose) polymerase 1. *J. Biol. Chem.* **276**, 47,664–47,670.

10. Dear, T. N., Hainzl, T., Follo, M., et al. (1997) Identification of interaction partners for the basic-helix-loop-helix protein E47. *Oncogene* **14**, 891–898.

11. Hassa, P. O. and Hottiger, M. O. (1999) A role of poly (ADP-ribose) polymerase in NF-kappaB transcriptional activation. *Biol. Chem.* **380**, 953–959.

12. Hassa, P. O., Covic, M., Hasan, S., Imhof, R., and Hottiger, M. O. (2001) The enzymatic and DNA binding activity of PARP-1 are not required for NF-kappa B coactivator function. *J. Biol. Chem.* **276**, 45,588–45,597.

13. Kannan, P., Yu, Y., Wankhade, S., and Tainsky, M.A. (1999) PolyADP-ribose polymerase is a coactivator for AP-2-mediated transcriptional activation. *Nucleic Acids Res*, **27**, 866–874.

14. Lee, D., Kim, J. W., Kim, K. et al. (2002) Functional interaction between human papillomavirus type 18 E2 and poly(ADP-ribose) polymerase 1. *Oncogene* **21**, 5877–5885.

15. Meisterernst, M., Stelzer, G., and Roeder, R. G. (1997) Poly(ADP-ribose) polymerase enhances activator-dependent transcription in vitro. *Proc. Natl. Acad. Sci. USA* **94**, 2261–2265.

16. Mendoza-Alvarez, H. and Alvarez-Gonzalez, R. (2001) Regulation of p53 sequence-specific DNA-binding by covalent poly(ADP-ribosyl)ation. *J. Biol. Chem.* **276**, 36,425–36,430.

17. Nirodi, C., NagDas, S., Gygi, S. P., Olson, G., Aebersold, R., and Richmond, A. (2001) A role for poly(ADP-ribose) polymerase in the transcriptional regulation of the melanoma growth stimulatory activity (CXCL1) gene expression. *J. Biol. Chem.* **276**, 9366–9374.

18. Oei, S. L. and Shi, Y. (2001) Poly(ADP-ribosyl)ation of transcription factor Yin Yang 1 under conditions of DNA damage. *Biochem. Biophys. Res. Commun.* **285**, 27–31.

19. Santilli, G., Cervellera, M. N., Johnson, T. K., Lewis, R. E., Iacobelli, S., and Sala, A. (2001) PARP co-activates B-MYB through enhanced phosphorylation at cyclin/cdk2 sites. *Oncogene* **20**, 8167–8174.

20. Simbulan-Rosenthal, C. M., Rosenthal, D. S. ,Luo, R., and Smulson, M. E. (1999) Poly(ADP-ribose) polymerase upregulates E2F-1 promoter activity and DNA pol alpha expression during early S phase. *Oncogene* **18**, 5015–5023.

21. Newman, R. E., Soldatenkov, V. A., Dritschilo, A., and Notario, V. (2002) Poly(ADP-ribose) polymerase turnover alterations do not contribute to PARP overexpression in Ewing's sarcoma cells. *Oncol. Rep.* **9**, 529–532.

22. Tulin, A., Stewart, D., and Spradling, A. C. (2002) The *Drosophila* heterochromatic gene encoding poly(ADP-ribose) polymerase (PARP) is required to modulate chromatin structure during development. *Genes Dev.* **16**, 2108–2119.

23. Tulin, A. and Spradling, A. (2003) Chromatin loosening by poly(ADP)-ribose polymerase (PARP) at *Drosophila* puff loci. *Science* **299**, 560–562.

24. Ullrich, O., Diestel, A., Eyupoglu, I. Y., and Nitsch, R. (2001) Regulation of microglial expression of integrins by poly(ADP-ribose) polymerase-1. *Nat. Cell. Biol.* **3**, 1035–1042.

25. Vyas, D. R., McCarthy, J. J., Tsika, G. L., and Tsika, R. W. (2001) Multiprotein complex formation at the beta myosin heavy chain distal muscle CAT element correlates with slow muscle expression but not mechanical overload responsiveness. *J. Biol. Chem.* **276**, 1173–1184.

26. Zhang, Z., Hildebrandt, E. F., Simbulan-Rosenthal, C. M., and Anderson, M. G. (2002) Sequence-specific binding of poly(ADP-ribose) polymerase-1 to the human T cell leukemia virus type-I tax responsive element. *Virology* **296**, 107–116.

27. Bauer, P.I., Chen, H. J., Kenesi, E., et al. (2001) Molecular interactions between poly(ADP-ribose) polymerase (PARP I) and topoisomerase I (Topo I): identification of topology of binding. *FEBS Lett.* **506**, 239–242.

28. Kirsten, E., Minaga, T., and Kun, E. (1982) Coincidence of subnuclear distribution of poly(ADP-ribose) synthetase and DNA polymerase beta in nuclei of normal and regenerating liver. *FEBS Lett.* **139**, 117–120.

29. Simbulan-Rosenthal, C. M., Rosenthal, D. S., Hilz, H., et al. (1996) The expression of poly(ADP-ribose) polymerase during differentiation-linked DNA replication reveals that it is a component of the multiprotein DNA replication complex. *Biochemistry* **35**, 11,622–11,633.

30. Kun, E., Kirsten, E., and Ordahl, C. P. (2002) Coenzymatic activity of randomly broken or intact double-stranded DNAs in auto and histone H1 trans-poly(ADP-ribosylation), catalyzed by poly(ADP-ribose) polymerase (PARP I). *J. Biol. Chem.* **277**, 39,066–39,069.

31. Bauer, P. I., Buki, K. G., Hakam, A., and Kun, E. (1990) Macromolecular association of ADP-ribosyltransferase and its correlation with enzymic activity. *Biochem. J.* **270,** 17–26.

32. Pion, E., Bombarda, E., Stiegler, P., et al. (2003) Poly(ADP-ribose) polymerase-1 dimerizes at a 5′ recessed DNA end in vitro: a fluorescence study. *Biochemistry* **42,** 12,409–12,417.

33. Cilento, G. and Tedeschi, P. (1961) Pyridine coenzymes. IV. Charge transfer interaction with the indole nucleus. *J. Biol. Chem.* **236,** 907–910.

34. Kim, H., Jacobson, M. K., Rolli, V,. et al. (1997) Photoaffinity labelling of human poly(ADP-ribose) polymerase catalytic domain. *Biochem. J.* **322,** 469–475.

35. Bauer, P. I., Buki, K. G., and Kun, E. (1990) Evidence for the participation of histidine residues located in the 56 kDa C-terminal polypeptide domain of ADP-ribosyl transferase in its catalytic activity. *FEBS Lett.* **273,** 6–10.

36. Kameshita, I., Matsuda, Z., Taniguchi, T., and Shizuta, Y. (1984) Poly (ADP-Ribose) synthetase. Separation and identification of three proteolytic fragments as the substrate-binding domain, the DNA-binding domain, and the automodification domain. *J. Biol. Chem.* **259,** 4770–4776.

37. Gradwohl, G., Menissier de Murcia, J. M., Molinete, M., et al. (1990) The second zinc-finger domain of poly(ADP-ribose) polymerase determines specificity for single-stranded breaks in DNA. *Proc. Natl. Acad. Sci. USA* **87,** 2990–2994.

38. Yoshihara, K., Hashida, T., Yoshihara, H., Tanaka, Y., and Ohgushi, H. (1997) Enzyme-bound early product of purified poly(ADP-ribose) polymerase. *Biochem. Biophys. Res. Commun.* **78,** 1281–1288.

39. Ueda, K., Kawaichi, M., Okayama, H., and Hayaishi, O. (1979) Poly(ADP-ribosy)ation of nuclear proteins. Enzymatic elongation of chemically synthesized ADP-ribose-histone adducts. *J. Biol. Chem.* **254,** 679–687.

40. Miwa, M., Saito, H., Sakura, H., et al. (1977) A 13C NMR study of poly(adenosine diphosphate ribose) and its monomers: evidence of alpha-(1″ leads to 2′) ribofuranosy1 ribofuranoside residue. *Nucleic Acids Res.* **4,** 3997–4005.

41. Ferro, A. M. and Oppenheimer, N. J. (1978) Structure of a poly (adenosine diphosphoribose) monomer: 2′-(5″-phosphoribosyl)-5′-adenosine monophosphate. *Proc. Natl. Acad. Sci. USA* **75,** 809–813.

42. Inagaki, F., Miyazawa, T., Miwa, M., Saito, H., and Sugimura, T. (1978) NMR analyses of conformation of ribosyl adenosine 5′,5″-bis(phosphate) in aqueous solution. *Biochem. Biophys. Res. Commun.* **85,** 415–420.

43. Kun, E., Kirsten, J., Mendeleyev, J., and Ordahl, C. P. (2004) Regulation of the enzymatic catalysis of poly(ADP-ribose) polymerase by dsDNA, polyamines, Mg^{2+}, Ca^{2+}, histones H1 and H3, and ATP. *Biochemistry* **43,** 210–206.

12

Multigenerational Selection and Detection of Altered Histone Acetylation and Methylation Patterns

Toward a Quantitative Epigenetics in Drosophila

Mark D. Garfinkel, Vincent E. Sollars, Xiangyi Lu, and Douglas M. Ruden

Summary

Quantitative epigenetics (QE) is a new area of research that combines some of the techniques developed for global quantitative trait loci (QTL) mapping analyses with epigenetic analyses. Quantitative traits such as height vary, not in a discrete or discontinuous fashion, but continuously, usually in a normal distribution. QTL analyses assume that allelic *DNA sequence* variation in a population is partly responsible for the trait variation, and the aim is to deduce the locations of the contributing genes. QE analyses assume that epigenetic variation in a population is partly responsible for the trait variation, and the aim is to associate inheritance of the trait with segregation of informative epigenetic polymorphisms, or *epialleles*. QTL and QE analyses are thus complementary, but the latter has several advantages. QTL mapping is limited in resolution because of meiotic recombination and population size, placing quantitative traits on genomic regions that are each typically several megabase-pairs long, and requires DNA sequence variation. In contrast, QE analysis can make use of powerful emerging mapping techniques that allow the positioning of epialleles defined by chromatin variation to individual genes or chromosomal regions, *even in the absence of DNA sequence variation*. In this chapter, we present a case study for QE analysis—epigenetic mapping of enhancers of the Kr^{If-1} ectopic eye bristle phenotype in an isogenic strain of *Drosophila melanogaster*.

Key Words: Epigenetic inheritance; epialleles; quantitative inheritance; chromatin remodeling; microarrays; chromatin immunoprecipitation; DNA methylation; histone methylation; histone acetylation; *Drosophila*.

1. Introduction

Variable expressivity and variable penetrance are two of the most perplexing (and frequently annoying) properties of mutant phenotypes. They challenge experimentalists using genetic analyses in model organisms and

From: *Methods in Molecular Biology, vol. 287: Epigenetics Protocols*
Edited by: T. O. Tollefsbol © Humana Press Inc., Totowa, NJ

clinicians attempting to counsel, diagnose, and treat patients with hereditary diseases or disease predispositions, even in situations in which the principal cause of a phenotype or disorder is a single-gene mutation. Traditionally, variable expressivity and variable penetrance are thought to arise from four main sources: (1) variation in genetic background, generally defined as allelic variation in DNA sequences present within a population, that had remained outside the control of the experimenter; (2) variation in environmental factors, which can be systematically altered by the experimenter but not without at least some residue of uncontrolled variation; (3) epistatic interactions among distinct genetic components; (4) and a potentially complex interaction between genetic and environmental components.

Another source of variation, which was recognized long ago but only recently has become amenable to direct experimental manipulation, is epigenetic in origin. This type of variation in the genome can occur by alterations in chromatin structure, or postreplicative chemical modification of DNA such as methylation. Epigenetic phenomena include mating-type silencing (reviewed in **ref. 1**) and telomere position effect in yeast (reviewed in **ref. 2**), position effect variegation in *Drosophila* (reviewed in **ref. 3**), paramutation in a variety of plant species (reviewed in **ref. 4**), and imprinting in mammals, which affects expression of more than 60 genes (reviewed in **ref. 5**).

These phenomena arise from sequential accumulation and posttranslational modification of specialized proteins on the chromatin. At the first level are the core histones, which are subject to covalent posttranslational modifications such as methylation, phosphorylation, acetylation, and ubiquitinylation. Some of these modifications are associated with active or accessible chromatin; others are associated with inactive or condensed chromatin. On each core histone, certain amino acid residues may be susceptible to more than one posttranslational modification, and thus they are mutually exclusive. Significantly, modification-susceptible residues cluster at the amino-terminal "tails" of each histone protein, sites that are involved in the interactions between adjacent nucleosome cores (reviewed in **ref. 6**). The lysine-9 residue of histone H3, for example, is acetylated on active chromatin and promotes the binding of TAFII250 to gene promoters *(6)*. This residue, in contrast, is methylated during heterochromatin formation in yeast and *Drosophila (6,7)* and during DNA elimination in the ciliate *Tetrahymena (8)*. Both histone acetyltransferases (HATs) and histone deacetylases (HDACs) are encoded by small-to-medium-sized gene families in a wide variety of eukaryotes.

HDAC activity, which falls into three subclasses based on sequence and enzymology, is necessary to remove acetyl moieties from active chromatin prior to histone methylation. Once bound to particular chromatin locations, HDACs may specifically facilitate binding of histone methyltransferases

(HMTs) to these chromatin sites *(6,7)*. Sequential activity and association of HDACs and HMTs, in combination with the resulting lysine-9-methylated histone H3, triggers accumulation of HP1, which is a critical component in assembling stably inactivated heterochromatin *(6)*. Other proteins involved in stably inactivated heterochromatin include ATP-dependent chromatin-remodeling proteins of the chromo-domain and bromo-domain families, several of which were first identified by mutations in the *trithorax* group of *Drosophila* developmental control genes *(9,10)*. Since no histone lysine demethylase activity has yet been discovered in any organism, regulation of histone deacetylation and the subsequent histone lysine-residue methylation assumes grave import in the life of a cell.

Along with these mutually exclusive antagonistic modifications on lysine-9, several other amino acid side chains on histones H3, H4, and H2B are susceptible to posttranslational modification in a combinatorial fashion. Among these are H3 serine-10, which can be phosphorylated, and H3 lysine-14, which can also be acetylated. Neither of these modifications is entirely independent of the other, or of the modification state on lysine-9. Thus, several H3, H4, and H2B protein isoforms exist within each cell. Jenuwein and Allis *(11)* recently proposed a histone code that recognizes the combinatorial possibilities that correlate with different chromatin states. Antibodies and antisera reagents designed to detect distinct histone modification variants are available from over a half-dozen commercial suppliers and will facilitate a variety of studies to test the histone code hypothesis.

Although identification of histone modification enzymes and in vitro characterization of their reactions are important steps in understanding epigenetic regulation, as is the in vivo assessment of histone modification state using individual cloned genes, newly developed methods allow testing of the histone code hypothesis in vivo on a genome-wide scale. Chromatin immunoprecipitation (ChIP), alone or followed by microarray analysis of the associated DNA (so-called ChIP-chip experiments), is a powerful emerging technique for determining global changes in genomic DNA element association with particular chromosomal proteins as a function of physiological condition or genotype. In one approach to performing ChIP, nuclei isolated from cells or tissues are subjected to chemicals that reversibly crosslink genomic DNA with its associated chromosomal proteins (other authors omit formaldehyde crosslinking; *see* Chap. 3). Immunoprecipitation with a specific antibody brings down complexes that contain both the target protein and a subset of genomic DNA. In the ChIP-chip procedure, after reversing the chemical crosslinkages, polymerase chain reaction (PCR) amplifies and labels the genomic DNA, the sequence content of which is determined by hybridization to microarrays.

Using the ChIP-chip approach, Robyr et al. *(12)* conducted a global examination of histone acetylation state changes in the budding yeast, *Saccharomyces cerevisiae*, under various nutrient conditions. *S. cerevisiae* has an extremely small and compact genome, from which the complete set of intergenic upstream spacer DNAs (where most *cis*-acting transcription control regions reside in this organism) can be arrayed for hybridization. These authors found that large domains of the yeast genome undergo changes in acetylation state dependent upon the carbon source provided to the cells. Many of the genes detected by increased chromatin acetylation were previously known to be transcriptionally induced by alternate sugars. Simple gene-disruption techniques allowed these authors to construct yeast strains that are isogenic except for the ablation of single HDAC family members. Robyr et al. *(12)* thus demonstrated that different large contiguous regions of the yeast genome are sensitive to histone deacetylation in an HDAC-type–specific fashion and that each HDAC has a distinct repertoire of target chromatin (or, alternatively, target genes).

Not all chromatin proteins are immunogenic, and ChIP-chip techniques do not work well for these chromatin-associated proteins, so Henikoff and colleagues *(13)* have devised a clever alternative called DamID They discovered that the *Escherichia coli* DNA adenine methyltransferase (Dam), encoded by the *dam* gene, can be fused to the DNA binding domain of an arbitrary eukaryotic chromosomal protein, resulting in a chimeric protein that can methylate eukaryotic DNA in vivo. The principle of DamID is that the Dam enzyme modifies double-stranded DNA on the adenine residue of the 5'-G-A-T-C-3' tetramer, thereby generating 5'-G-6mA-T-C-3' tetramer, which is sensitive to cleavage by the restriction enzyme *Dpn*I. The spacings between successive 5'-G-A-T-C-3' tetramers in long complex DNA sequences are dependent on the GC content and nearest neighbor frequencies but is approximated by a Poisson distribution with average spacing of 256 bp (4n). Nonmethylated sequences will be resistant to *Dpn*I cleavage and fall into a much higher molecular weight class determined by the random-shear propensities of the DNA extraction method. Sequences methylated directly owing to their native *dam* recognition sites or to proximity to recognition sites for an arbitrary chromosomal protein will be sensitive to *Dpn*I cleavage and can be size-selected by centrifugation. The genomic identities and relative abundance of these methylated sequences are determined by microarray hybridization after PCR amplification and labeling. van Steensel et al. *(13)* showed that *Drosophila* tissue culture cells transfected with plasmid constructs bearing the *dam* protein-coding region alone had a background methylation pattern, consistent with the general tetramer-recognition properties of Dam. Fusing three different transcription-regulatory proteins (a member of the GAGA-binding factor family, HP1, and a member of the Sir2 family of HDAC) to the Dam-coding region yielded chimeric proteins that methylated DNAs with sequence content distinctive to each transcription-regulatory protein.

DamID is a general method of identifying genomic DNA accessible to Dam-tagged DNA-binding proteins. It can in principle, like the histone acetylation mapping technique of Robyr et al. *(12)*, be used to probe chromatin accessibility changes in response to experimental manipulations. Use of DamID in *Drosophila* cell culture, intact transgenic *Drosophila* animals, or other higher organisms has an obvious limitation at present compared with yeast: microarrays representing all possible transcription regulatory regions are unavailable and may be unfeasible owing to the different architecture of these regions in metazoan genomes (an alternative, whole-genome–sequence tiling-path microarrays, has recently been proposed for *Drosophila [14,15]*). Nevertheless, DamID *(13)* and histone acetylation mapping *(12)* have tremendous potential for studying epigenetic regulation.

Several recent research reports argue that epigenetic variation can, under certain circumstances, be the *sole* basis for *heritable* phenotypic variation in multicellular organisms. Different mice from a single nearly isogenic strain carrying an intracisternal-A-particle–like (IAP) retrotransposon insertion in the promoter of the *agouti* gene (the A^{vy} allele) can display a range of coat pigmentation *(16)*. These authors showed that the phenotypic variation results from variation in the amount of ectopic transcription from the A^{vy} allele stimulated by the IAP insertion that correlates inversely with variation in cytosine (CpG) methylation state of the retrotransposon *(16)*. Furthermore, these authors showed that the expression status of the A^{vy} allele, which is "read out" in somatic epidermal tissues, is transmissible through the maternal germline but not through the paternal germline. This is remarkable in light of conventional imprinting in mammals, in which DNA methylation is "erased" during gametogenesis and is reestablished in early embryogenesis; in mouse, DNA copies of retrotransposons appear to be at least partly resistant to demethylation. A second example of inherited variation in expressivity of a retrotransposon insertion in mice, the $Axin^{Fu}$ allele, differs from the A^{vy} case in that both paternal and maternal inheritance was observed *(17)*. Rakyan et al. *(17)* also observed that different mouse strains can differ in their capacity to erase methylation at the $Axin^{Fu}$ allele and the A^{vy} allele differentially.

Studying "metastable epialleles" *(18)* in mice is limited by the time required to follow the inheritance pattern through many generations, which also constrains the ability to test for response to artificial selection. Both limitations are absent when one is working with the more rapidly breeding organisms such as the flowering plant *Arabidopsis thaliana (19)*, the nematode worm *Caenorhabditis elegans*, or the dipteran fly *Drosophila melanogaster*. We and our colleagues *(20)* constructed an isogenized *D. melanogaster* strain sensi-

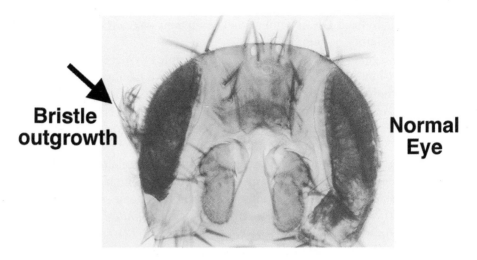

Fig. 1. Disrupting Hsp90 function induces heritable epialleles that cause homeotic transformation in a sensitized *Drosophila melanogaster* strain. Ectopic leg-like bristle outgrowth (arrow) from one eye of an adult *D. melanogaster* fly carrying Kr^{If-1} that had been treated with the Hsp90 inhibitor geldanamycin. The other eye of this individual shows only the "irregular facets" characteristic of the Kr^{If-1} mutation. The ectopic leg-like bristle outgrowth phenotype is initially a consequence of epigenetic alterations in geldanamycin-treated Kr^{If-1} animals and is both heritable and selectable for increased penetrance in subsequent, non-drug-treated, generations *(20)*.

tized for homeotic transformation in the eye owing to the presence of the "irregular facets" allele of the *Krüppel* gene (Kr^{If-1}). The Kr^{If-1} is spontaneous in origin, and thus potentially a transposable element insertion, but the Kr^{If-1} molecular lesion is unknown. In our isogenized Kr^{If-1}, strain we estimated that DNA sequence-level variation was reduced to a very low level, perhaps 5×10^{-5} polymorphisms per nucleotide position, during strain construction *(20)*. The isogenized Kr^{If-1} strain, which normally exhibits a severe disruption of the ommatidial array in each eye, was then induced to display a different defect in eye morphology—ectopic leg-like bristle-bearing outgrowths (**Fig. 1**). In one set of experiments Sollars et al. *(20)* had applied the potent and specific inhibitor of the chaperone protein Hsp90, geldanamycin. In other experiments we *(20)* transiently introduced any one of several mutations in the *trithorax* group of chromatin-remodeling-protein genes. Penetrance of the more severe eye defects induced by the Hsp90 antagonist geldanamycin and by the *trithorax* group mutation *verthandi* increased dramatically in response to selection following removal of the inducer, reaching a maximum level within a half-dozen generations *(20)*. We also demonstrated that drugs that inhibit histone deacetylation immediately reduced the penetrance of the ectopic leg-like eye

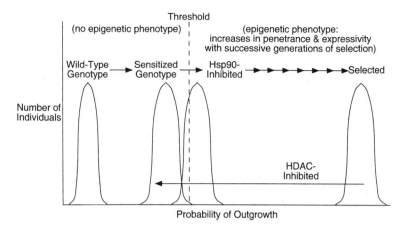

Fig. 2. Sensitization, induction, selection, and reversal of epialleles. Wild-type flies have very little or no propensity to undergo a particular homeotic transformation during eye development, whereas introduction of the Kr^{If-1} mutation increases that probability (rightward shift of the distribution). Hsp90 inhibition by geldanamycin increases this probability further, apparently through disruption of chromatin structures (formation of new epialleles), resulting in individuals that have a phenotype above threshold for selection in the experiment. Further rounds of selection (series of rightward arrows) result in a population in which many individuals display the homeotic transformation; germline-transmissible changes in chromatin conformation have thus occurred that manifest in somatic tissue. The selected epialleles can be erased—the chromatin states returned to normal—with histone deacetylase (HDAC) inhibitors *(20)*. (Modified from **ref. 21**.)

outgrowth, further implicating heritable but reversible changes in chromatin structure as the basis for the induced epigenetic phenotype (**Fig. 2**).

1.1. Future Prospects

Our selection experiments with the isogenized Kr^{If-1} strain provide a case study for *de novo* induction of epialleles—heritable variation not in DNA sequence, but in chromatin structures that confer altered regulatory properties on one or more underlying genes. We believe *D. melanogaster* is particularly well suited for *quantitative epigenetics*—to use the term coined by Rutherford and Henikoff *(21)*—the process of mapping epialleles using a combination of quantitative trait-locus methods and the growing armamentarium of chromatin-related biochemical methods and genome sequence-based microarray techniques such as ChIP-chip and DamID. The general experimental plan would be to take a highly inbred or, preferably, an isogenized strain sensitized for a phenotype of interest and divide the population into two groups. One group would

Table 1
Comparing and Contrasting QTL and QE Mapping Procedures

QTL analysis	QE analysis
Maps genetic (DNA-sequence) variations throughout the genome	Maps epigenetic (chromatin-structural) variations throughout the genome
Requires two outbred strains or two inbred/isogenized strains	Can be performed with a single inbred/isogenized strain
Sensitization with a mutation allows the identification of *genetic* modifiers of the mutant phenotype	Sensitization with a mutation allows the identification of *epigenetic* modifiers of the mutant phenotype
Initially enormous regions (>>1 Mb) identified owing to limitations of meiotic recombination and DNA marker density	Immediately localized to individual genes or small (<10-kb) gene regions by bio chemical methods like chromatin immunoprecipitation and DNA microarray procedures

be passaged without any perturbation. The other group would be exposed, for a single generation, to an Hsp90 inhibitor. Disruption of chromatin structures owing to the decreased activity of this chaperone would be inferred from the rare appearance of progeny that had an enhanced phenotype. These flies would be crossed *inter se* and their offspring selected for further enhancement of the phenotype for several generations until a plateau had been detected. ChIP-chip assays would then be conducted using reagents that detect specific modified histone isoforms (*see* Chap. 9 for ChIP-chip methods of detecting acetylated and methylated histones), and the chromosomal distribution of these histone isoforms compared relative to the unselected control strain. We would expect that variations in the penetrance of the novel phenotype among selected lines would correlate with quantitative differences in the abundance (or perhaps identities) of DNA sequences detected in the ChIP-chip assays. A comparison of features of quantitative trait locus mapping and quantitative epigenetics is given in **Table 1**.

In the case of our studies with lines selected from isogenized Kr^{If-1}, had we done ChIP-chip assays on dissected third-instar eye-antennal imaginal discs, we might have detected altered histone acetylation at loci correlated with their ectopic expression: that is, we would predict novel *epialleles* of these genes' chromatin. We are pursuing this hypothesis by constructing isogenized *Droso-*

phila strains that carry both Kr^{If-1} and either a Dam-tagged *Drosophila* histone deacetylase or a Dam-tagged *Drosophila* histone methyltransferase. We will subject the resulting strains to Hsp90-inhibitor treatment and multigeneration selection of ectopic eye outgrowth, and we will monitor changes in adenine methylation in the selected lines. Altered distribution of adenine methylation will be inferred to represent altered distribution of the Dam-tagged histone modification enzymes, which in turn will be inferred to represent altered distributions of deacetylated, acetylated, methylated, or demethylated chromatin— the sites of *epialleles* generated in the initial Hsp90 treatment and subsequent selection.

Although our published experiments made use of the gain-of-function Kr^{If-1} allele to sensitize the *Drosophila* genome for a particular quantitative epigenetics selection experiment, it may be possible to use deficiencies that reduce gene activity for sensitization as well. In this regard it is exciting to note that a European consortium *(22)* of *Drosophila* researchers has undertaken to implement the Golic and Golic *(23)* rearrangement screen (RS) strategy of generating sequence-defined deletions in the isogenic background used for the *D. melanogaster* genome sequencing project. In the RS strategy, P-element transformation is used to introduce two different constructs that have FRT sites flanking either the 5'-half or a 3'-half of the *white*$^+$ eye-color marker gene. Thousands of individual insertions peppering the *Drosophila* genome have been generated by selecting for pigmented eyes (over 2500 were available at the time this review was completed; **ref. 22**). Crossing each of the insertions to an FLP-producing strain allows the recovery of *white*-mutant flies from which, depending on the inserted construct, either the 5'-half or the 3'-half of the *white*$^+$ gene has been excised. Each remnant half-gene has a chromosomal location that can be determined with nucleotide-level precision. Crosses are then used to introduce the 5'-remnant and 3'-remnant half-genes into flies that also harbor the FLP recombinase gene. FLP/FRT-mediated rejoining of the two half-genes into a functional w^+ gene allows for selection of chromosome deletions or inversions depending on the known relative orientation and distance separating the half-genes used in the crosses. At the time of writing, over 105 deletions have been constructed by consortium member labs *(22)*. As this number grows, we expect these strains to become an important resource to the broader *Drosophila* community for mapping a variety of genetic and epigenetic traits.

Although we concentrate in this chapter on our experiences with *Drosophila*, we believe quantitative epigenetics can also be performed in several other model organisms. Genetically sensitized strains of mice that carry mutations in homeo-box genes involved in limb-digit specification or eye development (e.g., *Pax6* mutations) may prove to be fruitful in identifying epialleles whose epigenetic state contributes to the formation of these organs.

2. Materials

2.1. Generation of Isogenic Drosophila Strains

Thousands of *D. melanogaster* strains are available from three main *Drosophila* Stock Centers (Bloomington, IN; Kyoto, Japan; and Szeged, Hungary), Berkeley *Drosophila* Genome Project participant labs (University of California-Berkeley; Baylor College of Medicine, Houston, TX), and from individual investigators throughout the world. Two online databases are indispensable for retrieving genetic and genomic information about *Drosophila*: FlyBase <http://flybase.bio.indiana.edu> and GADFly <http://www.fruitfly.org>. These sites include a tremendous volume of curated and contributed information regarding genes and mutant alleles, chromosome rearrangements, balancer chromosomes, transposable elements (both naturally occurring and synthetic), and strain lists from the main centers.

1. b^1 Kr^{If-1} (from the Bloomington Stock Center).
2. b^1 dac^1 pr^1 cn^1 wx^{wxt} bw^1 (from the Bloomington Stock Center).
3. $iso\text{-}w^{1118}$; $iso\text{-}2$; $iso\text{-}3$ (from the Bloomington Stock Center).
4. $iso\text{-}2$; $iso\text{-}3/TM6B$, Sb (from **ref. 20**).
5. Standard cornmeal/agar/sugar fly food (*see*, for example, **refs. 24–28**).

2.2. Genetically Sensitized Drosophila Strains

1. $iso\text{-}w^{1118}$; $iso\text{-}2\text{-}Kr^{If-1}$; $iso\text{-}3$ (from **ref. 20**).
2. Iso-1-derived collection of more than 2500 P-element insertions and a growing number of newly constructed sequence-defined chromosomal deletions generated from these elements using the Golic and Golic strategy *(22,23)*.
3. Standard cornmeal/agar/sugar fly food *(24–28)*.

2.3. Pharmacological Inhibition of Hsp90 Function

1. Geldanamycin (Sigma-Aldrich).
2. Geldanamycin stock solution: dissolve geldanamycin in double-distilled sterile water at a concentration of 356 μM immediately before use.
3. Formula 4-24® Blue *Drosophila* food (Carolina Biological Supply, Burlington, NC, cat. no. WW-17-3210). This powdered fly food mix does not require boiling for preparation, as does standard cornmeal/agar/sugar fly food, so inactivation of heat-labile drugs such as geldanamycin is not a concern.
4. Geldanamycin-containing fly food. We prepared Carolina Biological Formula 4-24 Blue *Drosophila* food according to the manufacturer's instructions and allowed it to cool to 45°C. Geldanamycin stock solution was added to a final concentration of 3.56 μM. Then 10-mL aliquots of drug-containing fly food were poured into each 2.3 × 9.5-cm plastic fly food vial (e.g., Applied Scientific; [*see* **Note 1**]).

2.4. Treatments That Increase Histone Acetylation In Vivo

1. Trichostatin A (TSA; Sigma-Aldrich).
2. Sodium butyrate (Sigma-Aldrich).
3. TSA stock solution: dissolve TSA in 50% (v/v) ethanol at a stock solution concentration of 900 μM. Stock solution may be used immediately or stored at –20°C.
4. Sodium butyrate stock solution: dissolve sodium butyrate in sterile double-distilled water at stock solution concentration of 1 M. Stock solution may be used immediately or stored at –20°C.
5. Formula 4-24 Blue *Drosophila* food (Carolina Biological Supply).
6. TSA-containing fly food: we prepared Carolina Biological Formula 4-24 Blue *Drosophila* food according to the manufacturer's instructions. After it cooled to 45°C, TSA stock solution was added to a final concentration of either 4.5 μM or 9.0 μM. Then 10-mL aliquots of drug-containing fly food were poured into each 2.3 × 9.5-cm plastic fly food vial (e.g., Applied Scientific; [*see* **Note 1**]).
7. Sodium butyrate-containing fly food: we prepared Carolina Biological Formula 4-24 Blue *Drosophila* food according to the manufacturer's instructions. After it cooled to 45°C, we added the sodium butyrate stock solution to a final concentration of either 10 mM or 20 mM. Then 10-mL aliquots of drug-containing fly food were poured into each 2.3 × 9.5-cm plastic fly food vial (*see* **Note 1**).

2.5. Detection and Quantitation of Acetylated Histones

A broad collection of antibody reagents is commercially available that recognize many of the diverse modified histone protein isoforms that have been discovered, as well as the unmodified proteins. Although many different manufacturers supply these reagents, our lab uses the rabbit antihistone antibody preparations from Cell Signaling Technology (Beverly, MA). For indirect immunodetection we used horseradish peroxidase (HRP)-linked goat antirabbit IgG from Cell Signaling Technology, and the SuperSignal West Pico chemiluminescence Western blotting reagent kit from Pierce (Rockford, IL).

3. Methods

3.1. Generation of Isogenic Drosophila Strains

There are two principal methods for generating isogenized *Drosophila* strains. One makes use of balancer chromosomes, a *Drosophila*-specific tool of transmission genetics that allows entire chromosomes that are free of recessive-lethal mutations to be inherited intact and undisturbed by meiotic recombination (*24–28*). An example of this technique, embodied in a six-generation crossing scheme, is in Brizuela et al. (*29*). The whole-genome-isogenized strain they produced, nicknamed Iso-1, was used to construct a series of cDNA and genomic DNA libraries *(9,10,30)* that were distributed widely in the *Drosophila* research community for use in individual investigator-driven gene cloning and analysis work. Iso-1 is the reference strain from which the complete *Drosophila* euchromatic genome sequence was obtained *(31,32)*. This strain is also being used for the identification and sequencing of full-length cDNA clones representing every *Drosophila* gene *(33)* and for the construction of chromosomal deletions with sequence-defined, P-element–engineered endpoints *(22,23)*.

The second method for generating isogenized *Drosophila* strains takes advantage of the fact that meiotic recombination between homosequential homologous chromosomes occurs in this species only in female flies. Suppose strain A contains a dominant visible mutation denoted D; that mutation can be introduced into the genetic background of strain B by mating the two strains and collecting F_1 virgin females carrying the dominant-visible mutation. The F_1 females are heterozygous for the D mutation and have half their genetic constitution from the strain A background and half from the strain B background. At fertilization, A-derived and B-derived genetic material is present *in trans* on the homologous chromosomes, but this relationship is scrambled during meiotic recombination when the adult females produce eggs. The proportion of strain-A-derived genetic background can be reduced by approx one-half by backcrossing these heterozygous females to males from parental strain B. Of the resulting F_2 hybrid progeny, only half carry the D mutation, and, owing to meiotic recombination in the F_1 mothers, on average three-fourths of their total genetic constitution is now derived from strain B. Taking virgin F_2 $D/+$ females and backcrossing them again to strain B males will result in an F_3 in which, again, only half the animals carry the D mutation and these have a further reduction in the amount of strain-A-derived genetic information.

Over the course of n generations, this iterative process of backcrossing virgin female progeny to strain B will result in replacement of strain-A-derived chromosomes by strain-B–derived chromosomes such that residual strain-A-derived material is given by 2^{-n}. Ten backcross generations should result in approx 0.1% residual strain-A-derived genetic material, most of which is expected to be tightly linked *in cis* to the D-mutant allele; 20 generations would take the residue of strain-A-derived material to a much lower level. In *Drosophila*, each generation takes approx 2 wk. The 10-generation backcross process can be accomplished in less than 5 mo, and the 20-generation scheme can be completed in under 10 mo. With mice, satisfactory inbreeding requires 20 generations, which would take over 5 yr owing to the much longer generation time. In addition to the substantial difference in breeding time between the two species, the difference in the costs for animal-rearing facilities, food, and labor is even more substantial; in all these areas *Drosophila* clearly has the advantage.

3.2. Genetically Sensitized Drosophila Strains

In the experiments we described *(20)*, a dominant-visible eye morphology mutation, Kr^{If-1}, was introduced into the $iso\text{-}w^{1118}$; $iso\text{-}2$; $iso\text{-}3$ genetic background by a hybrid of the above two procedures. In the first stage of the composite procedure, a third-chromosome balancer was used to monitor introduction of the $iso\text{-}w^{1118}$; $iso\text{-}2$; $iso\text{-}3$ third chromosome. The introduction of an intact $iso\text{-}w^{1118}$; $iso\text{-}2$; $iso\text{-}3$-derived X chromosome was accomplished by passing that chromosome through males. In this way, a multigeneration backcross scheme was used only to introduce second-chromosome derived material by recombination. Because Kr^{If-1} is located very near the telomere on the right arm of the second chromosome, we believe *(20)* that the residual non-$iso\text{-}w^{1118}$; $iso\text{-}2$; $iso\text{-}3$ genetic material was probably limited to a small region surrounding the Kr locus. Segregation of the ectopic bristle phenotype from the Kr^{If-1} allele in this strain is a further demonstration that the selected aberrant-eye phenotype was epigenetic in nature.

Below we outline genetic cross-schemes for generating strains in which particular sensitizing mutations are backcrossed into a standardized isogenic background, namely, the w^{1118}; $iso\text{-}2$; $iso\text{-}3$ strain. Cross-scheme 1 assumes that the mutation of interest arose from the insertion of an engineered $P[w^+]$ transposon, which can be followed directly by its eye color phenotype and mapped with single-nucleotide precision. Cross-scheme 2 assumes the case of a mutation induced by ethyl-methane-sulfonate (EMS) or some other chemical mutagen and also assumes that the DNA base change responsible has been determined.

3.2.1. Cross-Scheme 1: Mutant Allele Is Owing to a $P[w^+]$ Insertion

1. Mate w^{1118}; $iso\text{-}2$; $iso\text{-}3$ (a.k.a., Hoskin's isogenized strain) virgin female to $P[w^+]$/Balancer male (*see* **Note 2**).
2. Mate F_1 male: w^{1118}/Y; $iso\text{-}2/P[w^+]$; $iso\text{-}3/+$ to w^{1118}; $iso\text{-}2$; $iso\text{-}3$ females.
3. Mate F_2 virgin females (5–10): w^{1118}; $iso\text{-}2/P[w^+]$; $iso\text{-}3/+$ to w^{1118}; $iso\text{-}2$; $iso\text{-}3$ males (*see* **Note 3**).
4. Mate F_3 virgin females (5–10): w^{1118}; $iso\text{-}2/P[w^+]$; $iso\text{-}3/+$ to w^{1118}; $iso\text{-}2$; $iso\text{-}3$ males.
5. Mate F_4 virgin females (5–10): w^{1118}; $iso\text{-}2/P[w^+]$; $iso\text{-}3/+$ to w^{1118}; $iso\text{-}2$; $iso\text{-}3$ males.
6. Mate F_5 virgin females (5–10): w^{1118}; $iso\text{-}2/P[w^+]$; $iso\text{-}3/+$ to w^{1118}; $iso\text{-}2$; $iso\text{-}3$ males.
7. Mate F_6 virgin females (5–10): w^{1118}; $iso\text{-}2/P[w^+]$; $iso\text{-}3/+$ to w^{1118}; $iso\text{-}2$; $iso\text{-}3$ males.
8. Mate F_7 virgin females (5–10): w^{1118}; $iso\text{-}2/P[w^+]$; $iso\text{-}3/+$ to w^{1118}; $iso\text{-}2$; $iso\text{-}3$ males.
9. Mate F_8 virgin females (5–10): w^{1118}; $iso\text{-}2/P[w^+]$; $iso\text{-}3/+$ to w^{1118}; $iso\text{-}2$; $iso\text{-}3$ males.

10. Mate F_9 virgin females (5–10): w^{1118}; *iso-2*/$P[w^+]$; *iso-3*/+ to w^{1118}; *iso-2*; *iso-3* males.

11. Mate F_{10} virgin females (5–10): w^{1118}; *iso-2*/$P[w^+]$; *iso-3*/+ to w^{1118}; *iso-2*; *iso-3* males (*see* **Note 4**).

12. Mate one F_{11} w^{1118}; *iso-2*, $P[w^+]$/*iso-2*; *iso-3* male to a single w^{1118}; *iso-2*, *Pin*/*CyO*; *iso-3* female. Set up at least a half-dozen such single-pair matings (*see* **Note 5**).

13. Save stock: w^{1118}; *iso-2*, $P[w^+]$/*CyO*; *iso-3*.

3.2.2. Cross-Scheme 2: Mutant Allele Is a Chemically Induced Point Mutation

1. Find nearest $P[w^+]$ insertion based on examination of FlyBase/GADFly resources, and make *iso-$P[w^+]$* strain (w^{1118}; *iso-2*, $P[w^+]$/*CyO*; *iso-3*), as in Cross-scheme 1 (*see* **Note 2**).

2. Mate EMS/Balancer male to w^{1118}; *iso-2*, $P[w^+]$/*CyO*; *iso-3* females.

3. Mate F_1 male: w^{1118}/Y; EMS/*iso-2*, $P[w^+]$; *iso-3*/+ to w^{1118}; *iso-2*, $P[w^+]$/*CyO*; *iso-3* females.

4. Mate F_2 virgin females (5–10): w^{1118}; EMS/*iso-2*, $P[w^+]$; *iso-3*/+ to w^{1118}; *iso-2*, $P[w^+]$/*CyO*; *iso-3* males (*see* **Note 3**).

5. Mate F_3 virgin females (5–10): w^{1118}; EMS/*iso-2*, $P[w^+]$; *iso-3*/+ to w^{1118}; *iso-2*, $P[w^+]$/*CyO*; *iso-3* males.

6. Mate F_4 virgin females (5–10): w^{1118}; EMS/*iso-2*, $P[w^+]$; *iso-3*/+ to w^{1118}; *iso-2*, $P[w^+]$/*CyO*; *iso-3* males.

7. Mate F_5 virgin females (5–10): w^{1118}; EMS/*iso-2*, $P[w^+]$; *iso-3*/+ to w^{1118}; *iso-2*, $P[w^+]$/*CyO*; *iso-3* males.

8. Mate F_6 virgin females (5–10): w^{1118}; EMS/*iso-2*, $P[w^+]$; *iso-3*/+ to w^{1118}; *iso-2*, $P[w^+]$/*CyO*; *iso-3* males.

9. Mate F_7 virgin females (5–10): w^{1118}; EMS/*iso-2*, $P[w^+]$; *iso-3*/+ to w^{1118}; *iso-2*, $P[w^+]$/*CyO*; *iso-3* males.

10. Mate F_8 virgin females (5–10): w^{1118}; EMS/*iso-2*, $P[w^+]$; *iso-3*/+ to w^{1118}; *iso-2*, $P[w^+]$/*CyO*; *iso-3* males.

11. Mate F_9 virgin females (5–10): w^{1118}; EMS/*iso-2*, $P[w^+]$; *iso-3*/+ to w^{1118}; *iso-2*, $P[w^+]$/*CyO*; *iso-3* males.

12. Mate F_{10} virgin females (5–10): w^{1118}; EMS/*iso-2*, $P[w^+]$; *iso-3*/+ to w^{1118}; *iso-2*, $P[w^+]$/*CyO*; *iso-3* males (*see* **Note 4**).

13. Mate one F_{11} w^{1118}; *iso-2*, EMS/*iso-2*, $P[w^+]$; *iso-3*/+ male to a single w^{1118}; *iso-2*, *Pin*/*CyO*; *iso-3* female. Set up at least a half-dozen such single-pair matings (*see* **Note 5**).

14. Save stocks: w^{1118}; *iso-2*, EMS/*CyO*; *iso-3*.

15. Make sure that EMS-induced "point" mutation is still present by DNA sequencing and testing for recessive lethality (i.e., the absence of non-*Cy* segregants in the stock generated in **step 14**). This is one reason to establish multiple single-pair matings in **step 13**.

3.3. Pharmacological Inhibition of Hsp90 Function

Adult flies 1–3 d old were allowed to feed and lay eggs on geldanamycin-containing Formula 4-24 Blue food for 2 wk. Their progeny were thus subjected to chronic geldanamycin exposure throughout development. Adult progeny that had grown in the presence of geldanamycin were scored for eye phenotype. Selected pairs were used to establish lines on fresh fly food that lacked geldanamycin.

3.4. Treatments That Increase Histone Acetylation In Vivo

Adult flies were transferred to blue food containing either sodium butyrate or TSA, and were allowed to lay eggs for 1 wk. Progeny were thus exposed to each of these HDAC inhibitors chronically during embryonic, larval, and pupal development. Previous studies in our lab found that chronic exposure to these drugs killed >90% of the animals at concentrations of 20 mM for sodium butyrate and 9.0 μM for TSA, whereas concentrations of half those values were lethal to <10% of the animals *(20)*.

3.5. Detection and Quantitation of Acetylated Histones

We monitored the effects of sodium butyrate and TSA treatments on histone acetylation by Western blotting.

1. Eggs laid on HDAC inhibitor-containing food were allowed to hatch, and the larvae developed while consuming the inhibitor-laced food.
2. We harvested the white prepupae at the conclusion of the larval period of growth and feeding. We found that sufficient total protein could be extracted from just a single white prepupa, using a tissue grinder and a standard sodium dodecyl sulfate (SDS)/β-mercaptoethanol sample buffer *(33)*.
3. Proteins were separated using a standard SDS-polyacrylamide gel, with 12% acrylamide for best resolution of lower molecular weight proteins.
4. Electroblotting to nitrocellulose was performed using a Bio-Rad mini-Protean chamber and followed manufacturer's standard procedures. Immunological detection used reagents from the SuperSignal West Pico kit (Pierce, Rockford, IL) and generally followed the manufacturer's procedures.
5. Non-specific sites on the membrane were blocked by incubating it with a solution of TBS-T supplemented with 1% bovine serum albumin (blocking solution) on a gyratory shaker for 30 min at room temperature.
6. The antihistone antibody was added to the blocking solution and allowed to incubate for 1h at room temperature with gentle shaking.
7. The membrane was then washed for six 5-min periods with fresh batches of TBS-T.
8. HRP-linked secondary goat-antirabbit IgG was added to a fresh batch of blocking solution, and the filter was incubated for 1 h at room temperature with gentle shaking.

9. Unbound HRP-linked secondary antibody was removed by six 5-min washes with TBS-T as before.

10. During the washes, a 1-mL batch of detection reagent was prepared by mixing equal volumes of the stable peroxide solution and the Luminol-enhancer solution included with the SuperSignal West Pico kit. Given the small volume of detection reagent, it is very important to make sure that the membrane is completely wetted by it and does not dry out during the entire 5-min incubation.

11. After 5 min, wrap the membrane in a transparent plastic sheet-protector or Saran Wrap, making sure all bubbles have been forced out.

12. In a photographic darkroom, place the membrane against a sheet of X-ray film and develop after a 60-s exposure. Additional longer exposures may be necessary based on the first exposure. If one uses a PhosphorImager, longer exposure times will almost certainly be necessary. In our experience, blots remain chemiluminescent for up to 8 h, but the strongest signals appear within the first 2 h.

13. X-ray films were scanned and histone bands on the resulting image quantified using NIH Image.

4. Notes

1. We prepared small batches of drug-inhibitor-containing food and used them immediately. Other Hsp90 inhibitors such as radicicol (35) are also available, and they may be more stable than geldanamycin. See Chapter 8 for additional discussion of techniques using TSA.

2. In these cross-schemes, we suggest balancer chromosomes and marker mutations assuming (as in our work with Kr^{If-1}) that the mutation of interest maps to the second chromosome. If the mutation resides on another chromosome, different genotypes are necessary.

3. When performing mass-matings for backcrosses it is important to use good *Drosophila* husbandry techniques (24–28). For example, matings should be set up in half-pint milk bottles (i.e., Applied Scientific) containing approx 40-mL of standard agar/cornmeal/sugar fly medium. The adults should not be allowed to lay too many eggs, to avoid crowding of the larvae. Progeny should be collected promptly, to prevent contamination or confusion by succeeding generation offspring. Temperature and humidity should be well controlled.

4. If the experimenter deems it necessary to continue backcrossing for additional generations, the general procedure outlined in the previous steps can be continued.

5. Single-pair matings are conducted in 2.3 × 9.5-cm plastic fly food vials containing approx 10-mL agar/cornmeal/sugar fly food.

Acknowledgments

We regret that space limitations prevented us from citing more of the fascinating primary literature in this area. We thank our colleagues for comments on the manuscript, E. Whitelaw for sending preprints and reprints, and T. Tollefsbol for inviting us to participate in this publishing project. We appreciate the remarks made by two anonymous reviewers and the series editor-in-chief. Research in our lab was supported by NIH grants R01AA12276, R01GM63225, and R21ES11751 to D.M.R. and a UAB-CNRC grant to M.D.G.

References

1. Haber, J. E. (1998) Mating-type gene switching in *Saccharomyces cerevisiae*. *Annu. Rev. Genet.* **32**, 561–599.
2. Tham, W. H. and Zakian, V. A. (2002) Transcriptional silencing at *Saccharomyces* telomeres: implications for other organisms. *Oncogene* **21**, 515–521.
3. Wakimoto, B. T. (1998) Beyond the nucleosome: epigenetic aspects of position-effect variegation in *Drosophila*. *Cell* **93**, 321–324.
4. Alleman, M. and Doctor, J. (2000) Genomic imprinting in plants: observations and evolutionary implications. *Plant Mol. Biol.* **43**, 147–161.
5. Li, E. (2002) Chromatin modification and epigenetic reprogramming in mammalian development. *Nat. Rev. Genet.* **3**, 662–673.
6. Rice, J. C. and Allis, C. D. (2001) Histone methylation versus histone acetylation: new insights into epigenetic regulation. *Curr. Opin. Cell Biol.* **13**, 263–273.
7. Fischle, W., Wang, Y., and Allis, C.D. (2003) Histone and chromatin cross-talk. *Curr. Opin. Cell Biol.* **15**, 172–183.
8. Taverna, S. D., Coyne, R. S., and Allis, C. D. (2002) Methylation of histone H3 at lysine 9 targets programmed DNA elimination in *Tetrahymena*. *Cell* **110**, 701–711.
9. Tamkun, J. W., Kahn, R. A., Kissinger, M., et al. (1991) The *arflike* gene encodes an essential GTP-binding protein in *Drosophila*. *Proc. Natl. Acad. Sci. USA* **88**, 3120–3124.
10. Tamkun, J. W., Deuring, R., Scott, M. P., et al. (1992) *brahma*, a regulator of *Drosophila* homeotic genes structurally related to the yeast transcriptional activator SNF2/SWI2. *Cell* **68**, 561–572.
11. Jenuwein, T. and Allis, C. D. (2001) Translating the histone code. *Science* **293**, 1074–1080.
12. Robyr, D., Suka, Y., Xenarios, I., et al. (2002) Microarray deacetylation maps determine genome-wide functions for yeast histone deacetylases. *Cell* **109**, 437–446.
13. van Steensel, B., Delrow, J., and Henikoff, S. (2001) Chromatin profiling using targeted DNA adenine methyltransferase. *Nat. Genet.* **27**, 304–308.
14. Andrews, J., Ashburner, M., Cavalli, G., Cherbas, P., Russell, P. and White, K. Personal communication.
15. *Drosophila* Community Resources White Paper, August 2003. http://flybase.bio.indiana.edu/.data/news/announcements/drosboard/Whitepaper2003.html.
16. Morgan, H. D., Sutherland, H. G. E., Martin, D. I. K., and Whitelaw, E. (1999) Epigenetic inheritance at the agouti locus in the mouse. *Nat. Genet.* **23**, 314–318.
17. Rakyan, V. K., Chong, S., Champ, M. E., et al. (2003) Transgenerational inheritance of epigenetic states at the murine *AxinFu* allele occurs after maternal and paternal transmission. *Proc. Natl. Acad. Sci. USA* **100**, 2538–2543.

18. Rakyan, V. K., Blewitt, M. E., Druker, R., Preis, J. I., and Whitelaw, E. (2002) Metastable epialleles in mammals. *Trends Genet.* **18,** 348–351.

19. Queitsch, C., Sangster, T. A., and Lindquist, S. (2002) Hsp90 as a capacitor of phenotypic variation. *Nature* **417,** 618–624.

20. Sollars, V., Lu, X., Xiao, L., Wang, X., Garfinkel, M. D., and Ruden, D. M. (2003) Evidence for an epigenetic mechanism by which Hsp90 acts as a capacitor for morphological evolution. *Nat. Genet.* **33,** 70–74.

21. Rutherford, S. L. and Henikoff, S. (2003) Quantitative epigenetics. *Nat. Genet.* **33,** 6–8.

22. Ryder, E., Rasmuson-Lestander, A., Maroy, P., et al. Unpublished data: http://131.111.146.35/~pseq/drosdel/index.html.

23. Golic, K. G. and Golic, M. M. (1996) Engineering the *Drosophila* genome: chromosome rearrangements by design. *Genetics* **144,** 1693–1711.

24. Ashburner, M. (1989) *Drosophila, A Laboratory Handbook.* Cold Spring Harbor Laboratory Press, Cold Spring Harbor, NY.

25. Ashburner, M. (1989) *Drosophila, A Laboratory Manual.* Cold Spring Harbor Laboratory Press, Cold Spring Harbor, NY.

26. Ashburner, M. and Roote, J. (2000) Laboratory culture of *Drosophila*, in *Drosophila Protocols* (Sullivan, W., Ashburner, M., and Hawley, R. S., eds.), Cold Spring Harbor Laboratory Press, Cold Spring Harbor, NY.

27. Greenspan, R. J. (1997) *Fly Pushing: The Theory and Practice of Drosophila Genetics.* Cold Spring Harbor Laboratory Press, Cold Spring Harbor, NY.

28. Sullivan, W., Ashburner, M., and Hawley, R. S., eds. (2000) *Drosophila Protocols.* Cold Spring Harbor Laboratory Press, Cold Spring Harbor, NY.

29. Brizuela, B. J., Elfring, L., Ballard, J., Tamkun, J. W., and Kennison, J. A. (1994) Genetic analysis of the *brahma* gene of *Drosophila melanogaster* and polytene chromosome subdivisions 72AB. *Genetics* **137,** 803–813.

30. Smoller, D. A., Petrov, D., and Hartl, D. L. (1991) Characterization of bacteriophage P1 library containing inserts of *Drosophila* DNA of 75–100 kilobases. *Chromosoma* **100,** 487–494.

31. Adams, M. D., Celniker, S. E., Holt, R. A., et al. (2000) The genome sequence of *Drosophila melanogaster. Science* **287,** 2185–2195.

32. Celniker, S. E., Wheeler, D. A., Kronmiller, B., et al. (2002) Finishing a whole-genome shotgun: release 3 of the *Drosophila* euchromatic genome sequence. *Genome Biol.* **3,** 79.

33. Stapleton, M., Carlson, J., Brokstein, P., et al. (2002) A *Drosophila* full-length cDNA resource. *Genome Biol.* **3,** 80.

34. Sambrook, J., Fritsch, E. F., and Maniatis, T. eds. (1989) *Molecular Cloning, A Laboratory Manual*, 2nd ed. Cold Spring Harbor Press, Cold Spring Harbor, NY.

35. Roe, S. M., Prodromou, C., O'Brien, R., Ladbury, J. E., Piper, P. W., and Pearl, L. H. (1999) Structural basis for inhibition of the Hsp90 molecular chaperone by the antitumor antibiotics radicicol and geldanamycin. *J. Med. Chem.* **42,** 260–266.

13

Profiling DNA Methylation by Bisulfite Genomic Sequencing

Problems and Solutions

Liang Liu, Rebecca C. Wylie, Nathaniel J. Hansen, Lucy G. Andrews, and Trygve O. Tollefsbol

Summary

The surge of interest in DNA methylation during the last two decades has triggered an urgent need for an effective method to detect the methylation status of the cytosines in the genome. Bisulfite genomic sequencing is the most attractive choice so far for many laboratories. Various protocols have been established, but difficulties are often encountered, particularly by individuals who have limited experience in this field. This analysis presents a simple protocol that has consistently worked well in our laboratory. Discussions of potential technical problems and corresponding solutions are also included to facilitate the reproducibility of this protocol.

Key Words: DNA methylation; bisulfite genomic sequencing; epigenetics; polymerase chain reaction.

1. Introduction

Many studies over the past two decades have established that the occurrence of 5-methylcytosines, located in CpG dinucleotides, play a vital role in a variety of important cellular processes essential for normal development including differentiation, genomic imprinting, and X-chromosome inactivation. It has also been shown that DNA methylation has inhibitory effects on gene expression through the establishment and maintenance of a repressive chromatin structure, recruitment of methyl binding proteins, and interference with transcription factor binding *(1,2)*. Because of this significant influence on transcriptional regulation, inappropriate methylation has been closely linked to many human diseases, including cancer. Aberrant hypermethylation of the pro-

From: *Methods in Molecular Biology, vol. 287: Epigenetics Protocols*
Edited by: T. O. Tollefsbol © Humana Press Inc., Totowa, NJ

moters of tumor suppressors and global hypomethylation, which can alter the regulatory state of proto-oncogenes, have both been demonstrated as factors in carcinogenesis *(2,3)*. Because DNA methylation has significant effects on gene function, methylation detection has become essential for the elucidation of a broad spectrum of biological processes.

Several methods are currently available for the detection of 5-methylcytosine in genomic DNA, and numerous reviews have carefully examined and compared these various approaches *(2,4–6)*. The determination of which technique best fits a particular experiment depends on several factors, such as the level of sensitivity necessary and the specificity of acquired results *(6)*. One protocol that has been used for some time involves the use of methylation-sensitive restriction enzymes followed by Southern blot analysis. This method provides information about the relative occurrence and abundance of genome-wide 5-methylcytosine *(6)*. Several drawbacks are associated with this technique, however, including the fact that the consensus sequences for these restriction enzymes occur infrequently and thus allow analysis of only a limited proportion of methylation sites. There also is a requirement for relatively large quantities of DNA, and there is no detection of hemimethylation through this method *(5)*. Other common methods for methylation detection are based on genomic sequencing techniques involving chemical cleavage *(7)*. This type of protocol allows for site-specific methylation analysis but involves many of the same limitations encountered by Southern blotting techniques *(4)*. There is also the additional problem that these genomic sequencing methods rely on identification of a 5-methylcytosine residue by the absence of a band on a sequencing gel, leading to difficulty in analysis and frequent false positives *(8)*.

For more than a decade, bisulfite genomic sequencing has been the method of choice for the analysis of DNA methylation in complex genomes. This sensitive and direct approach has revolutionized the characterization of methylation patterns in genomic DNA, providing the most specific results of any technique currently used without many of the limitations *(2)*. Bisulfite genomic sequencing provides positive identification of 5-methylcystosine for the precise mapping of methylation sites on individual DNA molecules using very small amounts of genomic DNA *(9)*. The standard method for this technique is based on the modification of unmethylated cytosines to uracils by treatment of DNA with sodium bisulfite following denaturation (**Fig. 1**) *(10)*. The steps of this reaction are (1) sulfonation of the cytosine residue at the C-6 position, (2) hydrolytic deamination at C-4 to produce uracil-sulfonate, and (3) desulfonation under alkaline conditions *(6,11,12)*. 5-Methylcytosine remains unreactive to this process owing to interference of the methyl group with the access of bisulfite to the C-6 position *(13)*. Following bisulfite treatment, polymerase chain reaction (PCR) is carried out using primers specific for each

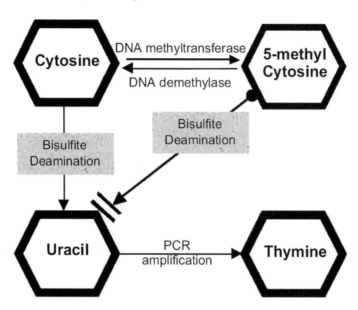

Fig. 1. Schematic depiction of the biochemical reaction pathways of cytosine in vivo and in vitro. Sodium bisulfite can convert cytosine into uracil through steps of sulfonation, hydrolytic deamination, and subsequent desulfonation with alkali. 5-Methylcytosine is, however, protected from this bisulfite reaction owing to the presence of the methyl group, which blocks the sulfonation by bisulfite.

modified strand of DNA (*see* **Notes 1–5**). The PCR yields products in which every 5-methylcytosine is displayed as a cytosine and each uracil, which originally was an unmethylated cytosine, is substituted by a thymine following amplification *(10)*. Direct sequencing can then be performed to generate an average methylation status of individual cytosine residues on multiple strands of DNA, or the PCR product can be cloned and then sequenced to analyze a specific individual molecule *(10)*.

Numerous modifications of the original bisulfite genomic sequencing method have been published over the last few years, allowing for a variety of technical improvements. A comprehensive investigation of several parameters, including the time/temperature combinations for bisulfite incubation and the determination of the degree of DNA degradation, have recently been performed *(14)*. Procedures that maximize the efficiency of denaturation, bisulfite conversion, and amplification *(9,15,16)*, and also increase the sensitivity of the technique to produce results using less than 100 cells, have also been reported *(9,17)*. The use of nested primers, reducing template degradation *(18)*, lowering PCR bias *(19,20)*, and eliminating artifacts *(21)* has also been a major improvement to bisulfite genomic sequencing, contributing to greater simplicity, speed, and success of the method.

Bisulfite genomic sequencing has proved to be an efficient and robust method for analyzing DNA methylation, having great advantages over previous techniques. Even though several technical improvements to the original method have solved many potential problems, this technique can be difficult to master, especially for those without previous exposure to the procedures. A modified bisulfite reaction protocol, which has proved to work with consistent efficiency, is described below. Discussion of technical details is also presented to facilitate troubleshooting for a laboratory with limited experience with this technique.

2. Materials

2.1. Equipment

1. 55°C Incubator, covered to provide a dark interior.
2. Vac-Man Laboratory Vacuum Manifold (Promega, cat. no. A7231).
3. Microcentrifuge at 4°C.

2.2. DNA Preparation

1. To start with isolated DNA: DNA isolation kit, Wizard genomic DNA purification kit (Promega, cat. no. A1125) and restriction enzyme and corresponding buffer.
2. To start with microdissected cells: 10 mg/mL proteinase K solution.

2.3. Bisulfite Treatment of DNA

1. Sodium bisulfite powder (Sigma, cat. no. S-8890).
2. Hydroquinone (Sigma, cat. no. H-9003).
3. 10 M NaOH solution, freshly prepared.
4. Mineral oil.

2.4. Purification of the Bisulfite-Treated DNA

1. 80% Isopropanol (2-propanol, reagent grade).
2. Wizard DNA clean-up system (Promega, cat. no. A7280).
3. Prewarmed (65–90°C) deionized water or TE buffer.
4. Disposable 3-mL syringes.
5. 6 M Ammonium acetate.
6. Absolute ethanol.

2.5. PCR, Cloning, and Sequencing of Targeted DNA Fragment

1. *Taq* DNA polymerase and associated PCR reagents and buffer.
2. pGEM-T Easy vector (Promega, cat. no. A1380).

3. Competent *E. coli* cells.
4. ABI Big-Dye DNA sequencing kit.

3. Methods

3.1. DNA Preparation

1. Tissues, cultured cells, or paraffin-embedded tissue sections can be used to isolate genomic DNA following the protocol provided by the manufacturer of the genomic DNA isolation kit (*see* **Note 6**). First, 0.5–10 µg of the isolated genomic DNA is digested by the appropriate restriction enzyme in 50 µL reaction volume to the optimal length, which leaves the target fragment intact. Proceed to **Subheading 3.2., step 1**.
2. For cells collected by laser-mediated microdissection, digest the cells in 2 mg/mL proteinase K solution at 55°C overnight, with the total reaction volume at 50 µL. Proceed to **Subheading 3.2., step 1**.

3.2. Bisulfite Treatment of DNA (see Note 7)

1. Dilute the fresh 10 *M* NaOH solution to 3 *M*, and prepare a 250 µL denaturing solution for each DNA sample by mixing 220 µL of water with 30 µL of 3 *M* NaOH.
2. Denature the DNA by adding this 250 µL of denaturing solution directly to the 50 µL DNA solution from either **step 1** or **step 2** of **Subheading 3.1.** (without any precipitation step).
3. Mix well and incubate at 55°C for 20 min. During this incubation period, make fresh bisulfite solution. The bisulfite solution has the following components, prepared in the order listed:
   a. Dissolve 5.4 g of sodium bisulfite in 10 mL water by mixing gently. (Invert the tube, do not vortex.)
   b. Dissolve 0.044 g hydroquinone in 10 mL water by vortexing. Add 666 µL of this freshly made solution into the sodium bisulfite solution.
   c. Add 400 µL of 10 *M* NaOH into the above sodium bisulfite solution, mixing well but gently.
4. Add 900 µL of the complete bisulfite solution directly to the 300-µL DNA sample from **step 3**, and cover the reaction mixture with a thin layer of mineral oil to diminish air contact.
5. Incubate the DNA/bisulfite solution at 55°C in the dark for 6 h.

3.3. Purifying the Modified DNA (see Note 6b)

The Wizard DNA clean-up kit and Vac-Man Laboratory Vacuum Manifold from Promega can be used to desalt and purify the bisulfite-treated DNA. The procedure is as follows (*see also* the protocol supplied by the manufacturer):

1. Attach a 3-mL syringe barrel into a Luer-Lok extension of each minicolumn, and insert the tip of the minicolumn into the vacuum manifold.

2. Add 1 mL of Wizard DNA clean-up resin into the syringe barrel.
3. Pipet the DNA-bisulfite sample into the syringe barrel and mix well with the resin by pipetting. Turn on the vacuum to draw the solution through the minicolumn. Turn off the vacuum to the minicolumn.
4. Add 1.5 mL of 80% isopropanol to the syringe barrel, and again turn on the vacuum to draw the solution through the minicolumn.
5. Repeat **step 4**.
6. Keep the vacuum on for an additional 30 s to dry the resin. Remove the syringe barrel and transfer the minicolumn to a new 2-mL microfuge tube.
7. Centrifuge the column at maximum speed for 2 min to remove the remaining isopropanol.
8. Transfer the minicolumn to a fresh 1.5-mL microfuge tube. Add 20 µL of prewarmed (70°C) water or TE buffer to the minicolumn and let it stand for 1 min. Centrifuge the minicolumn at maximum speed for 2 min. Save eluted DNA.
9. Repeat **step 8**. Save eluted DNA and add to the DNA from **step 8**.

3.4. Desulfonation and Precipitation of the DNA (see Note 6c)

1. Add 4 µL of 3 M NaOH to the eluted DNA solution from **Subheading 3.3., steps 8** and **9** (40 µL in total). Mix well with pipette and incubate for 15 min at 37°C to desulfonate the DNA.
2. Add 22 µL of 6 M ammonium acetate and 250 µL of absolute ethanol and precipitate the DNA at –20°C for at least 1 h. If the amount of DNA is very low, carrier DNA such as salmon sperm DNA (5–10 mg) can be added to facilitate the precipitation.
3. Pellet the DNA by centrifuging for 15 min in a microfuge at maximum speed at 4°C.
4. Carefully remove the supernatant and wash with 180 µL 70% ethanol; centrifuge as in **step 3**.
5. Remove the ethanol completely by aspirating. Let the DNA pellet dry at room temperature for 10 min. Resuspend in 10 µL deionized water.

3.5. PCR, Cloning, and Sequencing

1. PCR amplification of the bisulfite-treated DNA can be performed as with any other PCR reaction (*see* **Note 8**). A typical PCR reaction mixture using *Taq* DNA polymerase is as follows: 4 µL DNA, 5 µL 10x PCR buffer, 1 µL forward primer (10 µM), 1 µL reverse primer (10 µM), 1 µL 10 mM dNTPs mixture, 0.4 µL *Taq* DNA polymerase (5 U/µL), and 37.6 µL H_2O.
2. Following successful amplification, the PCR product can be gel-purified using a QIAquick Gel Extraction kit and directly sequenced. Alternatively, the PCR fragment can be ligated directly into the pGEM-T Easy cloning vector using *T4* DNA ligase (*see* **Note 9**). Competent *E. coli* cells can be transformed with the ligated DNA and plated on selective agar plates containing ampicillin and X-gal/IPTG to allow screening of positive transformants by the appearance of white colonies. The positive clones are selected and grown in LB medium. Plasmids containing the DNA insert of interest are extracted and subjected to sequence analysis (*see* **Note 10**).

4. Notes

1. Avoid CpG dinucleotides in the original sequence, since the methylation status of the C in the CpG dinucleotide is not known.
2. In case of extremely high CpG content in your target sequence, one may have to choose a primer sequence containing one or two CpGs. In this case you will need to design two sets of primers, one for amplifying the methylated sequence (keeping the C in the CpG dinucleotide as C for the forward primer and the G in the CpG as G for the reverse primer), and the other for amplifying the unmethylated sequence (replacing the C in the CpG dinucleotide with T for the forward primer and the G in the CpG with A for the reverse primer).
3. Proceed to design forward and reverse primers from the original sequence the same way as for ordinary PCR primers. Since the unmethylated cytosines should be converted by the bisulfite to thymine, you will need to replace all Cs (not located in the CpG dinucleotide) with Ts in the forward primer, and all Gs (not located in the CpG dinucleotide) by As in the reverse primer accordingly.
4. The optimal length of the oligos is between 25 and 32 nucleotides if possible, but not shorter than 20 nucleotides.
5. The length of the amplified sequence should not exceed 650 bp. A nested PCR reaction is normally required to obtain a sufficient amount of PCR product owing to the degradation of the DNA template during the bisulfite reaction. Alternatively, if no nested PCR primers are available, reamplification may be performed to increase the amount of PCR product.
6. No PCR amplification from the bisulfite-treated DNA: this represents the most common problem when trying to get the bisulfite method to work properly. The following factors may contribute to the problem:
   a. Starting with a very limited amount of DNA, such as a single cell or a small number of cells microdissected from tissue sections. To avoid losing DNA, we recommend that you first embed the cell(s) in low-melting-point agarose (mix one volume of cell solution with two volumes of 2% low-melting-point agarose solution, and pipet the mixture into prechilled mineral oil to form cell-agarose beads), and subject the cell-agarose beads to bisulfite treatment as described in **Subheading 3.2.**
   b. Loss of the DNA during recovery from the bisulfite solution. Make sure you follow the protocol exactly.
   c. Loss of the DNA when pelleting. This may be owing to the difficulty in pelleting a small amount of DNA. You can either add carriers (such as 10 μg glycogen or sheared yeast genomic DNA) when precipitating the DNA, or try the agarose-embedding method as mentioned above in **Note 6a**.
   d. Bisulfite-treated DNA may be too old. It is generally suggested that the bisulfite-treated DNA be used fresh, and not be older than 1 mo, at −20°C.
   e. Poor bisulfite reaction and highly inefficient conversion of the cytosine to uracil. Since the primers are designed to amplify converted DNA only, incomplete bisulfite reaction leads to mismatches between the primer sequence and the template sequence. *See* **Note 7** for suggestions on improving the bisulfite reaction efficiency.

f. Inappropriate PCR system. Given the large variability of the sequences to be investigated, most of which are high in GC content, you need to try different polymerases to find the one that may work the best with the specific sequence you are investigating. *See* **Note 8** for suggestions on improving the PCR reaction efficiency.

g. If no published primers are available for the gene of interest, include published primers for other genes as a control to make sure that the bisulfite modification procedure has worked properly before trying different primers.

7. Incomplete conversion of the unmethylated cytosine: If a stretch of cytosines or many cytosines not located in the CpG doublets are observed on the sequencing data sheet, the bisulfite reaction has not worked effectively.

a. The protocol of the bisulfite reaction needs to be followed strictly. Make sure that all reagents are fresh.

b. If you are sure that your genomic DNA is of good quality, try to lower the amount of DNA used; 0.5 µg of genomic DNA should normally be sufficient.

c. The NaOH solution must be freshly prepared each time prior to denaturing the DNA. In addition, boiling the genomic DNA for 10 min at 100°C before adding NaOH can improve the denaturing step.

d. Dissolving the bisulfite solution by vigorous shaking or vortexing should be avoided. Invert the tube gently to mix the bisulfite powder with water.

e. The incubator at 55°C needs to be insulated from light to keep the bisulfite solution stable.

8. Smearing PCR reactions: This problem is more encouraging than no amplification at all.

a. As a general rule in any PCR reaction, it is mandatory to optimize the annealing temperature and the salt concentrations of the PCR reactions, or add PCR facilitating reagents such as DMSO or Perfect Match® (Stratagene). If the problem persists, it is worthwhile trying a different PCR system. Remember that the newest PCR kit does not always guarantee satisfactory amplification of different specific sequences.

b. *Taq* DNA polymerase is the most commonly used enzyme for PCR amplification. In our laboratory, using SureStart *Taq* DNA polymerase from Stratagene helped us to solve the PCR smear problem associated with several other *Taq* DNA polymerases in the case of the specific sequences we studied (*see* **Fig. 2**). You will need to try different polymerases until you find one that produces a clean band with the specific sequence you are trying to amplify.

c. For agarose-embedded DNA, it may be a helpful practice to recover the DNA from the agarose using the QIAquick Gel Extraction kit if your experimental design can tolerate the partial loss of the DNA.

9. Cloning problem.

a. Gel purification of the PCR product is always recommended, even if your PCR reaction looks very specific from the agarose gel.

b. If you are using the T-A cloning system with the pGEM-T Easy vector, make sure that the DNA polymerase for your PCR system performs the function of

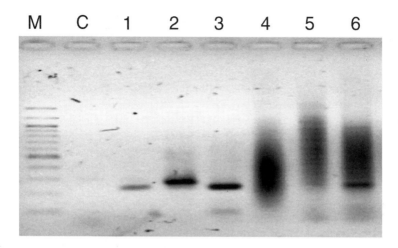

Fig. 2. Amplification of the hTERT promoter by nested primers using two different PCR systems: SureStart *Taq* DNA polymerase from Stratagene (lanes 1–3) and TITA-NIUM *Taq* DNA polymerase from Clontech (lanes 4–6). The rest of the PCR conditions are the same. Lane M, marker; Lane C, control.

adding one extra adenosine at the 5' end of both strands. Otherwise, either choose a blunt-end cloning strategy or incubate your PCR product with *Taq* DNA polymerase for 10 min at 72°C to add one extra adenosine at the 5' end of your PCR product before cloning.

10. Difficulty in sequencing the cloned PCR products: obtaining the clones of your PCR products does not mean that the hard work is over. Very often, people receive failed sequencing reports from automated sequencing machines. This problem is largely sequence specific: the higher the GC content in your target sequence, the harder it is to get the sequencing work done correctly.

a. Using consensus primers specific for the cloning vector is a good choice.

b. In the case of truncated sequencing results, you may have to use the primers for your PCR to perform "nested" sequencing to read through the entire sequence of interest.

c. For high GC content in the original sequence, using a kit for sequencing GC-rich sequences may be a good alternative, even though the actual sequence in your clones is AT-rich.

d. The cycling conditions of the sequencing reaction may also be optimized to solve the unsuccessful sequencing reactions, particularly if you use the primer for PCR reactions to sequence your PCR product.

Acknowledgments

This work was funded in part by grants from the National Institutes of Health, the Leukemia Research Foundation, the American Cancer Society, and the John A. Hartford Foundation.

References

1. Cirradi, M., Izzo, A., Badaracco, G., and Landsberger, N. (2002) Molecular mechanisms of gene silencing mediated by DNA methylation. *Mol. Cell. Biol.* **22,** 3157–3173.
2. Havlis, J. and Trbusek, M. (2002) 5-Methylcytosine as a marker for the monitoring of DNA methylation. *J. Chromatogr. B* **781,** 373–392.
3. Stirzaker, C., Millar, D. S., Paul, C. L., Warnecke, P. M., Harrison, J., Vincent, P. C., Frommer, M., and Clark, S. J. (1997) Extensive DNA methylation spanning the *Rb* promoter in retinoblastoma tumors. *Cancer Res.* **57,** 2229–2237.
4. Fraga, M. F. and Esteller, M. (2002) DNA methylation, a profile of methods and applications. *BioTechniques* **33,** 632–649.
5. Grigg, G. and Clark, S. (1994) Sequencing 5-methylcytosine residues in genomic DNA. *BioEssays* **16,** 431–436.
6. Rein, T., DePamphilis, M. L., and Zorbas, H. (1998) Identifying 5-mthylcytosine and related modifications in DNA genomes. *Nucleic Acids Res.* **26,** 2255–2264.
7. Church, G. M. and Gilbert, W. (1984) Genomic sequencing. *Proc. Natl. Acad. Sci. USA* **81,** 1991–1995.
8. Tommasi, S., LeBon, J. M., Riggs, A. D., and Singer-Sam, J. (1993) Methylation analysis by genomic sequencing of 5′ region of mouse *Pgk-1* gene and a cautionary note concerning the method. *Somat. Cell Mol. Genet.* **19,** 529–541.
9. Clark, S. J., Harrison, J., Paul, C. L., and Frommer, M. (1994) High sensitivity mapping of methylated cytosines. *Nucleic Acids Res.* **22,** 2990–2997.
10. Frommer, M., McDonald, L. E., Millar, D. S., et al. (1992) A genomic sequencing protocol that yields a positive display of 5-methylcytosine residues in individual DNA strands. *Proc. Natl. Acad. Sci. USA* **89,** 1827–1831.
11. Wang, R. Y. H., Gerhke, C. W., and Ehrlich, M. (1980) Comparison of bisulfite modification of 5-methyldeoxycytidine and deoxycytidine residues. *Nucleic Acids Res.* **8,** 4777–4790.
12. Grigg, G. W. (1996) Sequencing 5-methylcytosine residues by the bisulphate method. *DNA Sequence J. Sequencing Mapping* **6,** 189–198.
13. Hajkova, P., El-Maarri, O., Engemann, S., Oswald, J., Olek, A., and Walter, J. (2002) DNA-methylation analysis by the bisulfite-assisted genomic sequencing method, in *DNA Methylation Protocols* (Mills, K. I. and Ramsahoye, B. H., eds). Humana, Totowa, NJ, pp. 143–154.
14. Grunau, C., Clark, S. J., and Rosenthal, A. (2001) Bisulfite genomic sequencing, systematic investigation of critical experimental parameters. *Nucleic Acids Res.* **29,** 1–7.
15. Paulin, R., Grigg, G. W., Davey, M. W., and Piper, A. A. (1998) Urea improves efficiency of bisulphate-mediated sequencing of 5′-methylcytosine in genomic DNA. *Nucleic Acids Res.* **26,** 5009–5010.
16. Feil, R., Charlton, J., Bird, A. P., Walter, J., and Reik, W. (1994) Methylation analysis on individual chromosomes: improved protocol for bisulphate genomic sequencing. *Nucleic Acids Res.* **22,** 695–696.

17. McDonald, L. E. and Kay, G. F. (1997) Methylation analysis using bisulfite genomic sequencing: application to small numbers of intact cells. *BioTechniques* **22,** 272,273.
18. Raizis, A. M., Schmitt F., and Jost, J. P. (1995) A bisulfite method of 5-methylcytosine mapping that minimizes template degradation. *Anal. Biochem.* **226,** 161–166.
19. Voss, K. O., Roos, P., Nonay, R. L., and Dovichi, N. J. (1998) Combating PCR bias in bisulfite-based cytosine methylation analysis: betaine-modified cytosine deamination PCR. *Anal. Chem.* **70,** 3818–3823.
20. Warnecke, P. M., Stirzaker, C., Melki, J. R., Millar, D. S., Paul, C. L., and Clark, S. J. (1997) Detection and measurement of PCR bias in quantitative methylation analysis of bisulphate-treated DNA. *Nucleic Acids Res.* **25,** 4422–4426.
21. Warnecke, P. M., Stirzaker, C. , Song, J., Grunau, C., Melki, J. R., and Clark, S. J. (2002) Identification and resolution of artifacts in bisulfite sequencing. *Methods* **27,** 101–107.

14

Methylation-Sensitive Single-Strand Conformation Analysis

A Rapid Method to Screen for and Analyze DNA Methylation

Jean Benhattar and Geneviève Clément

Summary

The last few years have seen a growing interest in the study of DNA methylation because of its now acknowledged implication in cancer. The use of bisulfite to convert unmethylated cytosine to uracil, even as methylated cytosine remains unchanged, constitutes the basis for differentiating between methylated and unmethylated specific CpG sites in CpG islands. This technique therefore is critical to the success of this approach. Different parameters have to be considered in order to achieve a total conversion of cytosines to uracils. Several bisulfite-based methods are available for analyzing DNA methylation status. Methylation-sensitive single-strand conformation analysis (MS-SSCA) yields specific and semiquantitative data. The method is based on bisulfite treatment of DNA followed by polymerase chain reaction using primers without a CpG site to avoid selective amplification of either methylated or unmethylated DNA, and finally by single-strand conformation analysis (SSCA). The method allows one to establish clonal variations in the DNA methylation status for clones representing as little as 5–10% of the total cell population. MS-SSCA has, furthermore, a broad application field since it is the appropriate method for the analysis of frozen, fixed, and even microdissected tissues.

Key Words: APC; bisulfite modification; CDKN2A; CpG island; DNA methylation; single-strand conformation analysis; TIMP-3.

1. Introduction

Methylation of DNA is a heritable, enzyme-induced modification of the DNA structure without alteration of the specific sequence of the base pairs responsible for encoding the genome. Methylation of cytosine located within the dinucleotide CpG is in fact the main epigenetic modification in humans,

From: *Methods in Molecular Biology, vol. 287: Epigenetics Protocols*
Edited by: T. O. Tollefsbol © Humana Press Inc., Totowa, NJ

and it is now clear that abnormally methylated cytosine within a CpG dinucle-otide is a widespread phenomenon in cancer *(1)*. Two patterns of DNA methy-lation have been observed in the DNA of cancer cells: wide areas of global hypomethylation along the genome, and localized areas of hypermethylation at certain specific sites, the CpG islands, within the gene promoter regions *(2)*. The presence of 5-methylcytosine in CpG islands in the 5' promoter region of certain genes presumably interferes with the binding of transcription factors and/or promotes the interaction with methylation-dependent DNA binding pro-teins; this may result in gene silencing *(3,4)*.

As interest in DNA methylation mounted during the last few years, many new and powerful techniques were developed to facilitate its study. To gain a solid understanding of the DNA methylation patterns of the CpG islands in specific DNA sequences, the use of bisulfite-modified DNA is generally nec-essary *(5)*. Bisulfite converts unmethylated cytosine to uracil, while methy-lated cytosine, present at CpG sites, does not react. This reaction constitutes the basis for differentiating between methylated and unmethylated DNA se-quences. Total conversion of cytosines to uracils is a critical step in the success of this approach, which requires that particular attention be paid to several parameters, including total denaturation of the DNA, temperature, and reac-tion time with the sodium bisulfite *(6)*.

Several bisulfite-based methods are available. Sequencing of bisulfite-con-verted DNA provides a methylation map of single DNA molecules. Although this approach has been helpful in the study of the DNA methylation of genes associated with cancer, it is technically difficult and not sensitive enough *(7)*. Methylation-specific polymerase chain reaction (MSP) is an alternative qualita-tive method for studying the methylation of CpG islands *(8)*. MSP is the most widely used technique because of its high sensitivity, rapidity, and ease of execution. However, it can generate false-positive results owing to poly-merase chain reaction (PCR) overamplification. Furthermore, primer design is a critical and complex component of the procedure. MethyLight is an applica-tion of MSP that uses fluorescence-based real-time PCR technology *(9)*. Com-bined bisulfite restriction analysis (COBRA) constitutes a highly sensitive and semiquantitative method based on the creation or detection of a target for restric-tion endonuclease after bisulfite treatment *(10)*. This method also has the poten-tial to generate false-positive results if enzymatic digestion and/or bisulfite modification are incomplete. Unlike COBRA, methylation-sensitive single-nucleotide primer extension (Ms-SnuPE) uses bisulfite/PCR combined with single-nucleotide primer extension to analyze DNA methylation status quanti-tatively in a particular DNA region without using restriction enzymes *(11)*. The major disadvantage of this approach is the necessity of using radioactive tracers to obtain a high degree of sensitivity.

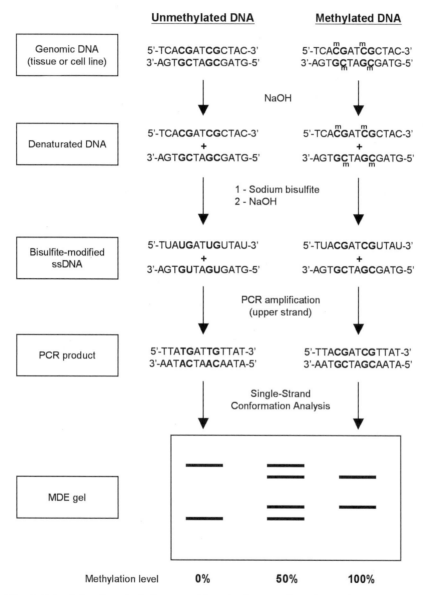

Fig. 1. Principle of methylation-sensitive single-strand conformation analysis (MS-SSCA). PCR, polymerase chain reaction; ssDNA, single-stranded DNA.

Methylation-sensitive single-strand conformation analysis (MS-SSCA) is based on bisulfite treatment of DNA followed by PCR using primers without CpG dinucleotides and complementary to the deaminated DNA strand, and finally by single-strand conformation analysis (SSCA) (**Fig. 1**) *(12,13)*. Indeed, bisulfite modification of DNA generates sequence disparities between methylated and unmethylated alleles and leads to the methylation-dependent alteration of single-strand conformation. MS-SSCA yields specific and semiquantitative data. By mixing methylated and unmethylated DNA of a known ratio, the percentage of methylation can be directly reflected by the ratio of intensity between the methylated and unmethylated bands. Five to ten percent of methylated alleles in a total cell population is the limiting detection rate of this technique. In addition, this approach not only allows the analysis of methylation status within a lesion but also gives further information about the clonality of the epigenetic alteration. The application field of MS-SSCA is wide since it can be applied to the analysis of frozen tissues as well as archival fixed tissues and even microdissected, formalin-fixed, paraffin-embedded tissues *(13,14)*.

2. Materials

2.1. Bisulfite Modification

1. 1 N HCl.
2. 3 M NaOH: 0.6 g sodium hydroxide (Merck, Dietikon, Switzerland), 5 mL nano-pure water.
3. 10 mM Hydroquinone: 11 mg hydroquinone (Fluka, Buchs, Switzerland), 10 mL nano-pure water.
4. 40.5% Sodium bisulfite pH 5.0: 9.1 g of sodium hydrogensulfite (Aldrich, St. Louis, MO), 1.6 mL of 3 M NaOH, 18.4 mL of nano-pure water.
5. Ethanol.
6. DNeasy Tissue Kit (Qiagen, Hilden, Germany).
7. Water-bath, 37°C.
8. Incubator, 55 and 70°C.

2.2. PCR Reaction

1. Thermocycler.
2. PCR reagents: 10X PCR buffer (200 mM Tris-HCl, pH 8.4, 500 mM KCl); 50 mM MgCl$_2$; 5 mM deoxynucleoside triphosphate mix (dNTP); 10 pmol/µL each primer; 5 U/µL of *Taq* DNA polymerase (Invitrogen, Basel, Switzerland).
3. Dimethyl sulfoxide (DMSO, Merck).
4. Primer sequences are listed in **Table 1**.
5. Standard agarose (Eurobio, Les Ulis, France).
6. 10X TAE buffer: 96.8 g of Trizma® Base, 40 mL of 0.5 M EDTA, pH 8.0, 22.84 mL of glacial acetic acid; add water up to 400 mL (pH 8.0–8.1).
7. 10 mg/mL Ethidium bromide, in water (Sigma, St. Louis, MO).
8. 20% Ficoll 400 (Amersham Biosciences, Buckinghamshire, UK): 2 g Ficoll 400, add water up to 10 mL. Rotate the tube to dissolve the solution.

Table 1
Sequence of PCR Primers Specific to the Bisulfite-Modified Upper DNA Strand and PCR Conditions for Amplification of the APC, CDKN2A, and TIMP-3 Promoter Gene Regions

Promoter gene	Primer	Sequence	PCR size (bp)	PCR conditions (T_m/DMSO)
APC	APC-forward	5'-GGGTTAGGGTTAGGTAGGTTGT-3'	159	53°C/yes
	APC-reverse	5'-CCCACACCCAACCAATC-3'		
CDKN2A	p16-forward	5'-GGGGGAGATTTAATTTGG-3'	194	54°C/yes
	p16-reverse	5'-CAACCCCTCCTCTTTCTT-3'		
TIMP-3	TIMP-3-forward	5'-GGTTTA*GTTTTTTTTTTGGAG-3'	154	50°C/no
	TIMP-3-reverse	5'-CCTACCTACTACCC*TCTCTAC-3'		

APC, adenomatous polyposis coli; DMSO, dimethyl sulfoxide; PCR, polymerase chain reaction; TIMP-3, tissue inhibitor of metalloproteinase 3.
*Corrected nucleotide (*see* **Note 8**).

9. 2X Ficoll loading dye: 450 µL of 20% Ficoll 400, 60 µL of 1% xylene cyanol; add water up to 1 mL. Store at 4°C.
10. 100 bp DNA ladder (Invitrogen): 25 µL of 100 bp DNA ladder + 475 µL H$_2$O + 500 µL 2X Ficoll loading dye.
11. Horizontal gel electrophoresis apparatus (e.g., Danaphor type 100, Danaphor, Grandvaux, Switzerland).
12. Ultraviolet (UV) transilluminator.

2.3. Single-Strand Conformation Analysis

1. MDE™ gel solution (BioWhittaker Molecular Applications, Rockland, ME).
2. 5X TBE buffer: 450 m*M* Tris-borate, 10 m*M* disodium EDTA, pH 8.0.
3. 10% Ammonium persulfate (APS) (Merck): 2 g water up to 20 mL, keep at 4°C.
4. *N,N,N',N'*-Tetramethylethylenediamine (TEMED) (Merck).
5. 500 m*M* NaOH/10 m*M* EDTA.
6. Formamide dye: 95% formamide, 10 m*M* EDTA, pH 8.0, 0.05% bromophenol, 0.025% xylene cyanol.
7. SYBR Gold stain (Molecular Probes, Eugene, OR).
8. 20-cm Vertical gel electrophoresis apparatus: SE600 series from Hoefer (San Francisco, CA).
9. Gel documentation system with a CCD camera (e.g., the AlphaImager from Alpha Innotech, San Leandro, CA).

2.4. Preparation of Markers

1. *Sss*I methylase (New England Biolabs, Beverly, MA).
2. Incubator, 37°C.
3. *Hpa*II and *Msp*I restriction enzyme (Roche, Rotkreuz, Switzerland).
4. Standard agarose (Eurobio).
5. 10X TAE buffer: 96.8 g of Trizma® Base, 40 mL of 0.5 M EDTA, pH 8.0, 22.84 mL of glacial acetic acid; add water up to 400 mL (pH 8.0–8.1).
6. 10 mg/mL Ethidium bromide, in water (Sigma).
7. 2X Ficoll loading dye: 450 µL of 20% Ficoll 400 (Amersham Biosciences), 60 µL of 1% xylene cyanol; add water up to 1 mL. Store at 4°C.
8. 1-kb DNA ladder (Invitrogen).
9. DNeasy Tissue Kit (Qiagen, Hilden, Germany).
10. GeneQuant Spectrophotometer (Amersham Biosciences).

3. Methods

3.1. Bisulfite Modification

Up to 2 µg of genomic DNA extracted from cell lines, frozen, formalin-fixed paraffin-embedded tissues, or the total amount of DNA obtained from microdissected tissues are used for the modification by sodium bisulfite (*see* **Note 1**).

1. Add 4 µL of 1 N HCl to 36 µL of genomic DNA preparation (*see* **Note 2**), maximum 2 µg of DNA in nano-pure water or Tris-HCl, pH 8.5, and incubate for exactly 2 min at room temperature (RT) (*see* **Note 3** for handling with fixed tissues).
2. Add immediately 4.3 µL of 3 M NaOH to neutralize the HCl and to denature the DNA. Vortex and incubate for 20 min at 37°C (*see* **Note 3**).
3. Add 28 µL of 10 mM hydroquinone followed by addition of 500 µL of 40.5% sodium bisulfite.
4. Vortex and incubate, light-protected for 4–6 h at 55°C.
5. Add 80 µL of nano-pure water and 365 µL of ethanol, mix well and load 500 µL of the mixture into a DNeasy column (column included in the DNeasy tissue kit) sitting in a collection tube. Spin for 2 min at 6000g. Discard the flowthrough and the collection tube.
6. Place the DNeasy column in a clean collection tube. Load the remaining 500 µL of the mixture into the column, and spin again for 2 min at 6000g. Discard the flowthrough and the collection tube.
7. Place the DNeasy column in a clean collection tube. Add 500 µL of buffer AW1 (solution contained in the DNeasy tissue kit), spin for 2 min at 13,000g. Discard the flowthrough and the collection tube.
8. Place the DNeasy column in a clean collection tube. Add 500 µL of buffer AW2 (solution included in the DNeasy tissue kit), and spin for 2 min at 13,000g. Discard the flowthrough and the collection tube.

9. Add 500 µL of freshly prepared 0.15 *M* NaOH/90% EtOH for desulfonation of the bisulfite-treated DNA, incubate for 10 min at RT and spin for 1 min at 13,000*g* (*see* **Note 4**). Discard the flowthrough and the collection tube.
10. Place the DNeasy column in a clean collection tube. Add 500 µL of buffer AW1, spin for 2 min at 13,000*g*. Discard the flowthrough and the collection tube.
11. Place the DNeasy column in a clean collection tube. Add 500 µL of buffer AW2, and spin for 2 min at 13,000*g*. Discard the flowthrough and the collection tube.
12. Place the DNeasy column in a clean collection tube. Rotate the column and spin again for 1 min to dry the column.
13. Place the DNeasy column in a clean microcentrifuge tube, add directly onto the column 50 µL of buffer AE (included in the DNeasy tissue kit), incubate for 15 min at 70°C, and then spin for 2 min at 13,000*g* to elute.
14. Store the bisulfite-modified DNA solution at –20°C (*see* **Note 5**).

3.2. PCR Reaction

1. Prepare the PCR master mix in a specially designated separate area. The volume prepared is based on the number of reaction tubes desired. For n reaction tubes (20 µL for each PCR reaction), add the following to a microcentrifuge tube: 12.3 × (n + 1) µL of nano-pure water, 2 × (n + 1) µL of 10X PCR buffer, 1 × (n + 1) µL of forward primer, 1 × (n + 1) µL of reverse primer, 0.6 × (n + 1) µL of 50 m*M* MgCl$_2$, 1 × (n + 1) µL of 5 m*M* dNTP, and 0.1 × (n + 1) µL of *Taq* DNA polymerase (*see* **Notes 6–8**).
2. Place 2 µL of each DNA solution in 0.5-mL microcentrifuge tubes on ice and aliquot 18 µL of the master mix into each tube. Include a negative control containing 2 µL of H$_2$O instead of DNA.
3. Prepare the program for amplification. Perform an initial denaturation step at 95°C for 5 min followed by a three-step profile: denaturation at 94°C for 30 s, primer annealing at optimal T_m (optimal T_m should be tested) for 45 s, and extension at 72°C for 45 s, for a total of 35 cycles (*see* **Note 9**). Perform a final incubation at 72°C for 10 min following the last PCR cycle. Store tubes at 15°C at the end of the last incubation. Conditions used for the amplification of the promoter region of the APC, CDKN2A, and TIMP-3 genes are listed in **Table 1**.
4. Start the thermocycler, and place the tubes in the block when the temperature reaches 95°C.
5. Perform amplification.
6. Control of PCR amplification:
   a. Prepare a 2% agarose gel in 1X TAE buffer containing 1 µg of ethidium bromide per ml. Use electrophoresis to separate the amplification products. Add 10 µL of PCR products to each well (5 µL of PCR product and 5 µL of 2X Ficoll loading dye), and add in one well 10 µL of a size marker (100-bp DNA ladder diluted 1:40) to confirm the correct size of the PCR products. Run at 100 mA until the xylene cyanol dye is approx 2 cm from the bottom of the gel.
   b. Place the gel on the UV transilluminator to visualize the PCR products.

3.3. Single-Strand Conformation Analysis

1. Prepare a 30% MDE gel. Use a 20-cm-long gel apparatus. Mix the following: 11 mL of H_2O, 2.2 mL of 5X TBE, 8.8 mL of MDE solution, 160 µL of 10% APS, and 15 µL of TEMED. Pour the solution rapidly in between the glass plates before it polymerizes, and remove potential air bubbles. Let the gel polymerize for 1 h at room temperature.
2. Denature the PCR products and the markers (*see* **Subheading 3.5.** and **Note 10**). Use 5 µL of PCR products and add 5 ml of denaturing mix (4 µL of H_2O + 1 µL of 500 mM NaOH/10 mM EDTA). Incubate at 50°C for 10 min.
3. After polymerization, wash each well of the gel with 0.5X TBE buffer.
4. Add 2 µL of formamide dye to the denatured PCR products and load onto the gel. Run the gel overnight at 150–200 V (7.5–10 V/cm) at 20°C in 0.5X TBE buffer.
5. After electrophoresis remove the gel carefully from the glass plates and stain for 20 min in the dark with a SYBR Gold gel stain diluted 1:10,000 in 1X TBE buffer (*see* **Note 11**).
6. Visualize by UV transillumination using a charge-coupled device (CCD) camera. Photograph the gel and save the image if necessary.

3.4. Interpretation of Data

1. Before screening a series of PCR samples, it is important to test the linearity of the amplification by a linear regression analysis. For each region of the gene to be studied, amplify the bisulfite-modified DNA from the methylation scale (*see* **Note 10** and **Subheading 3.5.**) and perform an SSCA (**Fig. 2**). Indeed, it is important to verify that an equal mixture of unmethylated and fully methylated DNA gives a similar level of amplification after analysis by MS-SSCA (*see* **Note 12**).
2. For each gene analyzed, interpretation of the methylation pattern of one sample should be done by comparing the ratio of intensity between the methylated and unmethylated bands with the methylation scale (**Fig. 3** and *see* **Note 13**).
3. In established cell lines three patterns of band mobility can be detected by MS-SSCA: no methylation (0%), full methylation (100%), and a mixture of both (50%) (*see* **Note 14**).
4. In tissues, an intermediate level of methylation reflects the ratio of the intensity between the methylated and unmethylated bands (**Fig. 3** and *see* **Note 14**).
5. If the band mobility pattern of the sample does not correspond to one of the markers, it could be interpretable either as an artifact of the PCR amplification or owing to the presence of partially methylated alleles in the tissues (methylation occurs in only some of the CpG sites within the analyzed region; *see* **Notes 15** and **16**).

3.5. Preparation of Markers

A methylation scale (markers) is prepared by methylating, with the *Sss*I methylase, all cytosine residues within CpG dinucleotides of a genomic DNA sequence. Methylated and unmethylated genomic DNAs can then be used as PCR templates for all the promoter gene regions that have to be analyzed.

APC promoter

Unmethylated	100	80	50	20	0
Fully methylated	0	20	50	80	100

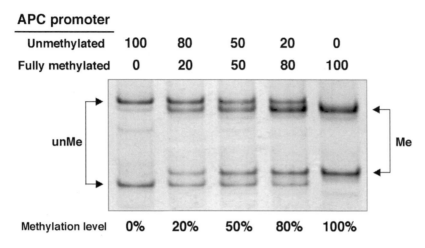

Methylation level	0%	20%	50%	80%	100%

Fig. 2. Determination of the semiquantitative methylation analysis by MS-SSCA. DNAs from a human colorectal tissue (unmethylated for the APC promoter or fully methylated at all CpG sites with the *Sss*I methylase) were mixed at various ratios, as indicated above the gel. After bisulfite modification, PCR amplification with primers specific for the APC promoter gene (*see* **Table 1**) and single-stranded conformation analysis, the percentage of methylation can be directed reflected by the ratio of intensity between the methylated (Me) and unmethylated bands (unMe).

1. Take 20 µg of genomic DNA isolated from normal frozen tissues.
2. Add to the DNA samples the following components supplied with the *Sss*I methylase: 5 µL of 20X S-adenosylmethionine (SAM; 3.2 m*M*), 10 µL of 10X NE buffer, 10 µL of *Sss*I methylase (20 U), and nano-pure water up to 100 µL.
3. Incubate at 37°C. After 3–4 h add 5 µL of 20X SAM and 2 µL of *Sss*I methylase. Continue the incubation overnight at 37°C.
4. Confirm complete CpG methylation by digestion with restriction enzymes *Hpa*II and *Msp*I. To 1 µL of the reaction mix add 7 µL of nano-pure water, 1 µL of 10X buffer L, and 1 µL of *Hpa*II or *Msp*I restriction enzyme.
5. Incubate at 37°C for 1–2 h.
6. Verify the digestion on a 1% agarose gel in 1X TAE buffer containing 1 µg of ethidium bromide per mL. Add 10 µL of 2X Ficoll loading dye to the 10 µL digestion mix and load 10 µL per well. Add in one well 10 µL of a size marker (1 µL of 1 kb DNA ladder, 4 µL of water, and 5 µL of 2X Ficoll loading dye).
7. Run the gel at 100 mA for approx 30 min in 1X TAE buffer.
8. Place the gel on the UV transilluminator to visualize the digestion product. Interpretation of the gel: *Hpa*II does not cut the methylated DNA, whereas *Msp*I cuts the methylated DNA—a smear is visible on the gel (*see* **Note 17**)
9. Purify the methylated DNA. Add 100 ml of buffer AL (buffer included in the DNeasy tissue kit), mix, and add 100 µL of 100% EtOH. Mix and transfer sample into a DNeasy minicolumn (column included in the DNeasy tissue kit) sitting in

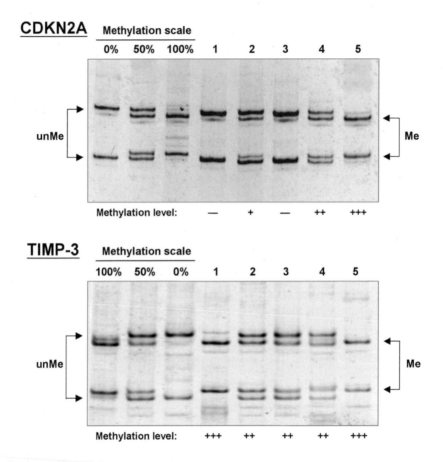

Fig. 3. Methylation analysis of the CDKN2A and tissue inhibitor of metalloproteinase 3 (TIMP-3) promoter gene regions by MS-SSCA. DNAs were extracted from paraffin-embedded fixed esophageal cancer tissues. After MS-SSCA with primers specific for either CDKN2A or TIMP-3, the level of methylation for each promoter gene region can be directly reflected by the ratio of intensity between the methylated (Me) and unmethylated bands (unMe). Level of methylation: −, no methylation; +, 10–40% of methylated DNA; ++, around 50% of methylated DNA; +++, around 100% of methylated DNA.

a collection tube. Spin for 1 min at 6000*g*. Discard the flowthrough and the collection tube.

10. Add 500 µL of buffer AW1. Spin for 1 min at 6000*g*. Discard the flowthrough and the collection tube.

11. Add 500 µL of buffer AW2. Spin for 1 min at 6000*g*. Discard the flowthrough and the collection tube.

12. Place the DNeasy column in a clean collection tube. Rotate the column and spin again for 3 min at 13,000*g* to dry the column.
13. Place the DNeasy column in a clean microcentrifuge tube, add directly onto the column 150 μL of 70°C prewarmed buffer AE (included in the DNeasy tissue kit), let stand for 2 min at RT, and then spin for 2 min at 13,000*g* to elute.
14. Quantify the purified methylated DNA at OD 260 nm with a spectrophotometer.
15. Prepare a methylation scale. Mix both unmethylated and purified methylated genomic DNA (total amount: 2 μg) to get different methylation ratios: 0, 20, 50, 80, and 100%.
16. Modify the mixture of DNA by sodium bisulfite, followed by PCR amplification and SSCA (*see* **Subheadings 3.1., 3.2.,** and **3.3.**).

4. Notes

1. Alternative procedures for DNA extraction can be used. Our experience indicates that recovery of DNA with the DNeasy tissue kit from Qiagen is comparable to that obtained by the standard phenol/chloroform extraction or by similar approaches. Furthermore, it offers the benefit of the recovery of higher size DNA molecules from fixed tissues.
2. This fragmentation step could also be done by enzymatic digestion.
3. The fragmentation step with HCl is not necessary when genomic DNAs obtained from fixed tissues have to be modified. To denature DNA, add 3 μL of 3 *M* NaOH to the DNA solution (40 μL) and incubate for 20 min at 37°C.
4. Parts of the bisulfite modification, mainly the washing steps and the final alkali treatment, are done on one unique column. This procedure is easy to perform, limits the risk of contamination, and yields a high amount of relatively pure modified DNA, which is essential for the following PCR amplification steps.
5. Many labs have noticed that bisulfite-modified DNA is no more amplifiable after a few weeks. Using our protocol, we observed that 1 yr or even older bisulfite-modified DNA is suitable for PCR amplification, but constant freezing-thawing should be avoided.
6. In preparing the master mix, it is useful to calculate the volume required by one or two additional reactions to allow for pipeting inaccuracies and other losses of volume. Prepare the master mix on ice and add the *Taq* DNA polymerase last, just before dispensing the mix into the individual tubes.
7. If necessary, DMSO can be added to the PCR master mix. For one reaction tube, add 1 μL of DMSO and adapt the volume of water.
8. Primer sequences for amplification of modified DNA should be chosen carefully. They should be specific for bisulfite-converted DNA. They also should not comprise any CpG sites, so that methylated and unmethylated DNA sequences are equally amplified, without favoring one or the other. Nevertheless, if the bisulfite-modified DNA sequence does not allow the selection of a primer set without CG sites, the primer sequence for the upper modified DNA strand has to be corrected by changing the C of the comprised CG for a G or an A (*see* **Table 1**, forward primer TIMP-3). Furthermore, PCR product size should not exceed

250 bp for the amplification of DNA from formalin-fixed, paraffin-embedded tissue.

9. When genomic DNA, extracted from fixed tissue, has to be amplified, it is necessary to perform 40 cycles with an extension time of 75 s in place of 45 s.

10. A methylation scale is necessary to determine the dynamic range of the semiquantitative methylation analysis by PCR-SSCP. Several approaches are possible for the preparation of the methylation scale. We propose to use *Sss*I methylase to methylate all the CpG sites of genomic DNA obtained from normal tissues (*see* **Subheading 3.5.**).

11. Numerous methods can be used to visualize the amplified products, such as ethidium bromide staining or ^{32}P labeling of PCR products. However, SYBR Gold staining is a rapid method, simple to perform, and provides good sensitivity and high resolution. SYBR Gold solution can be reused several times. It is, however, recommended to store the solution in a polypropylene container.

12. If a linear regression in the band intensity is not achieved with the amplification of the methylation scale, the primers specific for the bisulfite-converted DNA, or more likely the size of the amplified PCR product, have to be changed. Indeed, we noticed that when the PCR size was higher than 300–400 bp, a better amplification was observed with the unmethylated DNA.

13. The band migration pattern of methylated or unmethylated DNA varies from one DNA sequence to another. Indeed, the change of only one base is sufficient to create a new pattern of migration by SSCA. In addition, if electrophoresis are performed under the same conditions, the band migration pattern must always be identical for each DNA sequence.

14. In cell lines, a methylation pattern of 50% corresponds to the presence of both methylated and unmethylated alleles in equal amounts, suggesting a monoallelic methylation pattern. On the other hand, in tissues with a large majority of one particular cell type, a methylation pattern of 50% could suggest either a monoallelic methylation or a heterogenous methylation (e.g., hypermethylation occurring in a subpopulation of cells).

15. Duplicate amplifications should be performed for the confirmation of the results. With a nonconvincing result (weak amplification or nonreproducible bands), the analysis has to be repeated with newly bisulfite-modified DNA or even with newly extracted genomic DNA. If reproducible results are obtained, the detection of other band mobility patterns could be explained by the presence of partially methylated alleles in the tissues. (Methylation occurs in only some of the CpG sites within the analyzed region.) For this exceptional situation, sequencing of the PCR samples is recommended to determine the exact methylation pattern.

16. Some faint bands can be seen in **Fig. 3**. They probably correspond to artifacts of PCR amplification. Indeed, almost all of them are also present in the markers (*see* Methylation scale in **Fig. 3**).

17. Methylation of a genomic DNA at all CpG sites is incomplete if the DNA is cut by the restriction enzyme *Hpa*II. Should this be the case, it is necessary to repeat the reaction with the *Sss*I methylase.

References

1. Jones, P. A. and Laird, P. W. (1999) Cancer epigenetics comes of age. *Nat. Genet.* **21,** 163–167.
2. Wajed, S. A., Laird, P. W., and DeMeester, T. R. (2001) DNA methylation: an alternative pathway to cancer. *Ann. Surg.* **234,** 10–20.
3. Wade, P. A. (2001) Methyl CpG-binding proteins and transcriptional repression. *Bioessays* **23,** 1131–1137.
4. Jones, P. A. and Baylin, S. B. (2002) The fundamental role of epigenetic events in cancer. *Nat. Rev. Genet.* **3,** 415–428.
5. Clark, S. J., Harrison, J., Paul, C. L., and Frommer, M. (1994) High sensitivity mapping of methylated cytosines. *Nucleic Acids Res.* **22,** 2990–2997.
6. Grunau, C., Clark, S. J., and Rosenthal, A. (2001) Bisulfite genomic sequencing: systematic investigation of critical experimental parameters. *Nucleic Acids Res.* **29,** E65.
7. Esteller, M., Sparks, A., Toyota, M., et al. (2000) Analysis of adenomatous polyposis coli promoter hypermethylation in human cancer. *Cancer Res.* **60,** 4366–4371.
8. Herman, J. G., Graff, J. R., Myohanen, S., Nelkin, B. D., and Baylin, S. B. (1996) Methylation-specific PCR: a novel PCR assay for methylation status of CpG islands. *Proc. Natl. Acad. Sci.USA* **93,** 9821–9826.
9. Eads, C. A., Danenberg, K. D., Kawakami, K., Saltz, L. B., Blake, C., Shibata, D., Danenberg, P. V., and Laird, P. W. (2000) MethyLight: a high-throughput assay to measure DNA methylation. *Nucleic Acids Res.* **28,** E32.
10. Xiong, Z. and Laird, P. W. (1997) COBRA: a sensitive and quantitative DNA methylation assay. *Nucleic Acids Res.* **25,** 2532–2534.
11. Gonzalgo, M. L. and Jones, P. A. (1997) Rapid quantitation of methylation differences at specific sites using methylation-sensitive single nucleotide primer extension (Ms-SNuPE). *Nucleic Acids Res.* **25,** 2529–2531.
12. Bianco, T., Hussey, D., and Dobrovic, A. (1999) Methylation-sensitive, single-strand conformation analysis (MS-SSCA): A rapid method to screen for and analyze methylation. *Hum. Mutat.* **14,** 289–293.
13. Bian, Y. S., Yan, P., Osterheld, M. C., Fontolliet, C., and Benhattar, J. (2001) Promoter methylation analysis on microdissected paraffin-embedded tissues using bisulfite treatment and PCR-SSCP. *Biotechniques* **30,** 66–72.
14. Bian, Y. S., Osterheld, M. C., Fontolliet, C., Bosman, F. T., and Benhattar, J. (2002) p16 inactivation by methylation of the CDKN2A promoter occurs early during neoplastic progression in Barrett's esophagus. *Gastroenterology* **122,** 1113–1121.

15

SIRPH Analysis

SNuPE With IP-RP-HPLC for Quantitative Measurements of DNA Methylation at Specific CpG Sites

Osman El-Maarri

Summary

This chapter describes a detailed protocol using single-nucleotide primer extension (SNuPE) for quantitative analysis of DNA methylation on specific CpG sites. The first step DNA sample to be studied is treated with sodium bisulfite, which converts selectively unmethylated cytosines to uracil, while methylated cytosines remain unconverted. Subsequently, a SNuPE reaction is performed, with an oligo just flanking a CpG site, using a purified polymerase chain reaction product derived from bisulfite-treated DNA as a template. The oligo is extended by either ddCTP or ddTTP depending on whether the site is methylated or unmethylated, respectively. The reaction is quantitative and linear, and two to three sites can be studied simultaneously in a multiple reaction. The SNuPE product, without further purification, is separated by ion-pair reverse-phase (IP RP) high-performance liquid chromatography (using an alkylated nonporous polysterene-divinylbenzene cartridge) that allows an easy, semiautomated method for separation of the extended and unextended products and an accurate quantification of the extended products. The ratio of the ddCTP to the ddTTP gives the fraction of the methylated cytosines at that specific CpG site.

Key Words: Bisulfite; CpG methylation; SNuPE; DHPLC; ion pair reverse-phase HPLC; quantitative DNA methylation analysis.

1. Introduction

In the postgenome era, and after deciphering the human genome code, functional genomics has attracted a great deal of interest. This includes the functional analysis of proteins, and their interactions, and gene expression patterns. Another layer of information is the epigenetic modifications of DNA that influence the patterns of gene expression, including factors that affect chromatin structure, such as histone modifications and cytosine methylation. In mam-

From: *Methods in Molecular Biology, vol. 287: Epigenetics Protocols*
Edited by: T. O. Tollefsbol © Humana Press Inc., Totowa, NJ

mals, cytosine methylation occurs mainly in a CpG context. DNA methylation is involved in silencing genes in a tissue-specific manner and during specific developmental stages *(1,2)*. Moreover, alterations in normal patterns of methylation are associated with many human diseases such as imprinting diseases and tumors formation *(3,4)*. Hence there is great interest in the analysis and accurate quantification of methylation levels.

Many methods exist for analyzing DNA methylation patterns; these can be divided into two approaches (reviewed in **ref. 5**). The first is the total genome approach which gives the overall content of methylated cytosines in a given DNA, such as the enzymatic cleavage of DNA to individual nucleosides followed by separations on high-performance liquid chromatography (HPLC). The second is the sequence-specific approach which helps quantify methylation with a high degree of accuracy. This includes restriction enzyme analysis with methylation-sensitive enzymes and the widely used bisulfite analysis.

Bisulfite analysis was introduced by Frommer et al. in 1992 *(6)* and became the method most used to provide sequence-independent information (vs the use of methylation-sensitive restriction enzymes, which is restricted by the enzyme recognition sequence). Bisulfite analysis gives detailed information on methylation levels and patterns in a given region. It is based on the ability of sodium bisulfite to interact selectively with cytosines at their carbon 6 position to form sulfonated cytosine intermediates. These intermediates are then converted to uracil by pH-dependent deamination and desulphonation steps. 5-Methyl cytosine remains non-reactive under such conditions. The uracil in the bisulfite-converted DNA is replaced by thymine in the subsequent polymerase chain reaction (PCR). Several protocols and modifications of the original method have been published that allow analysis of only a few cells *(7–9)*.

After successful amplification of a region of interest (using bisulfite-treated DNA as a template), the ultimate aim is to quantify the methylated (CpG) and the unmethylated (TpG) portions of the PCR product. The literature is very rich in a wide variety of methods that vary in the accuracy of the methylation levels they provide and with the machines required for analysis. The traditional method of cloning and sequencing bisulfite PCR products provides the most detailed information. This approach, however, is very time-consuming and laborious, and large numbers of clones must be analyzed to provide statistically significant results. Therefore, several groups have developed alternative methods. One such method is combined bisulfite retriction analysis (COBRA), which is based on restriction enzyme digestion of bisulfite PCR products *(10)*. The use of this method is limited, however, since it only allows analysis of CpG methylation within (newly generated) restriction sites of the bisulfite PCR products. Another method is methylation-specific PCR (MSP), which is based on using two pairs of specific primers to amplify methylated or unmethylated alleles specifically, taking advantage of the sequence differences between methylated and unmethylated CpG sites that occur after bisulfite conversion *(11)*. Although MSP is very sensitive for low amounts of methylated or unmethylated product, it does not give a detailed picture of the methylation patterns and the exact quantity of methylated/unmethylated product. Recently a more flexible method, based on differential hybridization of bisulfite PCR fragments using oligonucleotide-containing chips, was introduced *(12)*. Although this method allows high-throughput screening, it requires a high technological laboratory standard and a sophisticated and laborious chip design and analysis tools.

More flexible methods are based on single-nucleotide primer extension (SNuPE) *(13)* techniques, whereby an oligo, just flanking the 5' end of a CpG site, is extended by either ddCTP or ddTTP for methylated and unmethylated templates, respectively. The SNuPE product is then detected and measured by various methods. Gonzalgo and Jones *(14)* were the first to apply such an approach for DNA methylation analysis by developing methylation-sensitive SNuPE (MS-SNuPE), which uses incorporation of radioactive nucleotides; the extended products are separated on acrylamide gels and quantified by autoradiography. A second method is MethyLight, a real-time PCR-based SNuPE technique, which is quantitative and highly sensitive but requires special fluorescently labeled oligonucleotides *(15)*. A third method is matrix-assisted laser desorption ionization (MALDI) mass spectrometry-based separation technique of the SNuPE reaction that is accurate but requires special modified primers *(16)*. Recently we and others *(17,18)* have developed an inexpensive, nonradioactive variation of such a SNuPE protocol using ion-pair reverse-phase HPLC *(19)* as a separation and detection method (SNuPE–IP RP HPLC or SIRPH). This protocol gives an accurate quantification of methylation at selected CpG sites.

The PCR product to be analyzed is purified to remove residual PCR oligos and dNTPs. Subsequently, unmodified primers immediately 5' to a CpG site are hybridized to the denatured single-stranded PCR product. The primers used are identical in sequence to the bisulfite-treated DNA strand that contains CpGs and/or TpGs (not GCs and/or ACs on the opposite strand), and thus it will hybridize to the opposite strand that contains GCs and/or ACs; this allows addition of ddCTP and/or ddTTP nucleotides at the 3' position of the primer (**Fig. 1**). Temperature cycling using Thermo Sequenase™ in the presence of both ddCTP and ddTTP extends the annealed primers. The ddTTP (for unmethylated CpG) or ddCTP (for methylated CpG; *see* **Fig. 1**) extended products are then directly loaded on an HPLC column (Wave DNA Fragment Analysis System, Transgenomics). Because of incorporation of the more hydrophobic ddTTP, the retention time of such an extended product is longer compared with that of

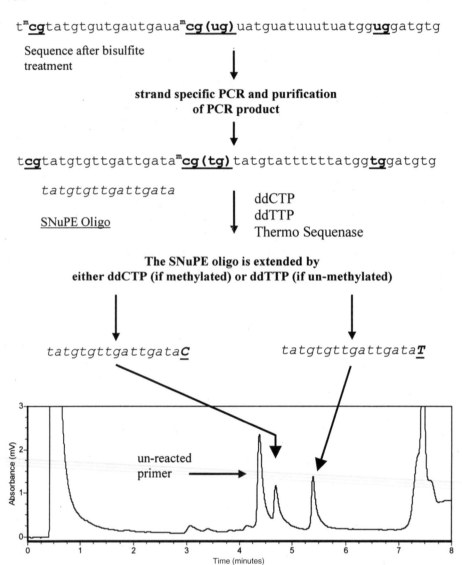

Fig. 1. General scheme of the SIRPH analysis.

products containing ddCTP (**Fig. 1**). The amount of the ddTTP and ddCTP extended products can then be quantified by measuring the height of the peaks and calculating their percentage ratios. The reaction produces highly reproducible results while maintaining linearity (**Fig. 2**).

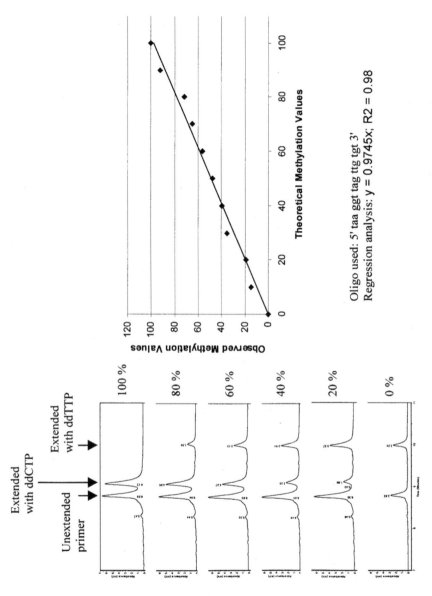

Fig. 2. Linearity of the reaction. A PCR product and a primer in the *SNRPN* gene was used with a serial mixes of methylated and unmethylated alleles in 10% increments.

2. Materials

2.1. Removal of Excess Primers and dNTPs

1. For gel extraction or direct PCR purification: QIAquick Gel Extraction kit, Qiagen, cat. no. 28704 or QIAquick PCR purification kit, cat. no. 28106.
2. A mixture of exonuclease I and shrimp alkaline phosphatase which will degrade the unreacted primers and inactivate dNTPs: ExoSap-IT, Amersham, cat. no. US78201.

2.2. SNuPE

1. ddTTP and ddCTP (Amersham, cat. no. 27-2081-01 and 27-2061-01).
2. Thermosequenase enzyme (Amersham, cat. no. E79000Y).
3. Standard unmodified oligos from *n*-1 secondary products. (Oligos by polyarcylamide gel electrophoresis [PAGE] are of sufficient quality.)

2.3. IP RP HPLC

1. For all HPLC analyses, we recommend the Wave system from Transgenomic together with the IP RP HPLC column, the DNASep (cat. no. DNA-99-3510, Transgenomic). The stationary phase in the column is made of alkylated nonporous polystyrene-divinylbenzene 2-µm beads particles (cat. no. PS/DVD-C18).
2. TEAA buffer (Transgenomic, cat. no. 553303).
3. Acetonitril (ROTH Art 8825.2).
4. HPLC-grade water (Merck, cat. no. 1.15333.2500).

3. Method

The SIRPH protocol can be divided into three parts: (1) generating the PCR product, (2) performing the SNuPE reaction, and (3) separating the products on HPLC and quantification of the peaks. In this chapter I describe the last two steps; protocols for bisulfite treatment can be found in Hajkova et al. *(8)* or El-Maarri et al. *(9)*.

3.1. Purification of PCR Product

The PCR product can be purified by one of two methods (*see* **Note 1**):

1. Run the product on 1% agarose gel until separation is optimal, excise the specific band, and recover the product by using a standard PCR-gel extraction kit (QIAquick Gel Extraction Kit, Qiagen), which yields very pure products with high rates of recovery. Alternatively, when there is no nonspecific PCR product(s), a PCR purification kit can be used directly without the need for separation on agarose (QIAquick PCR purification kit).
2. Add 2 µL of exonuclease I and shrimp alkaline phosphatase (ExoSap-IT, Amersham) to 5 µL of PCR product, and heat at 37°C for 15 min followed by 15 min at 80°C to deactivate the enzyme mixture.

3.2. SNuPE Reaction

1. Set up the SNuPE reaction in a total volume of 20 µL with the following components (*see* **Note 2**):
   a. 2 µL Reaction buffer (10 X buffer).
   b. 1 µL SNuPE Oligos (n) (12.5 pmole solution/for each oligo).
   c. SNuPE template:
      i. 1–5 µL PCR product (50–100 ng of 200–400 bp PCR product).
      ii. 1 µL ddCTP (1 m*M* solution).
      iii. 1 µL ddTTP (1 m*M* solution).
      iv. n µL Thermo Sequenase (diluted to 1 U/µL).
      v. Up tp 20 µL H$_2$O.
      vi. *n* = the number of oligos used for multiplex in the reaction.
   d. For SNuPE primers used in the reaction, *see* **Notes 3–8**.
2. Subject the above mix to the following thermocycles (*see* **Note 9**): cycle 1, 94°C for 2 min; cycle 2, 92°C for 10 s; cycle 3, 30°C for 1 min; cycle 4, 60°C for 1 min. Repeat **steps 2–4** 50 times.

3.3. Run the Products on HPLC

1. Load 10–15 µL of the PCR product directly on the HPLC machine (Wave, Transgenomics). Set the oven temperature to 50°C (*see* **Note 10**) and the elution gradient (mixture of buffers A and B) at 0.9 mL/min for 10 min:

Step	Time (min)	%A (0.1 *M* TEAA)	%B (0.1 *M* TEAA, 25% Acetonitril)
Loading	0.0	100-b1	b1
Start gradient	0.1	100-b1	b1
Stop gradient	10.0	100-b2	b
Start clean	10.01	0	100
Stop clean	11.1	0	100
Start equilibrate	11.2	100-b1	b1
Stop equilibrate	12.2	100-b1	b1

Where b1 is the start percentage of buffer B in the elution buffer that will steadily increase over a 10-min period to reach b2. The values of b1 and b2 are defined empirically for each set of SNuPE oligos (*see* **Note 11**).

2. Calculation of percent methylation: the percent of the methylated portion of the DNA can be calculated according to the formula: $M = [HC/(HC + HT)] \times 100$, where HC and HT are the peak heights of the ddCTP and ddTTP extended oligos, respectively (*see* **Notes 12–14**). The WaveMaker software automatically calculates the AC and AT.

4. Notes

1. Enzymatic treatment is more expensive but has the advantage that it is rapid and easier to perform, especially when analyzing large numbers of samples. Gel

extraction, on the other hand, is more laborious, but it has the advantage of concentrating a faint PCR product in a smaller volume. It also offers the possibility of isolating the specific product when nonspecific products are present.

2. The amount of template to be used is flexible; up to 1 µg could be used without affecting the quantification results, However, with less than 50 ng, the yield of the SNuPE reaction may not be high enough to give reproducible quantitative results. The oligos used in the SNuPE reaction should always be in excess; their corresponding band (on HPLC separation) can be used as a reference for the extended product(s) that should come shortly after.

3. The 3' end of the SNuPE oligo has to be just 5' (flanking) of the specific CpG site to be studied.

4. Avoid placing the oligo on a T-rich region, as this could increase mispriming and lead to inaccuracy in the methylation measurements; however, if possible, it is preferable to have the 3' end (region) of the oligo on a C to T (but not on an initial CpG) converted region so that the specificity to the bisulfite converted product is higher.

5. Oligos should not include a CpG site, as this will bias the linearity of measurements.

6. Oligos that are too short have a higher chance of mispriming. Oligos as short as 10 bases can still produce accurate data. However, for routine use we prefer oligos 15–18 bases long when possible.

7. For multiplex SNuPE reactions that are run simultaneously on the HPLC, the retention time of the individual oligos and their elongation products should be different. If, for practical reasons, two oligos have to be designed that give similar retention times on HPLC, we recommend extending one of the oligos by adding thymidine to its 5' end. In our experience this addition has no effect on the annealing to the template or on the SNuPE reaction. The number of Ts to be added has to be determined empirically; however, each additional T has a stepwise additional retardation effect in a linear fashion.

8. All oligos have to be tested for self-annealing and self-extension in the absence of a template.

9. The annealing temperature used is 30°C; there is no detectable change in either the yield of the reaction or the quantification results when using a range of 20°C (from 30 to 50°C) for the annealing. Therefore, as a standard procedure for all oligos used in the SNuPE reaction, a 30°C annealing is used. An extension time of 1 min should give a good reaction yield for most oligos; however, increasing the extension as well as the annealing times could give higher yields for some oligos. This has to be tested individually.

10. An oven temperature of 50°C (compared with 60, 70, and 80°C) was found to give the highest difference in retention time between the ddCTP and the ddTTP extended oligos.

11. When setting up a new assay, run with a wide gradient of 10% (b1) to 60% (b2) buffer B. Most short oligos of 10–20 bp should be eluted by this gradient. At a later stage, and depending on the retention time of the oligos, the gradient can be

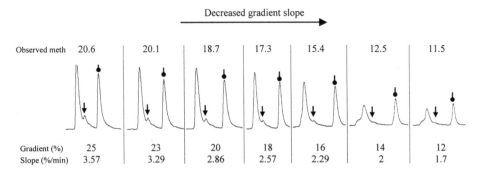

Fig. 3. Effect of the slope of the acetonitrile buffer on the separation of the minor allele (the methylated allele, in this case 12% methylated and 88% unmethylated) when it is too close to the unextended primer. The (↓) and (⬇) represent the ddCTP and ddTTP extended primers, respectively.

narrowed down from either the left side, the right side, or both sides simultaneously to give the best spatial resolution between the oligos.

12. If the unreacted primer, after HPLC separation, is close to the ddCTP extended primer, the integration of the area under the ddCTP extended primer curve may not be accurate. Therefore it is more accurate to use the peak height for measurements. The gradient used has great influence on both the separation efficiency and the accuracy of quantification, a slope of at least 2% increase of buffer B over 1 min gives a good separation (*see* **Fig. 3**). It is recommended to use the lowest slope that will still give a distinguishable peak for the minor allele (the ddCTP extended allele).

13. Reproducibility of the HPLC measurements: it is recommended that one test the accuracy of the measurement reproducibility on the HPLC machine. This can be done by injecting the same SNuPE product several times and calculating the standard deviation for each sample. Such measurements are shown in **Fig. 4**; for most oligos and at different ratios of ddCTP to ddTTP, the standard deviation ranges between 1 and 3%.

14. Limit of detection for the minor allele: this differs from one primer to another. Mainly two factors can have an influence: first, the yield of the SNuPE reaction, as some primers can be easily extended, giving a high yield that produces high peaks, whereas others are less efficient; and second, the separation between the unextended oligo and the ddCTP extended oligo, when the two peaks are partially overlapping, could lead to ambiguity in distinguishing the small peak of the ddCTP extended primer. However, for most oligos the limit of detection of the minor allele is between 5 and 10%.

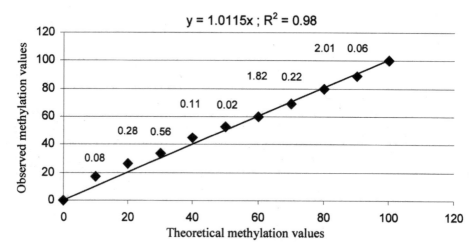

Fig. 4. Sensitivity and accuracy of HPLC measurements at different methylated/ unmethylated ratios. The same samples were reinjected three times; the standard deviation values are shown above each group of measurements.

References

1. Futscher, B. W., Oshiro, M. M., Wozniak, R. J., Holtan, N., Hanigan, C. L., Duan, H., and Domann, F. E. (2002) Role for DNA methylation in the control of cell type specific maspin expression. *Nat. Genet.* **31,** 175–179.
2. Ehrlich, M. (2003) Expression of various genes is controlled by DNA methylation during mammalian development. *J. Cell Biochem.* **88(5),** 899–910.
3. Walter, J. and Paulsen, M. (2003), Imprinting and disease. *Semin. Cell Dev. Biol.* **14,** 101–110.
4. Jones, P. A. and Baylin, S. B. (2002) The fundamental role of epigenetic events in cancer. *Nat. Rev. Genet.* **3(6),** 415–428.
5. Fraga, M. F. and Esteller, M. (2003) DNA methylation: a profile of methods and applications. *Biotechniques* **33,** 636–649.
6. Frommer, M., McDonald, L. E., Millar, D. S., Collis, C. M., Watt, F., Grigg, G. W., Molloy, P. L., and Paul, C. L. (1992) A genomic sequencing protocol that yields a positive display of 5-methylcytosine residues in individual DNA strands. *Proc. Natl. Acad. Sci. USA* **89,** 1827–1831.
7. Olek, A., Oswald, J., and Walter, J., (1996) A modified and improved method for bisulphite based cytosine methylation analysis. *Nucleic Acids Res.* **24,** 5064–5066.
8. Hajkova, P., El-Maarri, O., Engemann. S., Oswald, J., Olek, A., and Walter, J. (2002) DNA-methylation analysis by the bisulfite-assisted genomic sequencing method. *Methods Mol Biol.* **200,** 143–154.

9. El-Maarri, O., Kuepper, M., Oldenburg, J., and Walter, J. (2004) Quantitative DNA-methylation analysis by the bisulfite conversion method, in: *PCR Technology: Current Innovations* (Weissensteiner, T., Griffin, G. H., and Griffin, A., eds.), CRC Press, London, pp. 175–185.

10. Xiong, Z. and Laird, P. W. (1997) COBRA: a sensitive and quantitative DNA methylation assay. *Nucleic Acids Res.* **25**, 2532–2534.

11. Herman, J. G., Graff, J. R., Myohanen, S., Nelkin, B. D., and Baylin, S. B. (1996) Methylation-specific PCR: a novel PCR assay for methylation status of CpG islands. *Proc. Natl. Acad. Sci. USA* **93**, 9821–9826.

12. Adorjan, P., Distler, J., Lipscher, E., et al. (2002) Tumor class prediction and discovery by microarray-based DNA methylation analysis. *Nucleic Acids Res.* **30**, e21.

13. Syvanen A. C. (1999) From gels to chips: "minisequencing" primer extension for analysis of point mutations and single nucleotide polymorphisms. *Human Mutat.* **13**, 1–10.

14. Gonzalgo, M. L., and Jones, P. A. (1997) Rapid quantitation of methylation differences at specific sites using methylation-sensitive single nucleotide primer extension (Ms-SNuPE). *Nucleic Acids Res.* **25**, 2529–2531

15. Eads, C. A., Danenberg, K. D., Kawakami, K., et al. (2000) MethyLight: a high-throughput assay to measure DNA methylation. *Nucleic Acids Res.* **28**, e32.

16. Tost, J., Schatz, P., Schuster, M., Berlin, K. and Gut, I. G. (2003) Analysis and accurate quantification by MALDI mass spectrometry. *Nucleic Acids Res.* **31**, e50.

17. Matin, M. M., Baumer, A., and Hornby, D. P. (2002) An analytical method for the detection of methylation differences at specific chromosomal loci using primer extension and ion pair reverse phase HPLC. *Human Mutat.* **20**, 305–311.

18. El-Maarri, O., Herbiniaux, U., Walter, J., and Oldenburg, J. (2002) A rapid, quantitative, non-radioactive bisulfite-SNuPE- IP RP HPLC assay for methylation analysis at specific CpG sites. *Nucleic Acids Res.* **30**, e25.

19. Xiao, W. and Oefner, P. J. (2001) Denaturing high-performance liquid chromatography: A review. *Human Mutat.* **17**, 439–474.

16

Real-Time PCR-Based Assay for Quantitative Determination of Methylation Status

Ulrich Lehmann and Hans Kreipe

Summary

The best studied epigenetic modification in mammals is the methylation of cytosine. During the development and progression of malignant neoplasia, a global hypomethylation is often accompanied by a locus-specific increase in methylation. Also, during normal development specific alterations in DNA methylation patterns take place. In recent years it has become clear that in many situations only quantitative changes in methylation levels occur and that the pure qualitative detection of cytosine methylation misses important biological and pathophysiological information. Therefore, several protocols were developed for the quantitative detection of cytosine methylation. Here, we describe a real-time polymerase chain reaction-based assay for the sensitive and precise quantification of methylated and unmethylated alleles after bisulfite treatment of genomic DNA. In addition to providing quantitative methylation data, this methodology is suitable for high-throughput analysis.

Key Words: Real-time PCR; methylation-specific PCR; methylation; bisulfite conversion; DNA isolation.

1. Introduction

DNA methylation in mammalian cells occurs at the carbon atom 5 of cytosine within the dinucleotide CpG. The CpG dinucleotide displays a non-random distribution in the genome; the occurrence of 5-methylcytosine within this sequence also shows a nonrandom pattern. Short GC-rich sequences with enhanced frequency of CpG, called CpG islands (*1,2*), are interspersed throughout the otherwise CpG-poor genome. These CpG islands are very often found in the 5'-region of genes, and the methylation status of the cytosine residues affects the transcriptional activation of the gene. In general, high levels of methylation are tightly linked to transcriptional repression (*3*). Methylation patterns change not only during normal ontogenesis (*4*) but also during the

From: *Methods in Molecular Biology, vol. 287: Epigenetics Protocols*
Edited by: T. O. Tollefsbol © Humana Press Inc., Totowa, NJ

clonal evolution of cancer cells *(5)*. Therefore, there is a great interest in determination of methylation patterns and the quantitative assessment of methylation levels in tissue samples, preferentially with a technology that allows for the analysis of large sample series.

Nearly all protocols currently in use for the detection of methylation employ either methylation-sensitive restriction endonucleases (followed by Southern blotting or polymerase chain reaction [PCR]) or bisulfite treatment of DNA (followed by PCR). Incubation of genomic DNA with high concentrations of biulfite in acidic solution converts unmethylated cytosine to uracil (subsequently amplified as thymidine), whereas 5'-methylcytosine remains unaltered *(6)*. Thus, the epigenetic information of DNA methylation, which is lost during conventional cloning and amplification protocols, is translated into the primary sequence (*see* **Fig. 1**). After bisulfite treatment, the so-called converted DNA is amplified and analyzed employing a wide variety of methodologies.

To gain quantitative information on the methylation of a specific CpG site, several protocols have been developed (*see* **Subheading 3.6.**). Our approach is based on the following idea: after bisulfite treatment there exists a mixture of methylated and unmethylated "alleles," which can now be discriminated owing to the sequence differences introduced by the bisulfite treatment in analogy to the allelotyping already well described for the real-time PCR technology *(7)*. The CpG sites of interest are amplified with one flanking primer pair containing no methylation sites in their binding site. This ensures equal amplification of methylated and unmethylated DNA (equal efficiency has to be proved experimentally!). The discrimination between methylated and unmethylated DNA is achieved only on the level of the hybridization probes annealing in between the primers (one specific for methylated DNA and the other for unmethylated DNA). If equal reaction efficiency has been demonstrated for both primer/probe combinations, the detected fluorescence signals are a direct measure for the ratio of methylated and unmethylated DNA (*see* **Subheading 3.4.**).

In addition to the quantitative information provided by this new assay, further advantages are the speed and high throughput of the 96-well-based, real-time PCR system and the omission of all postamplification steps, which greatly reduces the work load and the risk of contamination. Also, the efficiency of individual reactions is accessible from the slope of the amplification plot in the logarithmic phase. This allows for the direct quality control of every amplification reaction and the identification of samples containing impurities or poor template that interfered with optimal amplification and thereby with the quantification.

1.1. Primer/Probe Design

The selection of new primer pairs for methylation-specific PCR and suitable hybridization probes for real-time PCR-based assays requires in the first step

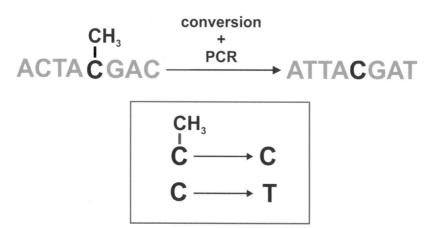

Fig. 1. Principal of bisulfite treatment of DNA. The epigenetic modification is converted into a difference in the primary sequence.

the identification of the CpG sites that are actually methylated. This is very often the most time-consuming step in the whole project. For some genes all relevant information is published, but often detailed analysis of the sample type that will be analyzed in larger series later on (e.g., breast cancer specimens) has to be performed. For this purpose genomic sequencing of bisulfite-treated DNA and/or sequencing of individual clones after amplification has to be employed. A general critical remark is that many primers described in the literature represent just a good guess of methylated sites, and often the results concerning cytosine methylation obtained within one cell type are transferred to a different cell type without actually demonstrating that this conclusion is justified.

If the CpG sites of interest have been identified, the major problem for primer selection is the considerably reduced sequence complexity after bisulfite treatment owing to the conversion of all non-CpG cytosines and all nonmethylated cytosines to uracil (equal to thymidine). Overall, there will be only three bases instead of four! The bisulfite treatment often generates long stretches of T alternating with very G- or CG-rich segments. This makes primer selection difficult and sometimes impossible.

The guidelines we try to follow are listed below:

1. The primer binding sites should include several cytosines in the original sequence to ensure specificity for converted DNA.
2. The 3'-end of the primer binding site should be a potentially methylated cytosine (to ensure maximal specificity for methylated or unmethylated DNA).
3. The annealing temperature of both primers should be similar (Unfortunately, in our experience every primer design program gives you a different optimal annealing temperature. The authors have had good experiences with

PrimerExpress© from Applied Biosystems, but internal consistency, i.e., always using the same program with identical parameters, is most important.)

4. The primer and probe sequences should include three to five potential methylation sites to maximize specificity.
5. Long repetitive stretches should be avoided.
6. The length of the primers should not exceed 30 nucleotides.
7. The PCR products should be as short as possible (60–80 bp), to maximize efficiency (especially important for the analysis of fragmented DNA isolated from formalin-fixed, paraffin-embedded biopsies).

1.2. Organization of the Laboratory

The enormous amplification power of PCR (up to 10^{13} times!), which is the basis for the exquisite sensitivity of this technology, also creates a serious problem: risk of contamination owing to the introduction of exogenous DNA into the reaction mixture. Since every PCR produces vast amounts of amplifiable molecules (usually much more than 10^9 molecules in a small volume of 15–25 μL) that can potentially contaminate subsequent amplification reactions of the same target sequence, the strict physical separation of the analysis of reaction products (after amplification) from all stages of sample preparation (before amplification) has to be implemented.

For these reasons, strictly enforced guidelines concerning the cleaning of instruments and the handling of samples before and after amplification need to be followed by all personnel involved. We perform all preamplification steps in a separate laboratory consisting of two rooms: one for setting up the PCR master mix (a "template-free" room) and the other for DNA extraction, bisulfite treatment, and adding converted DNA to the PCR mix.

Plastic labware and the benches are cleaned regularly using a 3% hypochlorite solution. The PCR products are analyzed in a separate laboratory. Under no circumstances should amplified samples or equipment from this working area be brought back to the pre-PCR area.

2. Materials

1. Proteinase K-buffer: 50 mM Tris-HCl, pH 8.1, 1 mM EDTA, 0.5% Tween-20.
2. Proteinase K, stock solution: 20 mg/mL in water, aliquots stored at –20°C (Merck, Darmstadt, Germany).
3. TE buffer: 10 mM Tris-HCl pH 8.1, 1 mM EDTA.
4. Phenol/chloroform/isoamylalcohol (25:24:1; Roth, Karlsruhe, Germany).
5. Sodium bisulfite: ACS reagent (Sigma, Deisenhofen, Germany, cat. no. S-8890), containing approx 75% metabisulfite according to the SO_2 content analysis performed by the manufacturer.
6. 4.1 M Sodium bisulfite pH 5,0, 1 mM hydroquinon: dissolve 8 g sodium bisulfite in 15 mL water (6 g metabisulfite and 2 g bisulfite, yielding 82.4 mmol bisulfite

when dissolved in water). For complete dissolving, the solution has to be heated to 50°C; also vigorous vortexing is often necessary. For adjusting pH to 5.0, approx 1 mL 10 M NaOH is required. Finally, 1 mL freshly prepared 20 mM Hydroquinone is added and the volume adjusted to 20 mL.

7. 20 mM Hydrochinone (Merck).
8. β-mercaptoethanol (Roth, Karlsruhe, Germany).
9. Sodium iodide: ACS reagent (Sigma, cat. no. S-9539).
10. 6 M Sodium iodide, 1 mM β-mercaptoethanol: dissolve 8.99 g NaI in 10 mL water and add 1 µL β-mercaptoethanol. The final β-mercaptoethanol concentration is approx 1.4 mM.
11. 3 M NaOH.
12. 20 mM NaOH, 90% ethanol.
13. "Glass milk" (QUIAEX suspension II, Quiagen, Hilden, Germany, cat. no. 20902).
14. *Taq*-polymerase: PlatinumTaq (Invitrogene, Karlsruhe, Germany).
15. PCR buffer: supplied with the enzyme.
16. Nucleotides for PCR: 10 mM dNTP-Mix (MBI, Fermentas, St. Leon-Roth, Germany).
17. ROX: passive reference dye, 100 µM stock solution (TibMolBiol, Berlin, Germany), stored at –20°C in the dark in small aliquots.
18. PCR tubes: optical tubes and caps (Applied Biosystems, Darmstadt, Germany).
19. PCR primers and probes for *p16INK4a*: PCR primers (Sigma-Ark, Darmstadt, Germany), and double-labeled hybridization probes (BioTeZ, Berlin, Germany).
    E5: 5'-CRTTATCTACTCTCCCCCTCTCC;
    E6 5'-GGTTGGTTATTAGAGGGTGGGG;
    M-probe: 5'-FAM-AACCGCCGAACGCACGC-TAMRA;
    U-probe: 5'-FAM-CAACCACCAAACACACACAATCCACC-TAMRA
    (R: A or G)
20. Tips with aerosol protection, DNase-, RNase-free (Sarstedt, Nümbrecht, Germany).
21. High-performance liquid chromatography (HPLC)-water (JT Baker, Deeventer, Holland, cat. no. 4218).
22. 3 M Sodium acetate, pH 7.0, containing 100 µg/mL Dextran T500 (Sigma, Taufkirchen, Germany).
23. Hypochlorite solution: use diluted 1:4 with tap water (Roth, Karlsruhe, Germany).
24. PCR bench with ultraviolet (UV) lamp, for decontamination of racks.
25. Real-time PCR instrumentation: SDS7700 (Applied Biosystems, Darmstadt, Germany).
26. Refrigerated table-top centrifuge for 0.2–2.0-mL tubes (max. 14,000g).
27. Vortex.
28. Thermoshaker with heated lid (CLF, Emersacker, Germany).

All PCR reagents are stored in aliquots to avoid repeated thawing and freezing and to minimize the risk of contamination.

The concentration of the TaqMan™ probes is checked by optical density (OD) measurement. When converting OD_{260nm} into probe concentration, the additional absorption owing to the two fluorophores has to be kept in mind.

Different suppliers give different numbers for the extinction coefficient of the same probe, but the calculated concentration differences are not really significant.

The dissolved probes are stored in small aliquots in the dark at –20ºC.

3. Methods

3.1. DNA Isolation

Methylation analysis relying on the bisulfite conversion of genomic DNA is compatible with DNA preparations of variable purity since the bisulfite treatment is a robust nonenzymatical chemical reaction.

More important for the success of the conversion is an efficient strand separation before addition of the bisulfite because this reagent reacts only with single-stranded DNA and not double-stranded DNA (*see* below).

In most instances we isolate DNA from frozen sections or formalin-fixed, paraffin-embedded samples by overnight incubation with proteinase K followed by extensive phenol/chloroform extraction and ethanol precipitation.

3.2. Bisulfite Conversion

The principal drawback of the bisulfite method is the fact that prolonged incubation of DNA with high concentrations of bisulfite in acidic solution destroys nucleic acids completely. Therefore the right balance between complete conversion and minimal damage of DNA has to be found.

3.2.1. Bisulfite Treatment of DNA

1. Incubate the DNA in a total volume of 50 µL of 200 mM NaOH at 42°C for 30 min for complete separation of both strands.
2. Add 275 µL 4.1 M bisulfite containing 1 mM hydroquinone (freshly prepared), and incubate the samples for 4 h at 55°C in the dark (*see* **Note 1**).
3. Add 375 µL 6 M sodium iodine containing 1 mM β-mercaptoethanol and 5 µL glass milk suspension (Quiagen, Hilden, Germany) and mix thoroughly.
4. After 10 min at room temperature, centrifuge the samples at 14,000g for 3 min at 4°C and discard the supernatant.
5. Wash the pellet three times with 70% ethanol.
6. Resuspend the pellet in 20 mM NaOH, 90% ethanol and incubate for 5 min at room temperature.
7. Wash the pellet twice with 90% ethanol (*see* **Note 2**).
8. Elute the air-dried pellet with 25 µL TE buffer for 15 min at 55°C (*see* **Note 3**).
9. Centrifuge again (14,000g, 3 min, 4°C) and transfer the supernatant to a fresh tube; 1–5 µL of this solution are used for methylation-specific PCR.
10. If the DNA is not used directly for PCR analysis, it is stored at –20°C (*see* **Note 4**).

We have also had good experience with the CpGenome modification kit from ONCOR (European supplier: QBIOGENE, Illkirch, France) for bisulfite conversion. However, this kit is quite expensive. To reduce the costs per sample it is possible to use only half the amount of reagents compared with the protocol provided by the manufacturer.

3.3. PCR

3.3.1. Master Mix

The PCR master mix contains all reaction components except the converted DNA, which is added in a separate area of the pre-PCR laboratory (*see* **Subheading 1.2.**). The primer and probe concentrations are 250 and 125 n*M*, respectively. For each reaction, 0.5 U *Taq*-polymerase (Platinum-Taq, Life Science Technologies, Karlsruhe, Germany) are used at a magnesium concentration of 2.5 m*M* in a total volume of 25 µL. The concentration of nucleotides (dNTPs) is always 200 µ*M*. We use ROX as an internal reference at a concentration of 1 µ*M*. The volume of the master mix is 20 µL per reaction, and the template DNA is always added in a volume of 5 µL in order to reduce volume errors during pipeting. For every primer/probe combination, a negative control is performed by adding water instead of DNA to the master mix.

3.3.2. Cycle Conditions

After an initial denaturation step at 95°C for 5 min, 45 cycles with 15 s at 95°C and 60 s at 60°C follow.

3.4. Assay Validation and Data Evaluation

As positive and negative controls, cell line DNA with a defined methylation status of the gene of interest is used. Preferably, the cell line DNA serving as positive control should be methylated completely and homogeneously, i.e., all cytosine residues in the region analyzed should be methylated in all cells. The negative control should be devoid of any methylation.

Alternatively, in vitro methylated DNA can be used as positive control. The advantage is that in vitro methylated DNA can serve as a positive control for all genes; the disadvantage being that the methylation reaction has to be performed regularly and may vary in its efficiency.

Real-time instrumentation provides the possibility of controlling the quality of every amplification reaction by carefully analyzing the amplification plot: the slope in the linear range has to be the same for all reactions compared.

As a caveat, we and others have found that the C_T values generated by different lots of the same probe are not identical. No German suppliers of hybridization probes guarantee absolute uniformity of different lots of the same sequence. Therefore, one has to compare the amplification plots of a newly purchased lot of a hybridization probe with amplification plots generated by aliquots from the former lot. In some cases we have observed differences of nearly two cycles.

Figure 2B shows the amplification plot for the analysis of a 1:1 mixture of methylated and unmethylated DNA. The degree of methylation for a given mixture is calculated as follows:

$$\%M = (1/R + 1) \times 100$$

with $R = (1 + E)^{\Delta Ct(M-U)}$, the measured reaction efficiency $E = 0.95$, and $\Delta Ct(M - U)$ is the difference in the Ct-values for the amplification of methylated (M reaction) and unmethylated (U reaction) alleles.

Equal efficiency for the amplification of both methylated and unmethylated DNA has to be shown in dilution experiments using several different preparations of converted DNA. If the efficiencies differ by more than a few percent, then new primers should be tested. A slightly different primer sequence can alter reaction efficiency to a significant extent. The efficiency of a PCR system is given by the slope of the regression line if the measured Ct values are plotted against DNA input:

$$E = 10^{-1/s} - 1$$

where E = reaction efficiency and S = slope of the regression line (Ct value/ DNA input-diagram). (For derivation, *see* **ref. 8**.)

3.4.1. Derivation of the Formula for the Calculation of the Degree of Methylation

Basic equation describing the PCR process:

$$X_n = X_0(1 + E)^n$$

where X_0 = template concentration at the beginning of the reaction, X_n = template concentration after n cycles, and E = reaction efficiency ($E = 1$ means a doubling in every cycle, for 100% reaction efficiency).

For the point of time (given as a cycle number) when the generated fluorescent signal crosses the threshold of detection, the so called C_T value, one can write:

$$M_T = M_0(1 + E)^{CT,M} = \text{constant}$$

for the amplification of methylated alleles and

$$U_T = U_0(1 + E)^{CT,U} = \text{constant}$$

for the unmethylated alleles.

It follows that:

$$M_T/U_T = M_0/U_0 \times (1 + E)^{[CT,M - CT,U]} = C'$$

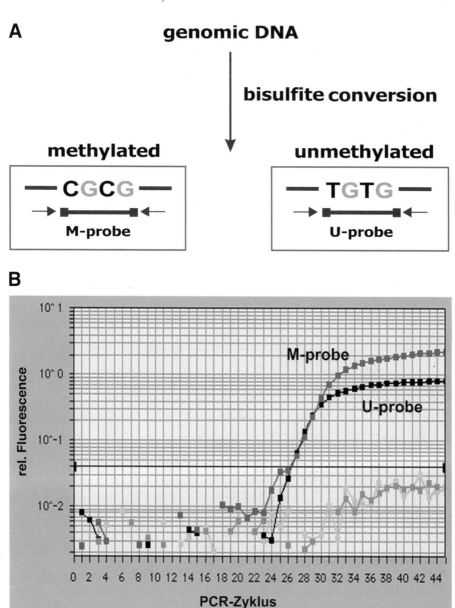

Fig. 2. (A) Principle of real-time MSP. A primer pair containing no potential methylation site in its sequences amplifies a short stretch of DNA containing the CpG sites for which the methylation status is to be determined. The very short length of the amplicon ensures identical amplification efficiencies for methylated and unmethylated alleles. **(B)** Amplification plots for a 1:1 mixture of methylated and unmethylated DNA, demonstrating equal reaction efficiencies.

or

$$C \times U_0/M_0 = (1 + E)^{\Delta CT(M-U)}, \text{ with } \Delta C_{T(M-U)} = C_{T,M} - C_{T,U}$$

Since we could show that $\Delta C_T = 0$ in case $U_0 = M_0$ (50% methylation), $C' = 1$ for this special case.

This means that for an unknown ratio between methylated and unmethylated alleles:

$$U_0{:}M_0 = R{:}1$$

where $R = (1 + E)^{\Delta CT(M-U)}$
where $U_0 + M_0 = 1$ it follows:

$$(1/M_0) - 1 = R$$

or

$$M_0 = 1/R + 1$$

or, as percentage:

$$M_0(\%) = (1/R + 1) \times 100$$

where $R = 1.9^{\Delta CT(M-U)}$, because the measured reaction efficiency is 0.95.

3.5. Supplementary Protocol for the Isolation of DNA From Microdissected Samples

The P.A.L.M. Laser-MicroBeam System (P.A.L.M., Bernried, Germany) is currently used at our institute.

1. Catapult the microdissected samples into the lid of a 0.5-mL reaction tube. Only the tubes offered by P.A.L.M. can be used for this, because for this application the distance between the section and the inner side of the lid is too great in the tubes made by other manufacturers.
2. Apply 30 – 50 µL proteinase K digestion buffer (50 mM Tris-HCl, pH 8.1, 1 mM EDTA, 0.5%, Tween-20, and 0.1 mg/mL proteinase K) to the lid and close the tubes in this inverted position. Leave the tubes to stand on their lids.
3. Incubate the samples overnight at 40°C in this inverted position in a small hybridization oven.
4. Centrifuge the tubes for 3 min at 14,000g, and incubate the samples at 95°C for 10 min in a thermoblock with a heated lid to inactivate the proteinase K (*see* **Note 5**).
5. Centrifuge the samples briefly and store at –20°C.

3.6. Further Reading

Original publications of real-time PCR-based protocols for quantification of DNA methylation are as follows:

1. Eads et al., 2000 *(10)*: The authors use an M-primer pair with an M-probe and compare signal intensity with a methylation-independent DNA input control.
2. Lehmann et al., 2001 *(11)*, described in here.
3. Lo et al., 1999 *(12)*: the authors use an M-primer pair in combination with an M-probe and a U-primer pair in combination with a U-probe. For quantification, an external standard is analyzed.
4. Muller-Tiedeow et al., 2001 *(13)*: the authors use an M-primer pair and a corresponding U-primer pair and one methylation-independent probe for both. For quantification, an external standard is analyzed.

4. Notes

1. The major modification we have introduced is the much shortened incubation time for the bisulfite treatment. Traditionally samples were incubated overnight (for ~16 h) to achieve complete conversion. It has been our experience that near complete destruction of DNA occurs after 16 h of incubation in the highly concentrated bisulfite solution at an acidic pH (pH = 5.0). This bisulfite-mediated degradation of DNA is a special problem when one is analyzing DNA isolated from archival specimens because the DNA is already highly fragmented. Real-time PCR was used to measure the DNA before and after bisulfite treatment. We demonstrated that after 3 h unconverted DNA is not detectable and the specific signals for the converted DNA have already reached their maximum (U. Lehmann, unpublished data). These observations have recently been confirmed by another group *(9)*. If small amounts of DNA are treated like that obtained by microdissection, we add 1 µg of an unspecific carrier nucleic acid (e.g., yeast DNA or tRNA, molecular biology grade) to minimize loss of material.
2. Careful purification of the bisulfite-treated DNA and complete separation of glass beads after elution is essential because traces of the chemicals used for the conversion can inhibit subsequent PCR amplifications and glass beads reduce the stability of nucleic acids during storage of DNA.
3. If larger amounts of DNA have been bisulfite-treated, the elution step can be repeated to increase recovery (but this reduces the concentration of the DNA in the final volume).
4. We did not perform systematic studies on the stability of bisulfite-treated DNA in the freezer. In our experience, starting with high-molecular-weight DNA isolated from fresh or fresh frozen material (cell pellets or biopsies), DNA is stable over several months after bisulfite treatment. This stability is clearly reduced if highly fragmented DNA isolated from formalin-fixed, paraffin-embedded biopsies is used for methylation studies.
5. If too much dye is present in the lysate or if several samples have to be pooled in order to increase the yield of DNA, a simple precipitation using ethanol and sodium acetate containing dextran as a carrier may be performed. For this purpose a 1:10 vol of sodium acetate, pH 7.0 containing 100 µg/mL dextran (MW: 500,000; Sigma, Deisenhofen, Germany) and 2.5 vol of absolute ethanol are added. After incubation at –20°C for at least 24 h, the samples are centrifuged (20 min, 14,000g, 4°C), washed once with 70% ethanol, air-dried, and dissolved in 20–50 µL TE-buffer (10 mM Tris-HCl, pH 8.0, 1 mM EDTA).

References

1. Bird, A. P. (1986) CpG-rich islands and the function of DNA methylation. *Nature* **321**, 209–213.
2. Gardiner-Garden, M. and Frommer, M. (1987) CpG islands in vertebrate genomes. *J. Mol. Biol.* **196**, 261–282.
3. Attwood, J. T., Yung, R. L., and Richardson, B. C. (2002) DNA methylation and the regulation of gene transcription. *Cell Mol. Life Sci.* **59**, 241–257.
4. Costello, J. F. and Plass, C. (2001) Methylation matters. *J. Med. Genet.* **38**, 285–303.
5. Esteller, M. (2002) CpG island hypermethylation and tumor suppressor genes: a booming present, a brighter future. *Oncogene* **21**, 5427–5440.
6. Frommer, M., McDonald, L. E., Millar, D. S., et al. (1992) A genomic sequencing protocol that yields a positive display of 5- methylcytosine residues in individual DNA strands. *Proc. Natl. Acad. Sci. USA* **89**, 1827–1831.
7. Sevall, J. S. (2001) Rapid allelic discrimination from real-time DNA amplification. *Methods* **25**, 452–455.
8. AppliedBiosystems (1997) User Bulletin #2, ABI Prism 7700 Sequence Detection System. Applied Biosystems.
9. Grunau, C., Clark, S. J., and Rosenthal, A. (2001) Bisulfite genomic sequencing: systematic investigation of critical experimental parameters. *Nucleic Acids Res.* **29**, E65–70.
10. Eads, C. A., Danenberg, K. D., Kawakami, K., et al. (2000) MethyLight: a high-throughput assay to measure DNA methylation. *Nucleic Acids Res.* **28**, E32–38.
11. Lehmann, U., Hasemeier, B., Lilischkis, R., and Kreipe, H. (2001) Quantitative analysis of promoter hypermethylation in laser- microdissected archival specimens. *Lab. Invest.* **81**, 635–638.
12. Lo, Y. M., Wong, I. H., Zhang, J., Tein, M. S., Ng, M. H., and Hjelm, N. M. (1999) Quantitative analysis of aberrant p16 methylation using real-time quantitative methylation-specific polymerase chain reaction. *Cancer Res.* **59**, 3899–3903.
13. Muller-Tidow, C., Bornemann, C., Diederichs, S., et al. (2001) Analyses of the genomic methylation status of the human cyclin A1 promoter by a novel real-time PCR-based methodology. *FEBS Lett.* **490**, 75–78.

17

Denaturing Gradient Gel Electrophoresis to Detect Methylation Changes in DNA

Masahiko Shiraishi

Summary

Denaturing gradient gel electrophoresis (DGGE) is a technique that fractionates DNA molecules on the basis of their melting behavior and thereby permits the separation of DNA fragments with local variations in base composition. The separation of DNA fragments by DGGE is determined by the nucleotide sequence, rather than size. This approach is effective when part of the molecule is relatively dense in G+C pairs. This separation is possible because of the pronounced drop in electrophoretic mobility in a polyacrylamide gel that occurs when a region of a DNA molecule melts, thereby forming a structure that is partly helical and partly random chain. The electrophoretic mobility of these partly melted DNA fragments is much lower than that of fully helical or fully dissociated molecules. The low residual mobility of the fragment restricts migration into more strongly denaturing regions of the gradient gel and results in focusing of the band. This property can be applied to detect the difference in melting temperature between methylated and nonmethylated DNA fragments after chemical treatment, or to enrich genomic regions in which aberrant methylation occurs. In this chapter, the application of DGGE to the analysis of genomic DNA methylation is reviewed.

Key Words: Bisulfite modification; CpG island; melting map; melting temperature; partial melting; segregation of partly melted molecules.

1. Introduction

Denaturing gradient gel electrophoresis (DGGE) is a technique used to separate DNA fragments on the basis of local variation in base composition within the DNA fragments (reviewed in **ref. 1**). Separation is made possible because of the pronounced drop in electrophoretic mobility (in a polyacrylamide gel) that occurs when a region of a DNA molecule melts and a structure forms that is partly helical and partly random chain. The electrophoretic mobility of these partly melted DNA fragments is much lower than that of fully helical or fully dissociated molecules. The low residual mobility of the fragment restricts mi-

From: *Methods in Molecular Biology, vol. 287: Epigenetics Protocols*
Edited by: T. O. Tollefsbol © Humana Press Inc., Totowa, NJ

gration into more strongly denaturing regions of the gradient gel and results in a sharp focusing of the band.

DGGE was originally developed to permit sequence-determined separation of DNA fragments *(2)* and was applied to the detection of variations in DNA sequences *(3)*. The underlying principle of DGGE is that two DNA fragments, which differ only by a single base pair, can vary in their melting temperature (T_m) and retard at different levels in a denaturing gradient gel *(4)*. This is effective when the single base change occurs in the domain that has the lowest T_m *(4)*.

In this article, two applications of DGGE to the study of DNA methylation are described. The first application exploits the difference in T_m of DNA fragments after chemical modification and PCR. Cytosine residues in single-stranded DNA are converted to uracil residues when they are treated with sodium bisulfite, whereas 5-methylcytosine reacts very weakly and remains largely unmodified (reviewed in **ref. 5**). Subsequent PCR produces a conversion of uracil (that was converted from cytosine) to thymine; 5-methylcytosine remains as cytosine. This difference results in different T_ms of the treated fragments. The second application of DGGE is for the isolation of DNA fragments associated with CpG islands owing to the reduced rate of strand dissociation of partly melted DNA fragments containing many CpG sites. This method is known as segregation of partly melted molecules (SPM) *(6)*.

2. Materials

1. Gradient Maker (SG30, Amersham Biosciences).
2. Electrophoresis apparatus: glass plates, spacers, combs, and so on (SE600 Standard Vertical Units, Amersham Biosciences). A spacer of 0.75 mm is preferred.
3. Tank: although a tank for the SE600 Standard Vertical Units is commercially available, an appropriate tank can be manually arranged supplemented with appropriate equipment such as a heater, stirrer, and thermostat.
4. Acrylamide (Wako).
5. Bis-acrylamide (Bio-Rad).
6. Urea (Gibco-BRL).
7. Formamide (Merck).
8. Ammonium persulfate (Wako).
9. TEMED (Wako).
10. Electrophoresis buffer (1× TAE): 40 mM Tris-HCl, 20 mM sodium acetate, 1 mM EDTA, pH 7.4.
11. Acrylamide stock solution (40% acrylamide): 37.5:1 acrylamide/bis-acrylamide.
12. Denaturant solution (0% denaturant): for 300 mL, 60 mL of 40% acrylamide stock solution, 15 mL of 20× TAE, and water to 300 mL.
13. Denaturant solution (90% denaturant): for 300 mL, 60 mL of 40% acrylamide stock solution, 15 mL of 20× TAE, 108 g of urea, 113 mL of formamide, and water to 300 mL. One hundred percent denaturant is 7 M urea and 40% formamide.

14. Peristaltic pump (Micro Tube Pump MP-3B, Tokyo Rikakikai) with tubing.
15. Power supply: any power supply that can provide 200 V and 200 mA will do.
16. 10 mg/mL Ethidium bromide solution.
17. Computer program MELT94: available at http://web.mit.edu/osp/www.melt.html. For more detailed information, contact Leonard Lerman (lslerman@mit.edu).
18. Restriction endonucleases: *Tsp*509I, *Mse*I, *Nla*III, and *Bfa*I (New England BioLabs).
19. Elution buffer: 0.5 M ammonium acetate, 10 mM manganese acetate, 1 mM EDTA, 0.1% sodium dodecyl sulfate (SDS).
20. SUPREC™01 (TaKaRa).

Materials and apparatus for DGGE are also described extensively elsewhere *(7,8)*.

3. Methods

The manner in which methylation changes are detected by DGGE is identical to the approach for the detection of sequence variation (*see* **Notes 1** and **2**) *(7,8)*. A similar system is also applied to the SPM method. In this section, two systems of DGGE are described. When a gradient of denaturant is parallel to the electric field, the system is called *parallel gradient gel*. Alternatively, when the gradient is perpendicular to the electric field, the term *perpendicular gradient gel* is used.

3.1. Preparation of a Denaturing Gradient Gel (Parallel Gradient Gel)

1. Prepare two 10-mL solutions having different denaturant concentration by mixing the appropriate volume of 0 and 90% denaturant solutions. The optimal concentration can be determined either by computation or empirically (*see* **Notes 3** and **4**). Add 100 µL of 10% ammonium persulfate solution and 4 µL of TEMED. Mix well and put on ice.
2. Slowly pour 8.2 mL of each solution down the wall of the chamber of the gradient maker. The solution with the higher denaturant concentration is in the right side chamber (**Fig. 1A**, output side). Take care not to block the connecting tube with air bubbles. Place a stirring bar in the higher concentration denaturant solution and begin vigorous stirring. Turn on the peristaltic pump, then immediately open the two stopcocks simultaneously, and transfer the solution into the frame.
3. Mark the top of the poured solution. Fill the remaining space with the solution that has a lower concentration of denaturant. Place a comb in the top of the acrylamide. Allow the gel to polymerize for at least 30 min. The gel can be left overnight at an ambient temperature.

3.2. Preparation of a Denaturing Gradient Gel (Perpendicular Gradient Gel)

1. Dispense (ice-cold) 10 mL of 0% (or other appropriate concentration) and 10 mL of 90% denaturant solutions. The gel-casting apparatus should be set up as shown in **Fig. 2**.

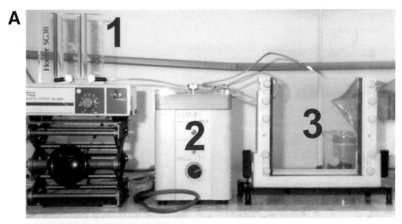

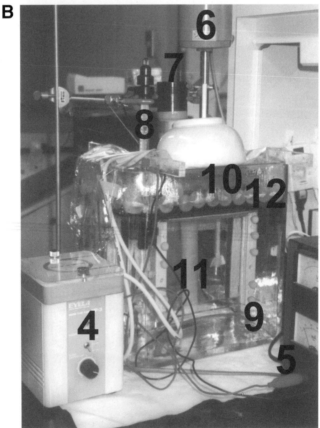

Fig. 1. (A,B) Electrophoresis apparatus and preparation of a denaturing gradient gel. 1, gradient maker on a magnetic stirrer; 2, peristaltic pump; 3, vertical gel-casting apparatus; 4, peristaltic pump; 5, power supply; 6, mixer; 7, heater; 8, thermostat; 9, tank (11 L); 10, upper buffer chamber; 11, immersed gel; 12, float.

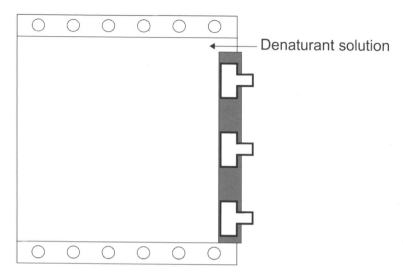

Denaturant solution

Fig. 2. Orientation of the gel frame for the preparation of a perpendicular gradient gel. The gel-casting apparatus is set up as shown in **Fig. 1A**. A spacer (gray bar) is attached to the top and turned to the right side. The acrylamide solution is poured at the edge of the spacer.

2. Follow **Subheading 3.1., steps 1** and **2**.
3. After polymerization, wash out the unpolymerized solution by rinsing with 1× TAE, and then fill the remaining space with 0% denaturant solution (or other appropriate concentration) with ammonium persulfate and TEMED. Allow the gel to polymerize for at least 30 min. The gel can be left overnight.

3.3. Denaturing Gradient Gel Electrophoresis (Parallel Gradient Gel)

1. Preheat the buffer in the tank to 60°C using an additional heater together with a rod heater, as shown in **Fig. 1B** (*see* **Note 5**).
2. Remove the comb and wash the slot twice with 1× TAE immediately prior to loading the samples. Fill the slot with 1× TAE. Any conventional gel loading solution can be used.
3. After loading the samples, place the gel in the tank. The tank shown in **Fig. 1B** accommodates 11 L of buffer. Fill the upper chamber with the buffer contained in the tank until the buffer drains out from the hole at the side of the chamber and begin circulation of the buffer.
4. Apply voltage at 10 V/cm (140 V for a gel of 14-cm length; *see* **Note 6**) and run the gel for an appropriate period with vigorous mixing of the buffer with circulation—4–6 h for a typical parallel gradient gel (*see* **Note 7**).
5. DNA fragments are visualized by a conventional ethidium bromide staining method *(9)*. Briefly, submerge the gel in an appropriate volume of water, then add a small volume of ethidium bromide solution (approx 100 µL or less volume for 200 mL of water), and shake gently for 15 min. Remove staining solution, rinse the gel several times with distilled water, and photograph the gel.

3.4. Denaturing Gradient Gel Electrophoresis (Perpendicular Gradient Gel)

1. Remove the spacer at the top and follow **Subheading 3.3., steps 2** and **3**. Load sample uniformly throughout the well.
2. Place the gel plate into the tank.
3. Apply voltage at 10 V/cm and run for 30 min at an ambient temperature with circulation of the buffer. This is to transfer all DNA fragments into the gel.
4. Using an additional heater together with a rod heater, shown in **Fig. 1A**, warm the bath temperature up to 60°C with vigorous mixing of the buffer. Upon reaching 60°C, remove the additional heater and resume run as in **Subheading 3.3.4**. The period of the run depends on the sample, typically 3–5 h.
5. Visualize DNA fragments by a conventional ethidium bromide staining method.

3.5. SPM Analysis

1. Digest cloned DNA fragments with three restriction endonucleases, *Tsp*509I (AATT), *Mse*I (TTAA), and *Nla*III (CATG). An additional digestion with *Bfa*I (CTAG), which is described in the original paper *(6)*, is optional. The DNA should not be contaminated with chromosomal DNA of the host.
2. Subject an aliquot of digested DNAs (0.5 μg for plasmid clones and 1–2 μg for cosmid and P1 clones) to parallel DGGE, as described in **Subheading 3.3.** The range of the gradient is 9–90% (*see* **Notes 8** and **9**). Run the gel for 12 h.
3. Stain the gel with ethidium bromide. Excise appropriate bands under UV (366 nm) irradiation using a razor blade.
4. Transfer the gel slice into a 1.5-mL Eppendorf tube, and cut to pieces of approximately 1–2 mm³. Add appropriate volume of elution buffer *(9)*, approximately equal or slightly greater to the volume of the gel. Incubate at 37°C overnight. For better yield of recovery, incubation at 50°C for several hours prior to a 37°C overnight incubation is recommended.
5. Transfer the supernatant to SUPREC™-01. Rinse the gel slice with half volume of elution buffer. Vortex well and transfer the supernatant to SUPREC-01.
6. Centrifuge at 12,000g for 2 min at ambient temperature. Add 2 vol of ethanol and recover DNA by a conventional procedure. Addition of carrier is not necessary. An aliquot of the recovered fragment can be subjected to cloning in an appropriate plasmid vector without further purification.

4. Notes

1. Addition of a G+C-rich sequence (G+C clamp) to the end of PCR fragments allows detection of sequence variation that cannot be detected otherwise *(10)*.
2. Since cytosine methylation stabilizes the DNA duplex *(11–13)*, it is expected that DNA fragments having the same nucleotide sequence but an altered methylation status will have a different T_m and therefore can be separated by DGGE. It is believed that methylation at C5 of cytosine possibly stabilizes the helix because of the incremental change in the hydrophobic interactions involved in base stack-

ing *(14)*. It has been shown that nonmethylated, hemimethylated, and symmetrically methylated fragments having the same nucleotide sequence can be separated by DGGE *(14)*. It has also been reported that the change in retardation level is approximately similar to that resulting from a base substitution *(14)*. These findings demonstrate that methylation influences T_m in a similar manner as a point mutation and that DGGE permits the detection of variations in methylation status. The relative retardation level potentially reflects the number of methylated CpG sites within the lowest melting domain of the fragment. This principle cannot be applied to the PCR and/or cloned fragments since methylation is erased in these fragments. This principle underlies the detection of methylation variation by hybridization methods that do not affect the original methylation status of genomic DNA fragments *(15,16)*. However, it is very difficult to specify the precise position of methylated cytosine residues by DGGE. Furthermore, since the mobility shift can only effectively be detected when sequence variation is observed in the domain having the lowest T_m, it is difficult to analyze the methylation status of a G+C-rich region, such as CpG islands, by conventional DGGE.

3. A melting map will help you to understand the melting profile and electrophoretic mobility of DNA fragments in a denaturing gradient gel *(17)*. Melting properties of DNA fragments can be calculated using the program MELT94. **Figure 3** shows representative melting maps. The contour shows the midpoint of melting equilibrium (neglecting strand dissociation) at each base pair. In **Fig. 3A**, the nucleotide sequence of exon 1 and promoter region of the human *CDH1* gene (positions 922–1193, accession no. L34545) is shown. If the sequence is not methylated, the sequence after bisulfite treatment (the details of which are described elsewhere in this book) will be as shown in **Fig. 3B**. If the sequence is fully methylated at CpG sites, the converted sequence will be as shown in **Fig. 3C**. Melting maps of putative PCR products with attachment of a clamp at the 5' end are shown in **Fig. 3D**. The melting temperature of the DNA fragment derived from the nonmethylated sequence (solid line) is lower by approx 5°C than that of the fragment derived from the fully methylated sequence (dotted line). This is expected since all Cs are converted to Ts in the former, whereas Cs at CpG sites remain unchanged in the latter. The difference results in retardation of the DNA fragments derived from the nonmethylated sequence at the lower denaturant concentration than that derived from the methylated sequence (**Fig. 3E**). This difference can be detected by conventional DGGE since a difference in T_m as small as 1°C can easily be detected. The validity of this simulation has been experimentally verified, although different sequences were analyzed *(18,19)*.

4. To determine optimal range of denaturant for the detection of sequence variation, running a perpendicular gradient gel will give a good estimation. Two different DNA fragments having a very similar sequence but differing in T_m can be resolved by perpendicular gradient gel electrophoresis (**Fig. 4**). Denaturant concentration corresponding to these T_m (indicated by dotted arrows) ±10% denaturant will be the choice of the denaturant range. A rule of thumb is that the effective T_m is given as the summation of bath temperature and the denaturing effect of

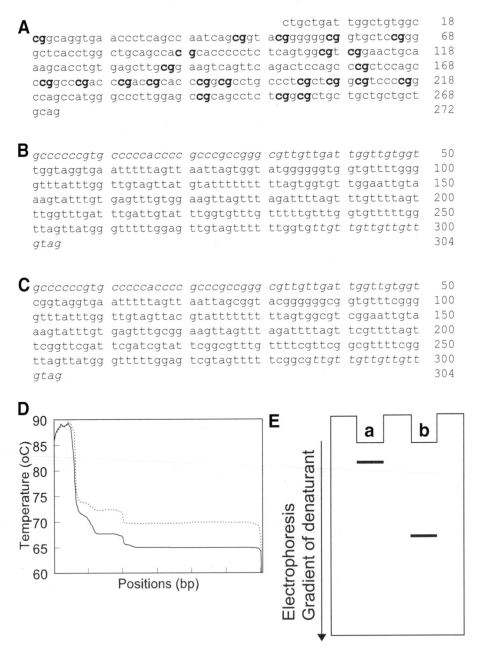

A
```
                                        ctgctgat tggctgtggc    18
cggcaggtga accctcagcc aatcagcggt acggggggcg gtgctccggg    68
gctcacctgg ctgcagccac gcaccccctc tcagtggcgt cggaactgca   118
aagcacctgt gagcttgcgg aagtcagttc agactccagc ccgctccagc   168
ccggcccgac ccgaccgcac ccggcgcctg ccctcgctcg gcgtccccgg   218
ccagccatgg gcccttggag ccgcagcctc tcggcgctgc tgctgctgct   268
gcag                                                     272
```

B
```
gcccccgtg ccccacccc gcccgccggg cgttgttgat tggttgtggt     50
tggtaggtga attttagtt aattagtggt atgggggtg gtgttttggg    100
gtttatttgg ttgtagttat gtattttttt ttagtggtgt tggaattgta   150
aagtatttgt gagtttgtgg aagttagttt agattttagt ttgttttagt   200
ttggtttgat ttgattgtat ttggtgtttg tttttgtttg gtgttttggg   250
ttagttatgg gttttggag ttgtagtttt ttggtgttgt tgttgttgtt    300
gtag                                                     304
```

C
```
gcccccgtg ccccacccc gcccgccggg cgttgttgat tggttgtggt     50
cggtaggtga attttagtt aattagcggt acggggggcg gtgtttcggg   100
gtttatttgg ttgtagttac gtattttttt ttagtggcgt cggaattgta   150
aagtatttgt gagtttgcgg aagttagttt agattttagt tcgttttagt   200
tcggttcgat tcgatcgtat tcggcgtttg ttttcgttcg gcgttttcgg   250
ttagttatgg gttttggag tcgtagtttt tcggcgttgt tgttgttgtt    300
gtag                                                     304
```

D
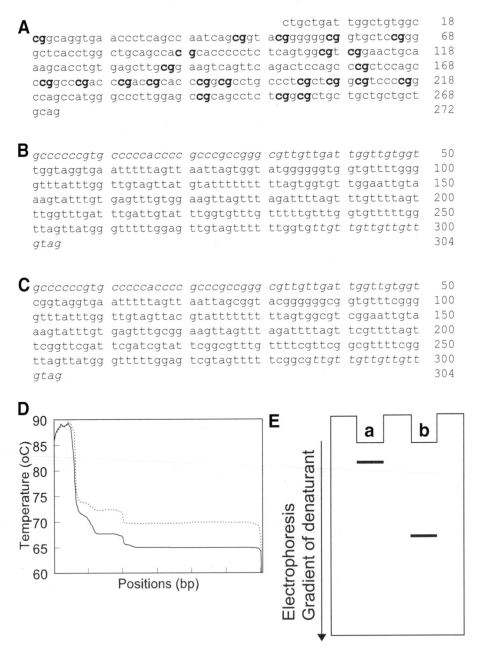

E

Fig. 3. Simulation of the analysis of genomic DNA methylation by DGGE. **(A)** Nucleotide sequence of exon 1 and the promoter region of the human *CDH1* gene (positions 922–1193, accession no. L34545). CpG sequences are shown in bold characters. After bisulfite modification and PCR, nonmethylated and fully methylated

Gradient of denaturant

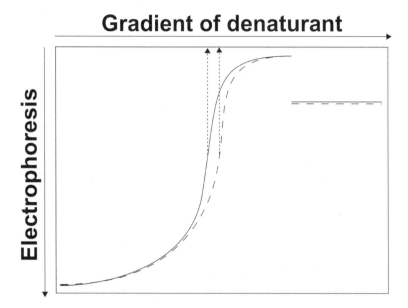

Fig. 4. A representative pattern of perpendicular gradient gel electrophoresis. Two DNA fragments that are very similar in sequence but different in T_m of the lowest melting domain can be separated. T_m of fragment A (solid line) is lower than that of fragment B (dashed line).

urea and formamide, which can be converted at the rate of $0.3°C/\%$ denaturant *(20,21)* since a linear gradient of chemical denaturant is equivalent to a temperature ramp.

5. The T_m of most melting domains derived from a human genomic sequence is above 60°C. However, the T_m of an A+T-rich domain, such as Alu repeated sequences, is sometimes below or close to 60°C *(22)*. A+T-rich property of DNA is enhanced in bisulfite-treated DNA. If the calculated T_m of the lowest melting domain is below 60°C, the bath temperature should be altered accordingly.

6. For the sake of reproducibility, the potential difference across the gel should be measured by a voltage meter. Place one probe into the upper chamber and the other to the lower tank. Adjust applied voltage constant, such as 10 V/cm.

Fig. 3. *(continued)* sequences are converted to (**B**) and (**C**), respectively. Positions of PCR primers are indicated in italicized characters. The PCR primer at the 5' end has a 32-bp G+C-rich sequence at the 5' end. (**D**) Melting maps of sequences (B) (solid line) and (C) (dashed line). The contour shows the midpoint of melting equilibrium neglecting strand dissociation. (**E**) A simulation of separation by parallel DGGE. The PCR fragment (B) (lane a) retards at lower denaturant concentration than the PCR fragment (C) (lane b).

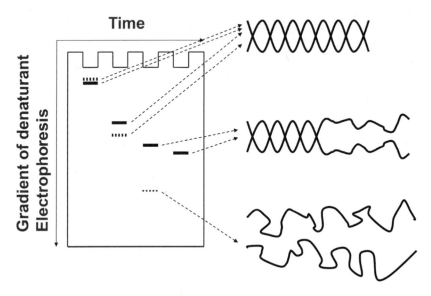

Fig. 5. Principle of the SPM method. A DNA fragment having a G+C-rich region (solid line) is persistently retained in a denaturing gradient gel after prolonged electric field exposure, whereas those without such a region (dashed line) become dissociated and are eluted from the gel.

7. It is critically important to keep the bath temperature constant during the run by vigorous mixing of the buffer in the tank.

8. DNA fragments having both a G+C-rich domain and a non-G+C-rich domain form a relatively stable, partly melted structure (helical at the G+C-rich domain and dissociated at the non-G+C-rich domain) in a denaturing gradient gel *(6,23– 25)*. The strand dissociation rate of these molecules is low, and such partly melted DNA fragments are retained in the gel if the stability of the remaining helical part of the fragment is sufficiently high. Such molecules are retained in the gel as a partly melted structure after prolonged electric field exposure, whereas other molecules disappear through strand dissociation. This is because the strongly denaturing conditions that influence retardation also tend to increase the rate of complete dissociation of the strand. It would be reasonable to speculate that DNA fragments derived from the edges of CpG islands consist of at least two different melting domains, because the G+C-rich nature of CpG island sequences results in high T_m, whereas flanking nonisland sequences are not G+C-rich and would have a lower T_m. Thus, preferential retention of DNA fragments derived from the edges of CpG islands after prolonged field exposure is predicted (**Fig. 5**). That DGGE can be used for the isolation of DNA fragments associated with CpG islands was implied when Fischer and Lerman *(4)* described the detection of point mutations by DGGE and showed that it depends on partial melting. Later on,

Myers et al. *(26,27)* proposed and showed that addition of a 300-bp G+C-rich sequence (GC-clamp) to DNA fragments lacking a high T_m domain would ensure partial melting. Sheffield et al. *(10)* also showed that addition of a short (40–45-bp) GC clamp was sufficient to protect the DNA fragment from strand dissociation and permit retention in a gel *(10)*. It can be expected that CpG island sequences would serve as "natural" G+C clamps, as demonstrated by attachment of one to the mouse β^{major}-globin promoter *(26,27)*. With the SPM analysis, it has been demonstrated that DNA fragments from the periphery of CpG islands, which have the features described above, are greatly enriched *(6,23–25)*. The combination of methyl-CpG binding domain column chromatography and the SPM method has been successfully applied to the comprehensive isolation of CpG islands methylated in human cancer, some of which correspond to novel tumor suppressor genes *(23,28)*.

9. For the SPM analysis, we usually apply a 9–90% denaturant gradient and run the gel for 12 h. However, these conditions can be further optimized depending on the purpose of the experiment.

Acknowledgments

This work was supported in part by a Grant-in-Aid from the Ministry of Health, Labor, and Welfare of Japan for the Second-Term Comprehensive 10-Year Strategy for Cancer Control.

References

1. Lerman, L. S., Fischer, S. G., Hurley, I., Silverstein, K., and Lumelsky, N. (1984) Sequence-determined DNA separations. *Ann. Rev. Biophys. Bioeng.* **13**, 399–423.
2. Fischer, S. G. and Lerman, L. S. (1979) Length-independent separation of DNA restriction fragments in two-dimensional gel electrophoresis. *Cell* **16**, 191–200.
3. Myers, R. M., Lumelsky, N., Lerman, L. S., and Maniatis T. (1985) Detection of single base substitutions in total genomic DNA. *Nature* **313**, 495–498.
4. Fischer, S. G. and Lerman, L. S. (1983) DNA fragments differing by single base-pair substitutions are separated in denaturing gradient gels: correspondence with melting theory. *Proc. Natl. Acad. Sci. USA* **80**, 1579–1583.
5. Shiraishi, M., Oates, A. J., and Sekiya, T. (2002) An overview of the analysis of DNA methylation in mammalian genomes. *Biol. Chem.* **383**, 893–906.
6. Shiraishi, M., Lerman, L. S., and Sekiya, T. (1995) Preferential isolation of DNA fragments associated with CpG islands. *Proc. Natl. Acad. Sci. USA* **92**, 4229–4233.
7. Myers, R. M., Maniatis, T., and Lerman, L. S. (1987) Detection and localization of single base changes by denaturing gradient gel electrophoresis. *Methods Enzymol.* **155**, 501–527.
8. Abrams, E. S. and Stanton Jr., V. P. (1992) Use of denaturing gradient gel electrophoresis to study conformational transition in nucleic acids. *Methods Enzymol.* **212**, 71–104.
9. Maniatis, T., Fritsch, E. F., and Sambrook, J. (eds.) (1982) *Molecular Cloning*, Cold Spring Harbor Laboratory, Cold Spring Harbor, NY.

10. Sheffield, V. C., Cox, D. R., Lerman, L. S., and Myers, R. M. (1989) Attachment of a 40-base-pair G+C-rich sequence (GC-clamp) to genomic DNA fragments by the polymerase chain reaction results in improved detection of single-base changes. *Proc. Natl. Acad. Sci. USA* **86,** 232–236.

11. Szer, W. and Shugar, D. (1966) The structure of poly-5-methylcytidylic acid and its twin-stranded complex with poly-inosinic acid. *J. Mol. Biol.* **17,** 174–187.

12. Gill, J. E., Mazrimas, J. A., and Bishop, Jr, C. C. (1974) Physical studies on synthetic DNAs containing 5-methylcytosine. *Biochim. Biophys. Acta* **335,** 330–348.

13. Ehrlich, M., Ehrlich, K., and Mayo, J. A. (1975) Unusual properties of the DNA from *Xanthomonas* phage XP-12 in which 5-methylcytosine completely replaces cytosine. *Biochim. Biophys. Acta* **395,** 109–119.

14. Collins, M. and Myers, R. M. (1987) Alterations in DNA helix stability due to base modifications can be evaluated using denaturing gradient gel electrophoresis. *J. Mol. Biol.* **198,** 737–744.

15. Uhlmann, K., Marczinek, K., Hampe, J., Thiel, G., and Nürnberg, P. (1999) Changes in methylation patterns identified by two-dimensional DNA fingerprinting. *Electrophoresis* **20,** 1748–1755.

16. Reindollar, R. H., Fusaris, K. W., and Gray, M. R. (2000) Methylation-dependent melting polymorphisms in genomic fragments of deoxyribonucleic acid. *Am. J. Obstet. Gynecol.* **182,** 785–793.

17. Lerman, L. S. and Silverstein, K. (1987) Computational simulation of DNA melting and its application to denaturing gradient gel electrophoresis. *Methods Enzymol.* **155,** 482–501.

18. Aggerholm, A., Guldberg, P., Hokland, M., and Hokland, P. (1999) Extensive intra- and interindividual heterogeneity of *p15INK4B* methylation in acute myeloid leukemia. *Cancer Res.* **59,** 436–441.

19. Daskalakis, M., Nguyen, T. T., Nguyen, C., et al. (2002) Demethylation of a hypermethylated P15/INK4B gene in patients with myelodysplastic syndrome by 5-aza-2'-deoxycytidine (decitabine) treatment. *Blood* **100,** 2957–2964.

20. Hutton, J. R. (1977) Renaturation kinetics and thermal stability of DNA in aqueous solutions of formamide and urea. *Nucleic Acids Res.* **4,** 3537–3555.

21. Nishigaki, K., Husimi, Y., Masuda, M., Kaneko, K., and Tanaka, T. (1984) Strand dissociation and cooperative melting of double-stranded DNAs detected by denaturant gradient gel electrophoresis. *J. Biochem.* (Tokyo) **95,** 627–635.

22. Lerman, L. S., Silverstein, K., and Grinfeld. (1986) Searching for gene defects by denaturing gradient gel electrophoresis. *Cold Spring Harbor Symp. Quant. Biol.* **51,** 285–297.

23. Shiraishi, M., Chuu, Y. H., and Sekiya, T. (1999) Isolation of DNA fragments associated with methylated CpG islands in human adenocarcinomas of the lung using a methylated DNA binding column and denaturing gradient gel electrophoresis. *Proc. Natl. Acad. Sci. USA* **96,** 2913–2918.

24. Shiraishi, M. and Sekiya, T. (1996) Isolation of CpG island fragments: a putative promoter region of the human prostacyclin synthase gene. *Proc. Jpn. Acad.* **77(B),** 101–103.

25. Shiraishi, M., Oates, A. J., Xu, L., et al. (1998) The isolation of CpG islands from human chromosomal regions 11q13 and Xp22 by segregation of partly melted molecules. *Nucleic Acids Res.* **26**, 5544–5550.
26. Myers, R. M., Fischer, S. G., Maniatis, T., and Lerman, L. S. (1985) Modulation of the melting properties of duplex DNA by attachment of a GC-rich DNA sequence as determined by denaturing gradient gel electrophoresis. *Nucleic Acids Res.* **13**, 3111–3129.
27. Myers, R. M., Fischer, S. G., Lerman, L. S., and Maniatis, T. (1985) Nearly all single base substitution in DNA fragments joined to a GC-clamp can be detected by denaturing gradient gel electrophoresis. *Nucleic Acids Res.* **13**, 3131–3145.
28. Shiraishi, M., Sekiguchi, A., Terry, M. J., et al. (2002) A comprehensive catalog of CpG islands methylated in human lung adenocarcunomas for the identification of tumor suppressor genes. *Oncogene* **21**, 3804–3813.

18

Photocrosslinking Oligonucleotide Hybridization Assay for Concurrent Gene Dosage and CpG Methylation Analysis

Risa Peoples, Michael Wood, and Reuel Van Atta

Summary

The phenotypic effects of aberrant gene expression are indistinguishable, regardless of whether the underlying mutation is one of gene copy number (deletion or duplication) or modification of differentially methylated CpG sites occurring in critical regulatory sequences in gene promoters. The XLnt photocrosslinking oligonucleotide technology provides for the hybridization-dependent covalent attachment of probe to target, allowing survival of the probe/target complex under otherwise denaturing conditions. Posthybridization wash stringency can be substantially higher than under standard techniques, leading to a marked increase in signal-to-noise ratios. In addition, the reduction in nonspecific background provides linearity to XLnt-based oligonucleotide assays comparable to that otherwise achieved only with very long probes. The technology is thus ideally suited for combining the high-throughput capacity of oligonucleotide hybridization platforms with accurate measurement of relative gene dosage. By integrating the XLnt system with an assay design separating probe/target immobilization and signal elaboration functions, relative gene dosage assessment can be applied to the quantitation of fractional resistance to methylation-sensitive restriction enzyme (MSRE) digestion. The method described below provides for the development of photocrosslinking oligonucleotide assays for relative gene dosage and fractional locus CpG methylation in a microtiter plate-based format.

Key Words: Gene dosage; deletion; duplication; methylation; imprinting; epigenetic; oligonucleotide hybridization; high-throughput; cancer diagnostic; photocrosslinking.

1. Introduction

High-throughput, cost-effective technologies for molecular diagnostics have been most successfully developed for analysis of sequence variants such as single-nucleotide polymorphisms (SNPs). However, in many cases, the most clinically relevant mutations are those that result in abnormal levels of gene transcripts of normal sequence. Aberrant transcript levels can result from either

From: *Methods in Molecular Biology, vol. 287: Epigenetics Protocols*
Edited by: T. O. Tollefsbol © Humana Press Inc., Totowa, NJ

abnormalities of gene dosage, such as whole-gene and larger deletions or duplications, or errors of CpG dinucleotide methylation. CpG methylation sites are frequently found clustered in gene promoter regions where their methylation status is tightly linked to regulation of gene expression. In certain instances, both gene deletions and methylation of promoter region CpG sites can underlie identical pathophysiological processes. The phenotypic effects are the consequence of abnormal transcript levels, and the underlying mutational mechanisms are not distinguishable. Examples of clinically relevant gene expression abnormalities of either etiology include (1) tumor suppressor gene mutations in cancer specimens and (2) chromosomal regions subject to gametic imprinting associated with developmental disorders. There is, therefore, a need in molecular diagnostics for tools that allow concurrent assessment of CpG methylation and overall gene copy number.

The XLnt technology is based on incorporating the coumarin-based photosensitive crosslinking agent into oligonucleotide hybridization probes. This molecule, specifically within the context of Watson-Crick hydrogen bonding to a complementary DNA sequence, and upon exposure to ultraviolet (UV) light of appropriate wavelength and intensity, will form a covalent bond, or crosslink, to the opposing nucleotide. The covalent bond established between the probe and target thus renders the complex completely resistant to disruption in what is otherwise a denaturing environment. It is therefore possible to perform posthybridization washing under the most stringent conditions, providing a marked reduction in nonspecific background hybridization levels not attainable under noncrosslinking conditions. The consequent improvement in signal-to-noise ratios provides significantly greater sensitivity and specificity for genetic assays.

The technology has been successfully applied to the development of assays for quantitative hepatitis B virus DNA detection from human serum *(1)*; SNP genotyping for the factor V Leiden variant *(2)* and the hereditary hemochromatosis C282Y and H63D alleles *(3)*; and fluorescent *in situ* hybridization-based detection of human papillomavirus type 16 from cervical swab specimens *(4)*. Both types of assays employ signal amplification for detection that maintains quantitivity. Elevation of signal-to-noise ratios conferred by the photocrosslinking technology enable the development of genetic assays using clinically realistic sample volumes without the need for prior target amplification (*see* **Note 1**).

The XLnt solution-based viral quantitation and genotyping assays employ differentially labeled crosslinker-containing oligonucleotides for ligand-based capture onto magnetic beads (capture probes) and antibody-mediated signal generation (reporter probes; **Fig. 1**). The XLnt technology allows high-stringency washing of posthybridization probe-target complexes, permitting accu-

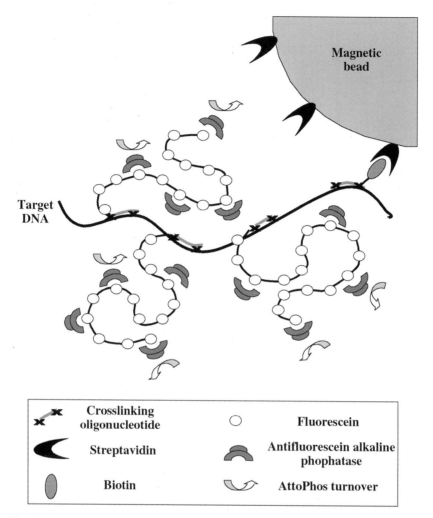

Fig. 1. The solution-based photocrosslinking assay design. Photocrosslinking oligonucleotides covalently bind target DNA. Biotinylated capture probes immobilize the complexes onto magnetic beads. Three polyfluoresceinated reporter probes are shown; for illustrative purposes, only 10–15 fluorescein molecules are indicated, although typical synthetic yields are generally higher. Reporter probes generate signal through sequential incubation with the antifluorescein antibody-alkaline phosphatase conjugate and alkaline phosphatase fluorescence-generating substrate AttoPhos. (Reproduced with permission from Clinical Chemistry, **ref. 6.**)

rate gene-dosage determination under conditions that also discriminate SNPs and other simple sequence variants (*see* **Note 2**). In addition, through incorporation of a prior methylation-sensitive restriction enzyme (MSRE) digestion

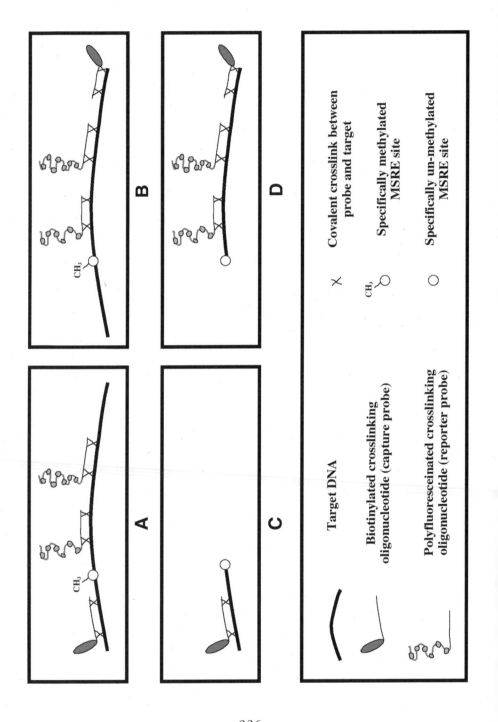

step, quantitative gene dosage determination can be applied toward assessment of fractional locus methylation *(6)* (**Fig. 2**).

2. Materials

1. 7-Hydroxy coumarin, 1-*O*-(4,49-dimethoxytri-tyl)-3-*O*-(7-coumarinyl)-2-*O*-(2-cyanoethyl-*N*,*N*-diisopropyl phosphoramidite) glycerol crosslinking reagent (Naxcor).
2. Expedite 8909 oligonucleotide synthesizer (Applied Biosystems).
3. Expedite synthesis reagents (Applied Biosystems).
4. Biotin TEG CPG (Glen Research).
5. FLUOS aminoreactive reagent fluorescein-NHS ester (Roche Applied Science).
6. Ammonium hydroxide.
7. 6 and 16% Denaturing polyacrylamide gels and electrophoretic equipment.
8. Sep-Pak C18 desalting columns (Waters).
9. Scanning UV spectrophotometer (Beckman-Coulter DU-7400).
10. DNA extraction kit (Gentra).
11. *Hpa*II (NEB).
12. Alkaline lysis solution: 281 m*M* NaOH, 7.5 m*M* Tris-HCl, pH 7.5, 0.75 m*M* EDTA, 0.1% bovine serum albumin.
13. 96-Well microtiter plates (Greiner).
14. Probe solution: 1.5 *M* NaCl, 35% formamide, 0.001% phenol red, 0.02% calf thymus DNA.
15. Neutralization solution: 234 m*M* citric acid, 308 m*M* NaH_2PO_4, 1.5 *M* NaCl, 0.4% Tween-20, 35% formamide.
16. Microtiter plate heating element (USA/Scientific).
17. UV crosslinking chamber (UVP model CL1000-L)with UV-A bulbs (UVP).
18. Pyrex 2-mm-thick filter.
19. Streptavidin coated magnetic beads (Dynabeads M-280, Dynal).
20. Magnetic bar assembly.

Fig. 2. *(opposite page)* Target DNA is assayed separately with each of two probe solutions; both utilize the same set of polyfluoresceinated crosslinking reporter probes in combination with either of a pair of biotinylated capture probes complementary to sequence on the same or opposite side of a methylation-sensitive restriction enzyme (MSRE) site from the reporter probes. The former capture probe is the methylation-insensitive capture probe (**B** and **D**) and the latter, the methylation-sensitive capture probe (**A** and **B**). If the CpG sites in question are methylated (A and B), the DNA survives digestion at that site, and each of the capture probe/target complexes remain contiguous with the target/reporter probe complex. In the alternate situation, in which the CpG sites are unmethylated (C and D), target is cleaved at these sites. In this instance, the methylation-insensitive capture probe/target complex retains signal elaboration properties (D), whereas the methylation-sensitive capture probe:target complex is incapable of developing signal (C).

21. Antifluorescein antibody-alkaline phosphatase conjugate (DAKO) diluted 1:20,000 final concentration in 100 mM Tris-HCl, pH 7.5, 112.5 mM NaCl, 0.5 X saline-sodium citrate, 0.025% sodium azide, 0.1 % Tween-20, 0.25% bovine serum albumin.
22. AttoPhos™ (Promega).
23. Wash 1: 0.1% sodium dodecyl sulfate (SDS), 0.1X SSC, 0.001% Tween-20.
24. Wash 2: 50% formamide, 0.5% Tween-20, 0.1X SSC.
25. Wash 3: 1X SSC, 0.1% Tween-20.
26. FluoroCount™ microplate reader (Packard).

3. Methods

The methods described include (1) oligonucleotide generation, (2) template DNA sample preparation, (3) assay performance, and (4) data interpretation.

3.1. Oligonucleotide Generation

The (1) design and (2) synthesis and modification of the photocrosslinker-containing oligonucleotides are described.

3.1.1. Oligonucleotide Design

Complete sequence information over a minimum of a few hundred contiguous nucleotides must be obtained from the locus of interest surrounding the CpG sites to be interrogated, as well as for an obligate two-copy unique region of the genome for use as a dosage control (*see* **Note 3**). Ideally, this information will include:

1. Fractional methylation status of all *Hpa*II sites in normal and diseased states.
2. Known sequence polymorphisms, in order to avoid their inclusion in probes.
3. Evaluation of potential homologies, in order to minimize crosshybridization of probes to external loci.

A panel of candidate probes is designed according to the illustrated scheme (**Fig. 3**). Candidate probe selection is empirical; ultimately, probes are screened and a subset selected for inclusion in the final panel, based on optimum signal-to-noise ratios demonstrated using PCR product templates. The nucleotide opposing the crosslinker moiety is variable, but optimum crosslinking occurs to thymidine and, therefore, probe design generally entails substitution of the XLnt molecule for adenosine. Specific requirements of probe design include:

1. Each capture-reporter probe set will recognize a total sequence region of no greater than 500 bp.
2. A crosslinker molecule can be incorporated into either or both of the penultimate 3' or 5' positions.
3. Optimal reporter and capture probe lengths are 15–30 bases and 30–50 bases, respectively (*see* **Note 4**).

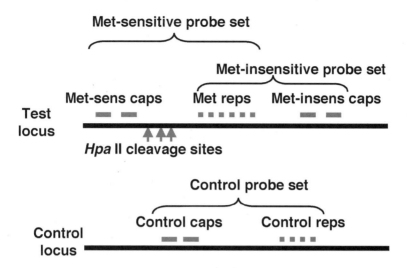

Fig. 3. Probe set design. Three separate probe sets must be created for this assay. Each probe set comprises fluoresceinated reporter probes and biotinylated capture probes, each containing the photocrosslinker molecule in one or two positions. The first two probe sets will generate signal from the test locus and will utilize the same panel of reporter probes (Met reps). The two capture probe sets described above will be designed for use with this reporter panel; the methylation-sensitive capture set (Met-sens caps) is designed on the opposite side of MSRE sites from the reporter panel, whereas the methylation-insensitive capture set (Met-insens caps) is designed from sequence on the same side as the reporter panel. A third set of probes comprises capture and reporter probes designed against sequence from a control locus (Control caps and control reps). (Reproduced with permission from Clinical Chemistry, **ref. 6**).

4. Optimal signal strength is achieved with the selection of a set of four to six reporter probes.
5. Optimal assay performance is achieved with two capture probes per probe set.

3.1.2. Oligonucleotide Synthesis and Modification

Oligonucleotides are synthesized on an Expedite 8909 Synthesizer (Applied Biosystems).

1. The crosslinker molecule is incorporated into the oligonucleotides during automated synthesis using a phosphoramidite derived from 7-hydroxy coumarin, 1-O-(4,49-dimethoxytri-tyl)-3-O-(7-coumarinyl)-2-O-(2-cyanoethyl-N,N-diisopropyl phosphoramidite) glycerol (patent pending).
2. Capture probe synthesis includes biotin incorporation directly into the 3' position of the oligonucleotide using Biotin TEG CPG during automated synthesis.
3. Reporter probe synthesis includes introduction of an (amino-spacer)$_{40}$ repeating unit to the 3' tail of the oligonucleotide backbone during automated synthesis.

4. Probes are cleaved from the solid support and deprotected by incubating the support in concentrated ammonium hydroxide for 16 h at 45°C (reporter probes) or 8 h at 55°C (capture probes).

5. Deprotected probes are purified by excision and elution from denaturing polyacrylamide gels (16% for biotinylated probes; 6% for amino-spacer–tailed probes).

6. Oligonucleotides are desalted with Sep-Pak C18 columns.

7. Reporter probes are fluoresceinated by incubating the polyamine probes with the amino-reactive reagent fluorescein-NHS ester FLUOS; excess FLUOS is removed through repeated rounds of centrifugal concentration under basic conditions.

8. Oligonucleotide concentrations and degree of fluorescein incorporation (for reporter probes) are quantified by UV spectroscopy. Typical fluorescein incorporation is 20–25 molecules per oligonucleotide.

3.2. Sample Preparation

Preparation of (1) sample DNA and (2) assay controls is described.

3.2.1. DNA Preparation

1. Sample DNA is isolated from mammalian cells using commercial reagents.
2. Purified DNA is quantified spectrophotometrically.
3. 200–300 µg of DNA is digested overnight with *Hpa*II at 1 U/µg (*see* **Note 5**).
4. DNA is ethanol-precipitated and resuspended in 900 µL of alkaline lysis buffer.
5. Samples are boiled for 20 min to shear the DNA (*see* **Note 5**).
6. Samples are centrifuged and aliquoted.

3.2.2. Control Sources

1. Positive control: sample DNA is isolated from known normal source as above; sample processing proceeds as above with the omission of the *Hpa*II digestion step (*see* **Note 6**).
2. Negative control: 250 µg of calf thymus DNA is precipitated and processed as for **steps 4–6** in **Subheading 3.2.1.** above (*see* **Note 7**).

3.3. Assay Performance

The XLnt solution-based assays utilize the same general method. The assay performance including (1) hybridization and crosslinking, (2) posthybridization washing, and (3) signal elaboration and detection is described (**Fig. 4**).

3.3.1. Hybridization and Photocrosslinking

1. Sample and control DNA is aliquoted into each of six wells of 125 µL apiece in a 96-well polypropylene plate.
2. Each sample or control well is assayed in duplicate with each of the three probe sets by addition of 50 µL of probe solution and probes, with the exception of the negative control wells (**Fig. 5**). These wells are assayed with probe solution and

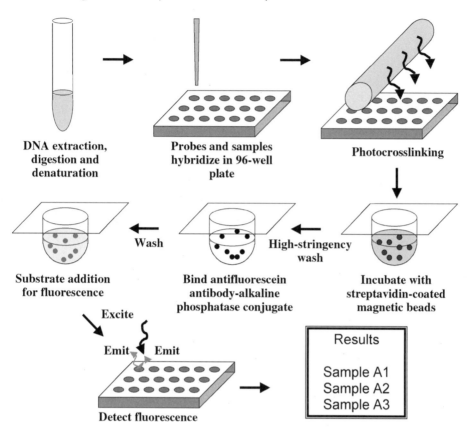

Fig. 4. Assay performance. Sample DNA is sheared, denatured, and aliquoted into microtiter plate wells. Target DNA is hybridized and crosslinked to photocrosslinker-containing oligonucleotides. Biotinylated capture probes are bound by streptavidin-coated magnetic beads for immobilization on a solid support during washing steps; fluoresceinated reporter probes generate fluorescent signal through sequential incubation with an antifluorescein antibody-alkaline phosphatase conjugate and the alkaline phosphatase substrate AttoPhos. (Reproduced with permission from Clinical Chemistry, **ref. 2**).

reporter probes only, with exclusion of the capture probes. Probe concentrations are determined by optimization but generally are successful with capture probes at 0.5 pmols apiece and reporter probes at 0.2 pmols apiece per 50-μL aliquot (*see* **Note 8**).

3. After a 5-min room temperature incubation, 50 μL of neutralization solution is added to each well with mixing (*see* **Note 9**).

4. A 2-mm Pyrex filter is placed on top of the plate and the covered plate is placed within the photocrosslinking chamber (**Fig. 6**).

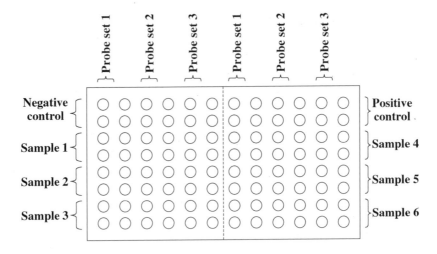

Fig. 5. The microtiter plate set-up. Six samples can be analyzed per plate. Alternate columns are used for compatibility with the magnetic bead capture apparatus.

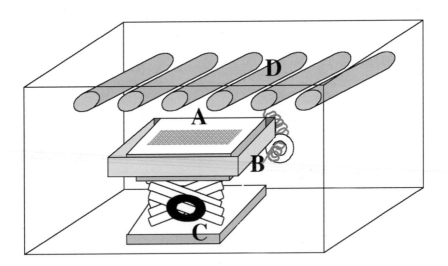

Fig. 6. The hybridization and photocrosslinking assembly is illustrated. The microtiter plate (**A**) is positioned on a microplate heating element (**B**) within the crosslinking chamber at 42°C. The heating element is then raised (**C**) to bring the plate cover to approx 2 cm from the UV source (**D**).

5. The plate is incubated for 20 min, following which the UV lamps are turned on with a further incubation for 30 min.
6. The plate is removed and cooled to room temperature for 5 min (*see* **Note 10**).

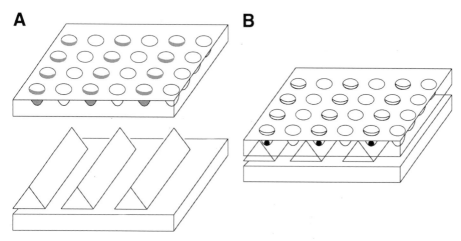

Fig. 7. Magnetic bead immobilization. A bar magnet assembly is created by affixing bar magnets to a solid support. The plate is oriented above the bar magnet assembly (**A**) and brought down upon it (**B**) before each aspiration such that the beads are pelleted tightly against one wall. Pellet formation takes about 30 s.

7. Streptavidin-coated magnetic beads are added without dilution at 7.5 µL per well with mixing. The plate is then incubated at room temperature for 30 min.

3.3.2. Bead Washing Procedure

Perform washing and resuspension steps as follows:
1. Magnetic beads are immobilized against the microtiter plate wall (**Fig. 7**).
2. Solution is aspirated from each well leaving the pelleted beads undisturbed (**Fig. 8**).
3. The beads are resuspended by forceful pipet evacuation of new solution (**Fig. 9**) (*see* **Note 11**).

3.3.4. Complete Signal Elaboration

1. Following bead addition and incubation, the plate is sequentially washed with 200 µL each of the following solutions: wash 1, wash 2, and wash 3.
2. Upon completion of the final wash, the beads are pelleted and wash solution removed as in **steps 1** and **2** in **Subheading 3.3.3.** above. 100 µL of the antifluorescein-alkaline phosphatase conjugate is added with mixing (*see* **Note 12**).
3. The plate is incubated at room temperature for 20 min.
4. The plate is sequentially washed four times with wash 3 (above).
5. The beads are again pelleted and the final wash removed. Then 100 µL of the alkaline phosphatase substrate AttoPhos is added with mild mixing to each well (*see* **Note 12**).
6. The filter cover is replaced and the plate incubated at 37°C in darkness for 1 h.
7. The fluorescent signal is read with a microplate fluorometer.

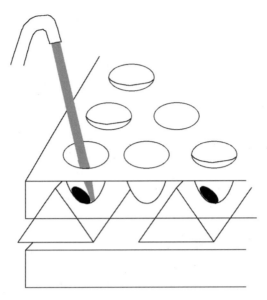

Fig. 8. Aspiration of noncaptured contents. A pipet tip (20–200 µL size) under constant suction attached to either of a vacuum pump or water aspirator is introduced sequentially to the bottom of each well; the solution is aspirated with care to avoid disrupting the pelleted beads.

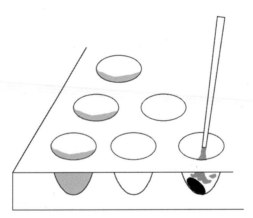

Fig. 9. Resuspension of pelleted beads. The plate is removed from the magnetic source and wash solution or reagent is introduced to each well by pipeting directly onto the pellet. Homogeneous resuspension of the beads should be demonstrated (*see* **Note 12**).

3.4. Data Interpretation

Results are obtained by comparing signals obtained from assaying sample DNA with pairs of probe sets. The relative gene dosage measurement for a

A

$$NSS = \frac{\text{Mean sample}}{\text{signal}} - \frac{\text{Mean negative}}{\text{control signal}}$$

B

$$SR = \frac{\text{Sample NSS Probe set 1}}{\text{Sample NSS Probe set 2}}$$

Dosage Ratio: Probe set 1 = Met-insens probe set
                     Probe set 2 = Control probe set

Methylation Ratio: Probe set 1 = Met-sens probe set
                      Probe set 2 = Met-Insens probe set

C

$$NSR = \frac{SR_{sample}}{SR_{positive\ control}}$$

Fig. 10. Data analysis. Each sample or control was assayed with each probe set in duplicate. The mean value is obtained for each duplicate pair, yielding three mean sample or control values, or one each per probe set. (**A**) For each mean sample value, the net sample signal (NSS) is obtained by subtracting the mean negative control value for that probe set. (**B**) For each dosage or methylation value determination, a signal ratio (SR) is derived from the ratio of the NSSs for the methylation-insensitive probe set to control probe set (dosage SR) or the ratio of the NSSs for the methylation-sensitive probe set to methylation-insensitive probe set (methylation SR). (**C**) The normalized signal ratios (NSRs) are obtained for each sample by dividing each of the dosage and methylation SRs by the appropriate SR calculated for the positive control specimen.

sample is determined by the normalized ratio of mean, background-corrected signal from the methylation-insensitive probe set divided by that derived from the control probe set. The fractional methylation value is determined by the normalized ratio of mean, background-corrected signal from the methylation-sensitive probe set divided by that derived from the methylation-insensitive probe set (**Fig. 10**).

Note that the gene copy number for the dosage control is two. Therefore, dosage normalized signal ratios (NSRs) are interpreted as relative to a diploid gene dose, that is, a dosage NSR of 1.0 corresponds to a two-gene copy number; 0.5, 1.5, and 2.0 are the values expected in the setting of a gene deletion, gene duplication, and tetrasomic state, respectively. The positive control used for the assay was not subject to MSRE digestion. Therefore, the control behaves as though all CpG sites were resistant to digestion, or as though the sample was 100% methylated. A sample methylation NSR of 1.0 indicates that the entirety of the CpG site interrogated is methylated, whereas a value of 0 is consistent with complete unmethylation. A value of 0.5 means that about 50% of the sites are unmethylated, a characteristic of imprinted regions of the human genome in which CpG methylation correlates with chromosomal parent-of-origin.

4. Notes

1. The factor V Leiden genotyping assay was recently studied at a large reference laboratory *(5)*. In this study, successful discrimination of wild-type homozygous, mutant homozygous and wild-type/mutant heterozygous samples was achieved using a minimum of 200 µL of anticoagulated whole blood, translating to a minimum extracted DNA specification of 2.5 µg without the need for target amplification.

2. Gene dosage determination is conveniently performed using a comparative hybridization approach whereby hybridization-dependent signal intensity correlates linearly with relative target amount. Such linearity is achieved using conditions demonstrating high signal-to-background ratios. Array comparative genomic hybridization (CGH; in which very long DNA sequences, usually from clones or PCR amplicons, are used as probes in a matrix platform allowing separate assessment of hybridization to target), has emerged as a powerful tool for multiplex dosage determination *(7)*. The quantitivity of the method is made possible by the relatively high posthybridization stringency conditions achievable with very long probe-target hybridization complexes. Oligonucleotide hybridization is a robust technique developed primarily for assessment of sequence variants. The utility of the method for determination of gene dosage is limited by the low-stringency conditions required in order for single-base pair differences between probes to demonstrate differential degrees of hybridization to target. Typically, oligonucleotide hybridization-based methods applied toward dosage determinations have called for mixtures of long probes interrogating multiple areas of a gene or transcript simultaneously. Because the XLnt technology converts short probe-target hybridization complexes into a covalently bonded molecule, high-stringency wash conditions are possible enabling accurate gene dosage quantitation in parallel with SNP-discriminating hybridization.

3. The control locus is selected from a relatively unique region of the genome demonstrating minimal homology with other DNA and expected to be invariably present in diploid copy number. Sequence from the nonpseudoautosomal X- and Y-chromosomal regions is excluded as dosage varies with gender, as are regions potentially subject to dosage polymorphisms, such as those from areas bounded by large repetitive DNA blocks. So-called housekeeping genes are good choices, as their products provide essential cell functions and are requisite for normal cell

growth. For evaluation of germline mutations, chromosomal aneuploidies compatible with life should be considered. Therefore, for instance, chromosomes 13, 18, and 21 should be excluded. Specifically for assays designed to evaluate somatic aberrations from heterogeneous cell populations, as in assays of tumor specimens, evidence for potential cell toxicity from over- or under-representation of gene dosage can be inferred by an examination of chromosomal aberrations in cancer cells (8). Cancer cells, having lost the normal controls over proliferation and DNA repair and being thus subject to the accumulation of mitotic errors, can indicate specific loci that are more likely to be cell-lethal when present in abnormal copy number. The scarcity of either deletions or duplications of a specific locus in tumor specimens can therefore be taken as evidence that the locus is toxic to cells in abnormal doses and, therefore, will be reliably present in diploid copy number in the vast majority of human cells.

4. Undefined polymorphisms affecting hybridization efficiency and stability are a risk of any oligonucleotide-based procedure. The chances of encountering this problem are greater when using sequence that is poorly characterized, as noncoding sequences often are, especially when obtained from high-throughput genome sequence sources. To mitigate this risk, we recommend using long capture probes, on the order of 30–50-mers. Reporter probes of 20 bases or more are also not significantly affected by a single base pair difference and using a minimum of four reporter probes also minimizes these risks.

5. Better sensitivity on the order of two- to fourfold is achieved by replacing the non-specific target shearing achieved by extensive boiling with specific restriction enzyme digestion concurrently with the *Hpa*II digestion step, if possible. To do this, restriction enzymes must be selected that produce fragments that are (1) completely inclusive of all probe sequences from both the test and control loci; (2) roughly a maximum of 500 bp for both test and control loci; and (3) optimally less than 500 bp on average for the rest of the genome, as determined by gel electrophoresis. If restriction enzyme digestion is done instead of shearing by boiling, the boiling step must still be performed for 3 min to denature the target DNA fully.

6. The user has the option of adding a positive control for *Hpa*II digestion. This would entail the addition of a separate normal control sample, ideally from the same source as the positive control described, which had been subject to *Hpa*II digestion assayed in parallel with each of the methylation-sensitive and methylation-insensitive test assay probe sets in each of four wells. The addition of this control would identify complete failure of enzymatic digestion across all samples. In order to incorporate a methodology allowing for evaluation of each sample, individually, for *Hpa*II digestion, it would be necessary to expand the assay to include evaluation of each sample with a fourth probe set in each of two further wells per sample. This probe set should be designed from a reliably fully unmethylated locus according to the design for a methylation-sensitive probe set, such that the expected result from an adequately digested sample would be the generation of negligible signal above background. The described embodiment

was developed for high-throughput applications in which minimizing the number of wells per plate was a high priority. Scouting experiments validated the reproducibility of enzyme digestion, and this control was, therefore, omitted from this protocol. However, the individual user may wish to incorporate either of these control approaches.

7. Multiple negative controls were assessed in designing this assay, including (1) solutions containing all probes and reagents but no target DNA, and (2) solutions containing all probes, reagents, and normal control DNA with the sample subsequently shielded from crosslinking under the UV light. The first formulation gave a background that was above signal obtained for a fully unmethylated sample, suggesting that DNA itself provides a significant background reduction factor. The second approach actually provides the closest assessment of "true background" but is very impractical to incorporate into the method, requiring a parallel vessel for each assay. The negative control that we use in which the capture probes are omitted provides the closest practical assessment of background.

8. At this time, no formal stability testing has been done on many of these reagents. In particular, probes are kept in water at 4°C and added to solutions containing all other reagents on the day of the test. Probe solutions are probably stable longer than this, but this has not been assessed.

9. Mixing of solutions within the wells is performed by repetitive pipeting up and down using the same tip, immediately following solution addition. In most cases, this is accomplished with two or three mixing steps. Because of the large volume and viscosity of the solutions, mixing following the neutralization step can take closer to five or six mixing steps. Phenol red is present in the probe solution to provide evidence of homogeneous mixing at this stage.

10. The assay components are quite stable at this point. This is the best place to leave the plate for an extended time (e.g., up to 2 h) if it is not possible to perform all assay steps at one time. After this step, it is necessary to complete the assay in the given times.

11. Complete aspiration and resuspension are very important. Effective aspiration requires a steady vacuum source that is neither too fast, which breaks the liquid column and leaves residual solution, nor too slow, which allows the beads to dry out. This is the one aspect of the assay that is something of an "art" that can be acquired in usually three or four practice runs. Resuspension is best performed by placing a pipet tip just below the rim of the well and pipeting forcefully, aiming directly at the pellet. We change pipet tips between each reagent addition; during aspiration and wash solution additions, a single pipet tip is used.

12. When resuspending the beads in the antifluorescein antibody-alkaline phosphatase conjugate, repeat pipeting up and down is necessary to mix the slightly viscous solution fully. The AttoPhos addition is easier and, if the pipet tip is appropriately positioned above the pellet, full mixing is usually achieved on direct addition of reagent. We always change pipet tips between wells for addition of either of these reagents. For AttoPhos addition, we use stuffed pipet tips and aliquot the reagent into a separate vessel for each assay to avoid contamination.

References

1. Chan, H. L. Y., Leung, N. W. Y., Lau, T. C. M., Wong, M. L., and Sung, J. J. Y. (2000) Comparison of three different sensitive assays for hepatitis B virus DNA in monitoring of responses to antiviral therapy. *J. Clin. Microbiol.* **38,** 3205–3208.
2. Zehnder, J., Van Atta, R., Jones, C., Sussmann, H., and Wood, M. (1997) Cross-linking hybridization assay for direct detection of factor V Leiden mutation. *Clin. Chem.* **43,** 1703–1708.
3. Wylenzek, C., Engelmann, M., Holten, D., Van Atta, R., Wood, M., and Gathof, B. (2000) Evaluation of a nucleic acid-based cross-linking assay to screen for hereditary hemochromatosis in healthy blood donors. *Clin. Chem.* **46,** 1853–1855.
4. Huan, B., Van Atta, R., Cheng, P., Wood, M. L., Zychlinsky, E., and Albagli, D. (2000) Photo-Cross-Linkable Oligonucleotide Probes for In Situ Hybridization Assays. *BioTechniques* **28,** 254–260.
5. French, C., Li, C., Strom, C., Sun, W., Van Atta, R., Gonzalez, B. and Wood, M. Detection of the factor V leiden mutation by a modified photo cross-linking oligo-nucleotide hybridization assay. *Clin. Chem.* **50,** 296–305.
6. Peoples, R., Weltman, H., Van Atta, R., Wang, J., Wood, M., Ferrante-Raimondi, M., Cheng, P., and Huan, B. (2002) High-throughput detection of submicroscopic deletions and methylation status at 15q11-q13 by a photo-cross-linking oligo-nucleotide hybridization assay. *Clin. Chem.* **48,** 1844–1850.
7. Snijders, A. M., Nowak, N., Segraves, R., et al. (2001) Assembly of microarrays for genome-wide measurement of DNA copy number. *Nat. Genet.* **29,** 263,264.
8. Mitelman, F., Johansson, B., and Mertens, F., eds. Mitelman Database of Chromosome Aberrations in Cancer. http://cgap.nci.nih.gov/Chromosomes/Mitelman).

19

Methylation-Specific Oligonucleotide Microarray

Pearlly S. Yan, Susan H. Wei, and Tim Hui-Ming Huang

Summary

The methylation-specific oligonucleotide (MSO) microarray is a high-throughput approach capable of detecting DNA methylation in genes across several CpG sites. Based on the bisulfite modification of DNA that converts unmethylated cytosines to uracil but leaves the 5'methylcytosine intact, the method utilizes short oligonucleotides corresponding to the methylated and unmethylated alleles as probes affixed on solid support and products amplified from bisulfite-treated DNA as targets for hybridization. MSO is suitable for examining a panel of genes across multiple clinical samples. This approach can generate a robust dataset for discovering profiles of gene methylation in cancer with aberrant DNA methylation in the neoplastic genome and widespread hypermethylation in tumor suppressor genes. MSO and other oligonucleotide-based arrays have been applied successfully for analyses of single genes and have been useful in delineating and predicting tumor subgroups using clustering methods (Gitan et al., [2002] *Genome Res.* **12,** 158–164; Adorjan et al, [2002] *Nucleic Acid Res.* **30,** e21; Balog et al., [2002] *Anal. Biochem.* **309,** 301–310). Here we focus on design criteria important to the interrogation of multiple CpG sites across several genes.

Key Words: DNA methylation; epigenetics; cancer; oligonucleotide microarray; high-throughput.

1. Introduction

DNA methylation of CpG islands, the postreplicative addition of the methyl group to the cytosine within the CpG dinucleotide, is an epigenetic modification pivotal to chromatin remodeling that often results in transcriptional repression *(1,2)*. In cancer cells in which aberrant methylation is a hallmark involving hypermethylation of multiple tumor suppressor genes and oncogenes, this molecular flag is increasingly viewed as having diagnostic utility as a biomarker, and the abnormal methylation process itself is viewed as an area for pharmacological intervention *(2,3)*. Offering varying degrees of specificity, sensitivity, and reliability, a number of techniques are available to assess CpG

From: *Methods in Molecular Biology, vol. 287: Epigenetics Protocols*
Edited by: T. O. Tollefsbol © Humana Press Inc., Totowa, NJ

methylation at different molecular levels *(4)*. These include, and are not limited to, methylayion-specific polymerase chain reaction (MSP) and MethyLight for interrogating CpG sites along single genes *(5,6)*, combined bisulfite restriction analysis (COBRA) and methylation-specific single-nucleotide primer extension (MS-SNuPE) for single sites of multiple genes *(7,8)*, and genome-wide scanning and profiling techniques *(9–12)*.

The recently developed methylation-specific oligonucleotide (MSO) microarray is a gene-specific, multiplex hybridization approach that can examine methylation across several CpG sites of numerous genes simultaneously *(13,14)*. It is based on the bisulfite modification of DNA that deaminates all unmethylated cytosines to uracil but is unreactive toward the 5'methylcytosine *(15)*. In the subsequent polymerase chain reaction (PCR) amplication step, as the uracil is copied as thymine and the 5'methylcytosine becomes cytosine in the daughter strands, methylation information of the gene is converted to sequence differences and hence are discriminating for annealing and hybridization.

The general strategy for the MSO microarray procedure is outlined in **Fig. 1**. The microarray slide is prepared to contain oligonucleotide probes of both methylated (M) and unmethylated (U) alleles for the CpG sites of interest, arrayed in multiplicates. Typically we test a range of 100–250 M and U oligonucleotide probes per panel set. The wild-type genomic DNA for analyzing methylation is treated with sodium bisulfite, and the modified DNA is the template for amplifying the region of interest. To ensure unbiased amplification of both the methylated and unmethylated alleles in the next step, primers covering 200–300 bp over the region are designed such that they do not contain CpG dinucleotides. The amplified products of the genes and CpG sites for interrogation, called the targets, are then pooled, purified, labeled with the fluorescence dye, and hybridized onto the probe microarray panel. Accordingly, the DNA targets form duplexes with the M or U oligonucleotide probes in proportion to the amount of methylated and unmethylated alleles present in the target population.

The MSO microarray method is both qualitative and quantitative for analyzing DNA methylation, with unique advantages. First, being a bisulfite-based strategy, the examination of CpG sites along a gene is not limited only to sequences whose motifs are restricted, as in the cleavage-based approaches. It has the power of resolution to distinguish even single-nucleotide differences; therefore, a vastly larger number of sites can be specifically probed by this method, which requires only nanogram quantities of DNA. Second, after calibrations for the M and U nucleotide pairs, the MSO microarray can be mended for measuring methylation levels and does not require cohybridization of a reference sample. However, as this method is a hybridization approach, it is

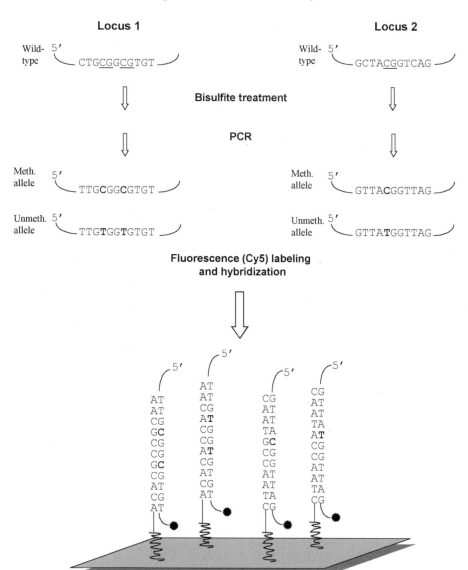

Fig. 1. Outline for the MSO microarray approach examining two loci. Briefly, the methylated and unmethylated alleles are equally amplified from a bisulfite-treated DNA template from primers flanking the sequence of analysis, labeled with fluorescent dye, and hybridized onto the slide that is arrayed with specially designed oligonucleotide probes distinguishing even single nucleotides.

somewhat hampered when one is interrogating CpG-dense sequences. Since it has been reported that the genes associated with transcriptionally repressive chromatins tend to be extensively methylated along the CpG island, one may focus primarily on less CpG-dense regions to determine the methylation status of genes *(16)*. For the study of cancer cells and tumors in conjunction with statistical analyses and a subgroup search algorithm, oligonucleotide-based microarrays have rapidly and reliably mapped the tumor suppressor gene *RASSF1A* in detail, have broadly classified and predicted human cancers *(13,17,18)*, and have established methylation patterns in cancer cell lines *(19)*.

2. Materials

1. Oligonucleotides representing the methylated and unmethylated alleles for arraying are synthesized with an amino-linked C6 ($NH_2[CH_2]_6$) attached to their 5' ends (IDT).
2. Microspotting solution (Telechem).
3. 96-Well plates.
4. Microarrayer.
5. Superaldehyde-coated glass slides (Telechem).
6. Water baths at 37°C, 50°C, and 95°C.
7. Sodium borohydride solution (prepared before use): 1.5 g NaBH4 in 450 mL phosphate-buffered saline (PBS) plus 133 mL 100% ethanol to reduce bubbling.
8. 0.2% Sodium dodecyl sulfate (SDS) solution.
9. Desiccated chamber.
10. CpGenome Kit (Serologicals).
11. Reagents for PCR amplification, e.g., AmpliTaq Gold (Applied Biosystems).
12. PCR purification kit (Qiagen).
13. Reagents for fluorescence dye labeling by terminal transferase, e.g., FluroLink Cy5-dCTP (Amersham).
14. Micro Bio-Spin P-30 Tris Spin Column (Bio-Rad).
15. UniHyb Solution (Telechem).
16. Cover slips.
17. Hybridization chamber (GeneMachines).
18. 2X SSC, 0.2% SDS solution (20X SSC: dissolve 175.3 g NaCl and 88.2 g Na citrate in water, adjust to pH 7.0 with NaOH, and bring volume to 1 L).
19. GenePix 4000A scanner and GenePix Pro software.

3. Methods

3.1. Principle for Designing MSO Probes

1. For the genes and CpG sites of interest, convert the DNA sequence information into methylated and unmethylated alleles. A program useful for this application is the CpG Ware from Serological (http://apps.serologicals.com/CPGWARE/dna_form2.html).
2. Obtain both the forward and reverse strands of these converted sequences, using another software program such as BioEdit.

3. Design oligonucleotide probes of 100% methylation and 100% unmethylation of the CpG sites of interest, examining up to three CpG sites.
4. Typically, we use the Oligo™ 6 software program to design the oligonucleotides with these guidelines:
   a. Probes are between 17–24 nucleotides long.
   b. The CpG site(s) interrogated is located preferably in the center of the probe.
   c. DNA sequences with four consecutive Ts, Gs, As, or Cs are not used.
   d. Oligonucleotides should have high melting temperatures (50–70°C).
   e. Probes forming hairpin loops or secondary structures are not used.
   f. If an optimal oligonucleotide pair for the forward strand cannot be found, the reverse strand can be used.
5. The methylated and unmethylated oligonucleotide pairs are sent off for synthesis with an amino-linked C6 attached to their 5' ends.

3.2. MSO Microarray Preparation

1. Prepare oligonucleotide stock solutions of the methylated and unmethylated alleles in 1 nmol/μL molecular-grade water and store at –20°C until use.
2. For printing as probes onto slides, suspend the oligonucleotides in 1X microspotting solution to a final concentration of 80 or 160 pmol/μL (*see* **Notes 1** and **2**).
3. Place the oligonucleotide suspensions into 96-well source plates and array in triplicate onto superaldehyde-coated glass slides (*see* **Notes 3** and **4**).
4. After printing, air-dry the slides in the desiccated chamber for at least 12 h before postprocessing.
5. For postprocessing, load the slides onto a slide carriage and rinse in 0.2% SDS and then water. Placing the slide carriage in a wash tank and rocking it back and forth is usually sufficient for rinsing and washing.
6. To denature any unreacted probe substrates, heat the slides in a 95°C water bath for 2 min.
7. To remove any free aldehydes, immerse the slides in freshly prepared sodium borohydride solution at room temperature for 5 min.
8. Rinse the slides three times in 0.2% SDS for 1 min each at room temperature.
9. Rinse the slides again one time in deionized water for 1 min at room temperature.
10. Dry the slides by centrifugation at 600 rpm for 5 min (65g on the microplate carrier T5-5.1-500 Rotor, Beckman Coulter TJ-25 Centrifuge).
11. After drying, store the slides in a desiccated chamber until use.

3.3. Target Preparation

1. Bisulfite-convert the genomic DNA using the CpGenome Kit according to the manufacturer's instructions.
2. A sample reaction mix to amplify the region of interest is as follows (*see* **Note 5**): 5 μL 10X PCR buffer, 4 μL 25 mM MgCl$_2$, 4 μL 10 mM dNTP, 0.5 μL 10 μM forward primer, 0.5 μL 10 μM reverse primer, 2 μL DNA template (0.02 μg/μL), 0.25 μL AmpliTaq Gold (Applied Biosystems), and 33.75 μL molecular-grade water, for a total volume of 50 μL.

3. The typical amplification program is (*see* **Note 6**):
   Step 1: Denature DNA at 95°C for 10 min → Step 2: 92°C for 1 min.
   Step 3: 50–60°C for 1 min → Step 4: 72°C for 1 min.
   Step 5: Go to Step 2 for 29 times → Step 6: 72°C for 5 min → Step 7: 4°C hold.
4. The PCR reaction mix is purified (Qiagen) and reconstituted in a 10 µL vol (*see* **Note 7**).
5. For any particular M and U oligonucleotide probe pair analyzing the CpG site(s) of interest, first test them for feasibility by hybridization over a range of methylation levels for calibrating a standard curve using controls (*see* **Note 8**).
6. Using the positive and negative controls, prepare four hybridization solutions of M and U samples at 0, 33, 66, and 100% methylation.
7. Label each of the four mixes for the standard curve with fluorescence dye as follows: 10 µL purified PCR products, 8 µL CoCl₂ (2.5 m*M*), 8 µL NEB4 buffer, 2 µL terminal transferase (20 U/µL), 1 µL Cy5-dCTP (25 nmol/25 µL), and 51 µL molecular-grade water for a total volume of 80 µL. Incubate the reaction at 37°C for 60–90 min.
8. Remove the unincorporated Cy5 dye from the targets by passing the reaction through a Micro Bio-Spin P-30 Tris Spin Column.
9. Vacuum-dry the labeled targets.
10. This labeling reaction is similarly used for control samples and the actual test samples.

3.4. Hybridization

1. Preheat the aluminum base of a hybridization chamber on a slide warmer.
2. Reconstitute the Cy5-labeled targets in 4 µL of molecular-grade water and mix thoroughly.
3. Add 16 µL of prewarmed UniHyb Solution to the target sample and mix gently to avoid forming bubbles.
4. Denature the target solution at 95°C for 2 min and quickly transfer to 50°C water bath to equilibrate.
5. With the MSO slide placed onto a prewarmed hybridization chamber, add 50–100 µL of 2X SSC to the channel underneath to retain humidity in the chamber during hybridization.
6. Pipet the denatured targets kept in the 50°C bath to the center of the arrayed area and gently place a cover slip over them, avoiding forming bubbles.
7. Secure the clear top plate of the hybridization chamber to the base plate, and place the whole assembly in the 50°C bath for 4–5 h.
8. After hybridization, remove the slides from the chamber and, to allow the cover slides to fall off, place the slides at a 60°-angle tilt in a wash tank containing 2X SSC, 0.2% SDS at room temperature.
9. Using the same wash solution that is now prewarmed to 50°C, wash the slide on a slide rack and tank for 15 min on the rocker.
10. Transfer the slide rack is to another wash tank containing 2X SSC and rock for another 5 min at room temperature.
11. To dry the slides, centrifuge at 65*g* (600 rpm) for 5 min.

3.5. Microarray Scanning and Data Analysis

1. Scan the slide with a GenePix 4000A scanner at a laser setting of 600 PMT.
2. Analyze the images acquired by the scanner with the software GenePix Pro 4.0.
3. For each sport on the image, determine the net signal by subtracting the local background from the mean average intensity.
4. Export the gpr file from GenePix software and compute further using Excel.
5. Before application to real test samples, assess each M and U oligonucleotide pair for its usefulness based on calibration of a regression curve. This is conducted by plotting the theoretical % methylation of the controls (i.e., 0, 33, 66, and 100%) vs the observed % methylation from signal intensities of the M and U spots. The observed % methylation is calculated by the equation: %methylation = [M/(M + U)] x 100% (*see* **Fig. 2** and **Note 9**).
6. The M and U oligonucleotide pair is satisfactory when the following criteria are met for the calibration:
   a. A difference of at least 40% in the observed methylation level (*y*-axis) between the 0% theoretical methylation and the 100% theoretical methylation (*x*-axis).
   b. A linear regression line with an R^2 value above 0.9.
   c. Signal intensities used to calculate the observed % methylation should be at least 30 U above the background value at each probe site.
7. Once standardization is established and deemed acceptable for a pair of MSO oligonucleotides, it becomes the calibration for the test samples (*see* **Note 10**).

4. Notes

1. The microspotting solution is quite viscous, requiring agitation and thorough mixing to disperse the probe solution evenly. This can be done by pipeting the solution up and down 10 or more times. This method of mixing is also required every time water is added back to replenish the arraying level in the original volume.
2. To evaluate probes giving varying weak and strong signal intensities owing to possibly different assay conditions and/or printing batches, the methylated and unmethylated oligonucleotide pairs can initially be spotted at more than one concentration.
3. To achieve reproducibility of the hybridization signals, the methylated and unmethylated oligonucleotide pairs of each CpG site interrogated are arrayed next to each other in a threefold redundancy. This also increases the likelihood of obtaining clean, undamaged signals.
4. The ambient humidity of the arraying chamber is of utmost importance for the spotted oligonucleotide probe solution to spread evenly, to give the best specific hybridization and removal of nonspecific targets during washes. Thus, humidity is monitored constantly and usually maintained at 65–70%.
5. The chemically altered DNA tends to be variously labile for amplification between samples and also the specific regions of interest. Therefore, the amount of template DNA in the PCR reaction might have to be adjusted to achieve good product yields.

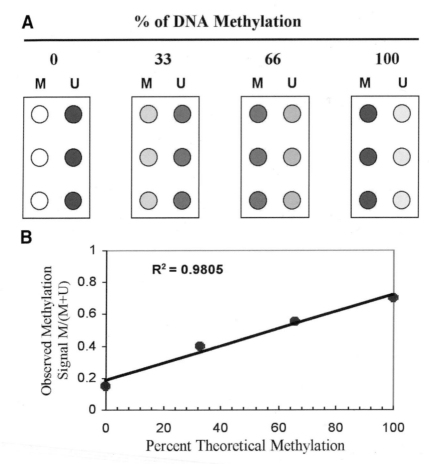

Fig. 2. A schematic example for hybridization and calibration curve for an M and U oligonucleotide pair using the MSO microarray. (**A**) Methylation controls are prepared and hybridized onto the MSO chip, giving a range of signal intensities in proportional to the amount of the M and U alleles in the target population. (**B**) Calibration curve for the specific M and U oligonucleotide pair. The signal intensity ratio (*y*-axis) of the detected methylation is plotted against the theoretical percent methylation (*x*-axis). A linear distribution would indicate that this particular pair of M and U oligonucleotide probes is effective and applicable for discriminating the M and U alleles in real test samples, providing the other criteria are met (*see* **Subheading 3.5., step 6**).

6. The precise PCR conditions will be different for the different primer sets and PCR systems used. Thus, the user will probably need to optimize the amplification programs accordingly (e.g., whether for single-primer annealing temperature, annealing over a gradient, nested PCR, or even the number of amplification cycles).

7. To attain high-throughput of the MSO technique, the many CpG sites and genes are interrogated all at once by combining target products from the PCR reactions

and processed further together. As crosshybridization between unmatched target and probes can sometimes occur, the MSO is not 100% efficient, and not all oligonucleotide pairs in the panel are applicable for data analysis of real samples. This is not a problem because when the spots are quantified and the standard curves calculated, the grossly crosshybridizing oligonucleotide pairs could be eliminated and rendered not applicable in the final analysis of the whole microarray panel.

8. DNA sources as positive control for 100% methylation may be genomic DNA treated with *Sss*I methylase (NEB), universally methylated DNA (Serologicals), or laboratory clones whose methylation status are known to be natively methylated for the gene. For the negative unmethylated control samples, materials such as DNA of white blood cells of the blood buffy coat or sperm DNA are suitable.

9. In principle, the observed methylation level, at which the regression curve crosses the y-axis for the 0% methylation, should be zero. The fact that it often is not is an indication of low levels of nonspecific binding probably caused by the lower melting temperature of the U probe. We have found from experience and validations from other methylation analyses that such an oligonucleotide pair is nevertheless effective for qualitative and quantitative assessments of methylation, given the criteria described in **Subheading 3.5., step 6** are met.

10. This protocol has the flexibility to increase research throughput by arraying oligonucleotide probes designed to interrogate the methylation patterns of multiple CG dinucleotides in many genes in the same panel. This multiplex format was tested in our laboratory in a panel containing 250 M and U probes spanning the promoter and the first exon regions of five genes (data not shown). The hybridization condition and the washing condition were not altered since the design criteria outlined in **Subheading 3.1., step 4** were followed in this larger panel. This study produced informative methylation data. We do notice, however, that as we included large numbers of amplified fragments in the hybridization pool, more nonspecific hybridization occurred, so that some probes did not meet the criteria in **Subheading 3.5., step 6**. An easy solution to this problem is to redesign the affected probes.

References

1. Bird, A. (2002) DNA methylation patterns and epigenetic memory. *Genes Dev.* **16**, 6–21.
2. Jones, P. A. and Baylin, S. B. (2002) The fundamental role of epigenetic events in cancer. *Nature Rev. Genet.* **3**, 415–428.
3. Plass, C. (2002) Cancer epigenomics. *Hum. Mol. Genet.* **11**, 2479–2488.
4. Mills, K. I. and Ramsahoye, B. H., eds. (2002) *Methods in Molecular Biology*, vol. 200: *DNA Methylation Protocols*. Humana, Totowa, NJ.
5. Herman, J. G., Graff, J. R., Myohanen, S., et al. (1996) Methylation-specific PCR: a novel PCR assay for methylation status of CpG islands. *Proc. Natl. Acad. Sci. USA* **93**, 9821–9826.

6. Eads, C. A., Danenberg, K. D., Kawakami, K., et al. (1999) CpG island hypermethylation in human colorectal tumors is not associated with DNA methyltransferase overexpression. *Cancer Res.* **59,** 2302–2306.

7. Xion, Z. and Laird, P. W. (1997) COBRA: a sensitive and quantitative DNA methylation assay. *Nucleic Acids Res.* **25,** 2532–2534.

8. Gonzalgo, M. L. and Jones, P. A. (1997). *Nucleic Acids Res.* **25,** 2529–2531.

9. Costello, J. F., Fruhwald, M. C., Smiraglia, D. J., *et al.* (2000) Aberrant CpG-island methylation has non-random and tumor-type specific patterns. *Nat. Genet.* **24,** 132–138.

10. Toyota, M., Ho, C., Ahuja, N., et al .(1999) Identification of differentially methylated sequences in colorectal cancer by methylated CpG island amplification. *Cancer Res.* **59,** 2307–2312.

11. Huang, T. H., Perry, M. R., and Laux, D. E. (1999) Methylation profiling of CpG island in human breast cancer cells. *Hum. Mol. Genet.* **8,** 450–470.

12. Yan, P. S., Chen, C. M., Shi, H., et al. (2001) Dissecting complex epigenetic alterations in breast cancer using CpG island microarray. *Cancer Res.* **61,** 8375–8380.

13. Gitan, R. S., Shi, H., Chen, C. M., et al. (2002) Methylation-specific oligonucleotide microarray: a new potential for high-throughput methylation. *Genome Res.* **12,** 158–164.

14. Shi, H., Maier, S., Nimmrich, I., et al. (2003) Oligonucleotide-based microarray for DNA methylation analysis: principles and applications. *J. Cell. Biochem.* **88,** 138–143.

15. Frommer, M., McDonald, L. E., Millar, D. S., et al. (1992) A genomic sequencing protocol that yields a positive display of 5-methylcytosine residues in individual DNA strands. *Proc. Natl. Acad. Sci. USA* **89,** 1827–1832.

16. Widschwendter, W. and Jones, P. A. (2002) DNA methylation and breast carcinogenesis. *Oncogene* **21,** 5462–5482.

17. Adorjan, P., Distler, J., Lipscher, E., et al. (2002) Tumor class prediction and discovery by microarray-based DNA methylation analysis. *Nucleic Acids Res.* **30,** e21.

18. Yan, P. S., Shi, H., Rahmatpanah, F., *et al.* (2003) Differential Distribution of DNA Methylation Within the RASSF1A CpG Island in Breast Cancer. *Cancer Res.* **63,** 6178–6186.

19. Balog, R. P., Ponce de Souza, Y. E., Tang, H. M., et al. (2002) Parallel assessment of CpG methylation by two-color hybridization with oligonucleotide arrays. *Anal. Biochem.* **309,** 301–310.

20

Methylation-Specific PCR *In Situ* Hybridization

Gerard J. Nuovo

Summary

Methylation-specific polymerase chain reaction (PCR) *in situ* hybridization, using paraffin-embedded, formalin-fixed tissues or formalin-fixed cell preparations, allows one to determine which specific cells have silencing of a given gene owing to hypermethylation of the promoter. Standard *in situ* hybridization, after conversion of nonmethylated bases, would not have sufficient sensitivity to detect the one or two copies of the promoter region of interest. The framework of the methodology is the same as solution-phase methylation-specific PCR. However, when working with intact tissue or cell preparations, adequate formalin fixation and protease digestion are essential for satisfactory results. Furthermore, since one often uses an oligoprobe, probe size (at least 40 bp), labeling method (3' end tailing), probe concentration, and posthybridization stringency conditions can all have an impact on the final results.

Key Words: PCR; *in situ* hybridization; hypermethylation; formalin; protease.

1. Introduction

It has been over 10 yr since the first peer-review paper described the polymerase chain reaction (PCR)-based amplification of DNA and RNA in intact tissue samples *(1,2)*. This breakthrough was driven by a drawback of *in situ* hybridization that continues to the present day—the inability to detect routinely 1 to a few copies of target in a given cell *(3,4)*. Indeed, the method was driven in its infancy by the pathogenesis of HIV-1 infection, marked by the integration of typically one provirus in a target cell, which can remain dormant for many years. Only PCR *in situ* hybridization was able to demonstrate that 30% of CD4 cells were infected by the provirus prior to clinical disease, which became the basis for aggressive antiretroviral therapy at the earliest possible time point of disease *(5–7)*.

Given the surge of interest in hypermethylation silencing of genes *(8–11)*, it is not surprising that PCR *in situ* hybridization would be used as a tool in this area. This is because hypermethylation-induced gene silencing typically

From: *Methods in Molecular Biology, vol. 287: Epigenetics Protocols*
Edited by: T. O. Tollefsbol © Humana Press Inc., Totowa, NJ

involves only one to two alleles per cell, which is too low for detection with standard *in situ* hybridization. With methylation-specific PCR *in situ* hybridization, one can amplify the DNA promoter region of interest by several hundred-fold using methylation-specific primers and then easily detect the product after *in situ* hybridization with the corresponding probe. The first use of methylation-specific PCR *in situ* hybridization in a peer-review format occurred in 1999, when it was demonstrated that, in cancers of the lung and cervix, hypermethylation-induced silencing of *p16* occurred routinely in squamous cell lesions but rarely in glandular lesions *(11)*. The methylation-specific PCR *in situ* hybridization method also allowed one to ascertain easily something that could not possibly have been known from solution-phase methylation-specific PCR. Specifically, in low-grade squamous cell dysplasias, only a variable percentage of the dysplastic squamous cells showed hypermethylation-induced silencing of *p16*, and these cells often did not have E6 or E7 human papillomavirus RNA; the latter is involved with Rb inactivation and thus involves the same pathway as *p16* *(11)*.

It has been my experience that most people who do solution-phase methylation-specific PCR have little experience working with tissue sections. This is unfortunate, as a good base in tissue-interpretative molecular methods, such as in situ hybridization or immunohistochemistry, is essential for achieving success with methylation-specific PCR *in situ* hybridization. Indeed, I would stress that one should learn basic *in situ* hybridization and immunohistochemistry before attempting to do methylation-specific PCR *in situ* hybridization.

Most of the major procedures with methylation-specific PCR *in situ* hybridization are the same as with the solution-phase counterpart. One can conceptualize each cell as a small Eppendorf tube in which thousands of individual PCR reactions are taking place. However, because one is working with intact tissues that are formalin-fixed and paraffin-embedded, or cell preparations, several other variables also become part of the major procedure list: this includes protease digestion, probe size, method of synthesis, probe concentration, and posthybridization stringency conditions.

2. Materials

1. Paraffin-embedded, formalin-fixed tissue or formalin-fixed cell preparation.
2. Xylene and 100% ethanol.
3. Pepsin solution (DAKO, Carpinteria, CA).
4. 1 M NaOH solution.
5. 3 M Sodium bisulfite and 10 mM hydroquinone solutions (Sigma, St. Louis, MO).
6. PCR reagents, including Ampligold (Applied Biosystems, Carpinteria, CA).
7. Thermal cycler.

8. Methylated and unmethylated specific primers and probes.
9. 3' End tailing probe labeling kit (biotin or digoxigenin; Enzo Biochemicals, Farmingdale, NY).
10. Probe dilution solution (Enzo Biochemicals).
11. Hot plate (95°C).
12. Stringency wash: 1 XSSC with 2% bovine serum albumin.
13. Alkaline phosphatase conjugate (either strepavidin or antidigoxigenin; Enzo Biochemicals).
14. Nitroblue tetrazolium/5-bromo-4-chloro-3-inodolyl phosphate (NBT/BCIP) chromogen solution (Enzo Biochemicals).
15. Counterstain (nuclear fast red).
16. Permount.

3. Methods

The methods described below outline (1) the preparation of the tissue for methylation-specific PCR *in situ* hybridization, (2) the PCR step, (3) the hybridization step, and (4) the detection step.

3.1. Preparation of the Sample for Methylation-Specific PCR In Situ *Hybridization*

Those who routinely perform *in situ* hybridization or immunohistochemistry can skip this section.

3.1.1. Removal of the Paraffin Wax

Deparaffinization is performed by placing the formalin-fixed, paraffin-embedded tissue in fresh xylene for 5 min, followed by incubation in 100% ethanol for 5 min, and then air drying.

3.1.2. Protease Digestion

Protease digestion is essential for successful methylation-specific PCR *in situ* hybridization, just as it is for standard *in situ* hybridization *(3,11,13)*. Formalin fixation creates protein–DNA crosslinks that sterically hinder access of the probe to the DNA target of interest. Protease digestion removes these crosslinks and thus permits the probe to hybridize to its complementary target. However, the protein-protein crosslinks induced by formalin-fixation are what keep the tissue morphologically intact, much like the scaffolding of a building. Too much protease digestion and the cell basically crumbles on itself; it then becomes impossible to determine what cell type it was originally. Thus, the goal is to digest in the protease for sufficient time to allow entry of the probe to the target but not for such a long a time as to destroy the skeletal support of the cell (*see* **Note 1**). Fortunately, most biopsies have been adequately fixed (for at least 4 h) in buffered formalin, allowing for a wide range of protease digestion times for successful methylation-specific PCR *in situ* hybridization. Pepsin digestion (2 mg/mL prepared by adding 9.5 mL sterile water to 0.5 mL 2 *N* HCl and 20 mg pepsin) for 20 min at room temperature will suffice for most biopsies. The pepsin can be removed by simply washing the slide in tap water for 1 min, followed by 100% ethanol for 1 min, and then air-drying. The pepsin can be stored at –20°C for 1 mo, thawed, and used immediately when ready.

3.1.3. Bisulfite Treatment

One follows the exact same protocol that would be used if performing methylation-specific solution-phase PCR. The one difference—of course—is that tissue or cells on slides are being used. This actually makes this step a bit easier, as one only needs to rinse the slides in tap water between the different steps. The protocol for sodium bisulfite treatment is as follows:

1. After protease digestion, incubate tissues in 0.2 *M* NaOH for 10 min at 37°C.
2. Prepare 50 µL of a 0.2 *M* NaOH solution to which is added 30 µL of a 10 m*M* hydroquinone solution and 500 µL of a 3 *M* sodium bisulfite solution. Add at least 25 mL to each tissue section, overlay with a polypropylene cover slip, and then incubate at 50°C for 15 h.
3. Rinse in tap water for 2 min, and then in 100% ethanol for 1 min, and air-dry.

3.2. The PCR Step

It has been well established that the sensitivity of PCR is highly dependent on the inhibition of competing, nonspecific DNA pathways. Specifically, primers can anneal to themselves (primer oligomerization) or to nonspecific DNA (mispriming), and each may serve as the initiation point of DNA synthesis during PCR *(2,14,15)*. Although these two pathways are nongeometric, compared with target-specific PCR amplification, they can quickly overwhelm the latter at the onset of PCR and reduce, or even eliminate, the target-specific PCR amplification pathway. The fact that the melting temperature (T_m) of primer oligomerization and mispriming is much lower than for target-specific annealing is the basis of hot-start PCR. By not allowing the DNA polymerase to be active until the temperature is at least 50°C, which is above the melting temperatures of primer oligomerization and mispriming, one ensures that the reaction will be optimal and that there will be robust target-specific amplification (*see* **Note 2**). The simplest way to achieve hot-start PCR is to withhold the DNA polymerase from the reaction mixture until the thermal cycler reaches 50°C. The other option is so-called chemical hot start, in which an anti-DNA polymerase antibody (AmpliTaq Gold) or other chemical (such as single-stranded DNA binding protein) is added that prevents polymerase activity until the temperature reaches 50°C, after which the chemical itself is deactivated *(2,14,15)*.

The hot-start maneuver is essential for successful methylation-specific PCR *in situ* hybridization. The anti-DNA polymerase method (e.g., AmpliGold) is perhaps the simplest way to do hot-start PCR. The cycling parameters are very similar with methylation-specific PCR *in situ* hybridization and solution-phase PCR: an initial denaturation for 3 min at 95°C, one cycle at 60°C for 1.5 min, and one cycle at 94°C for 45 s (*see* **Note 3**). In terms of the composition of the PCR mixture, besides the methylation-specific and unmethylation-specific primers (used at 20 µ*M*), the other reagents are the same as for solution-phase PCR, with two important exceptions. First, a higher concentration of magnesium is needed, perhaps reflecting sequestration on the glass slide or in the tissue. Second, one adds 2% bovine serum albumin, which blocks adsorption of the polymerase on the glass slide. The specific recipe is: 5 µL of the polymerase buffer, 9 µL 2.5 m*M* $MgCl_2$ solution, 8 µL of the dNTP solution (20 m*M* each of dATP, dCTP, dGTP, and dTTP), 1.6 µL of 2% bovine serum albumin, 3 µL of the two primers (20 µ*M* each), 21.4 µL of sterile water, and 2 µL of the DNA polymerase (AmpliGold). After 30 cycles, the tissue is ready for the hybridization step.

3.3. The Hybridization Step

It is important to stress that in situ hybridization is best done with a probe 80–120 bp in size. Probes larger than that have a difficult time accessing the target in the labyrinth of the DNA-protein complexes of the nucleus, and probes smaller than that do not have sufficient numbers of base pair matches to ensure hybridization during the poststringency wash step, which is essential if background is to be reduced to an acceptable level *(3)*. Furthermore, it should be noted that primer oligomerization does not appear to be operative under any conditions with *in situ* PCR *(3,15)*. One may theorize that this reflects the high concentration of protein inside a cell, as many proteins can inhibit primer-dimer formation during solution-phase PCR. Whatever the explanation, this allows one to use a probe that includes part or all of the region of the primers. This is very advantageous as it allows for a probe that is as long as possible. If at all possible, use a probe that is at least 40 bp in size, labeled by the 3' end tailing method (*see* **Note 4**). Use the probe at a concentration of 25 nmol/mL. The probe can be diluted in a commercially available solution that contains formamide, a salt solution, and dextran sulfate. Hybridization time should be 15 h at 37°C (*see* **Note 5**).

3.4. The Detection Step

After the hybridization step, one hopefully has the probe-target DNA tightly complexed in the nucleus (that is, where the promoter region of interest is located). Inevitably, there will also be target bound to nonspecific cellular targets, such as cell proteins and nucleic acids. The goal is to wash the slides in such a manner as to remove the latter while not allowing the probe-target complex to denature. With full-length probes (that is, 80–120 bp) this is easily achieved, as the T_m of the probe-target complex will be at least 25°C higher than for the nonspecific target complexes. The situation is much less advantageous for oligoprobes: for example, the differences in T_ms for a 20-mer bound to the target vs bound to cellular proteins may be only 10°C. Thus, the window of signal-to-background noise with small oligoprobes is narrow; one risks the situation where background is eliminated, but the signal is weak to nonexistent, even after PCR amplification. Start with a posthybridization wash using 1X SSC with 2% bovine serum albumin at 45°C for 10 min (*see* **Note 5**).

The last parts of the detection step are well known by anyone with experience using either immunohistochemistry or *in situ* hybridization. When using a biotin probe, one incubates the tissue in streptavidin-alkaline phosphatase for 20 min at 37°C followed by development in the chromogen NBT/BCIP for 1–3 h (*see* **Note 6**). It is recommended to monitor the reaction under the microscope before stopping it, by placing the slides in water to ascertain when the signal-to-background ratio is satisfactory.

After terminating the chromogen step, the slides should be rinsed in tap water for 1 min, placed in nuclear fast red for 1 min (this will stain the negative nuclei a light pink), and then coverslipped in Permount after 5-min incubations in 100% ethanol and xylene.

3.5. Final Comments

Methylation-specific PCR *in situ* hybridization has been used to document that the promoter of p16 is hypermethylated routinely in squamous cell cancers and their precursors in the cervix and lung but less commonly so in adenocarcinomas from these sites (**Fig. 1**) *(11)*. Furthermore, p16 hypermethylation has been documented as an event that can occur very early in the evolution of breast cancer, before any cytologic changes are evident (**Fig. 2**) *(12)*. Finally, methylation-specific PCR *in situ* hybridization showed that age-related hypermethylation of the 5' region of MLH1 in normal colonic mucosa is associated with microsattelite-unstable colorectal cancer development (**Fig. 2**) *(13)*. Clearly, these latter two observations raise the interesting question as to whether hypermethylation-induced gene silencing may occur prior to any cytologic or molecular event that is associated with oncogenesis; further work in this area using methylation-specific PCR *in situ* hybridization and other methodologies will surely provide interesting results.

4. Notes

1. For those with experience examining tissues under the microscope, especially in conjunction with immunohistochemistry or *in situ* hybridization, it is easy to rec-

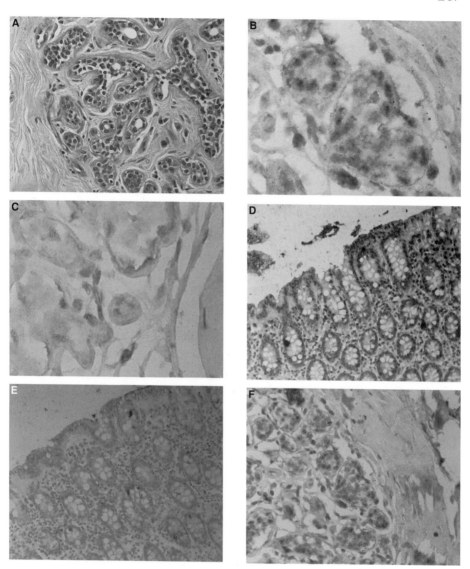

Fig. 1. Detection of hypermethylated p16 in lung and cervical neoplasms. Hypermethylated p16 was routinely detected in squamous cell carcinomas of the lung and cervix, but much less so in adenocarcinoma *(11)*. The results can be compared with p16 mRNA and protein detection. (**A**) Detection of p16 mRNA by RT *in situ* PCR in an adenocarcinoma of the lung; note the strong signal. (**B**) The area was negative for p16 hypermethylated DNA. (**C**) Similarly, p16 protein was detected by immunohistochemistry. (**D**) Histologic features of a dysplasia of the cervix that contained HPV 16 (not shown). (**E**) Many of the cells had hypermethylated p16 promoter. (**F**) the corresponding section on the same slide was negative for the nonmethylated promoter, which is an important negative control.

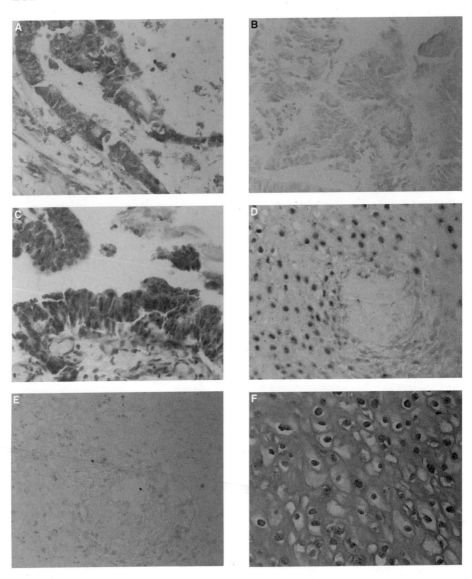

Fig. 2. Detection of hypermethylation in histologically unremarkable breast and colon tissues. (**A**) An area of normal breast tissue in a woman with no evidence of breast cancer. (**B** and **C**) A few histologically normal acini had hypermethylated p16 promoter. (**D**) One of the negative controls, showing the loss of signal with the omission of the DNA polymerase. (**E** and **F**) Similar results in histologically normal colon; note the signal for the hypermethylated MLH 1 promoter (E) and loss of signal using the nonmethylated primers/probe from the same region (F).

ognize over protease digestion. The nuclear and cytoplasmic detail is lost, and the more resistant cellular structures (such as the basement membranes) stand out (**Fig. 1**). For those with little experience, it is very helpful to take advantage of the counterstain nuclear fast red. After counterstaining for 1 min in a fresh solution of nuclear fast red, if one holds the slide up to the light a strong pink color should be evident. If the color is light pink to light blue, then most likely the protease digestion was too long. This is more problematic with certain types of tissues (for example, lymph nodes) and with tissues that have been fixed for less than 1 h. Tissues that are unfixed, or fixed in solutions that contain picric acid or a heavy metal, will usually not support successful methylation-specific PCR *in situ* hybridization *(3)*.

2. It is important to realize that there is one other nonspecific DNA synthesis pathway operative during *in situ* amplification. This is DNA repair, which is primer-independent. It operates much like nick translation for synthesizing DNA probes. Heating (during the paraffin-embedding process) causes nicks in the DNA. During the PCR step, the polymerase displaces the strand at the point of the DNA nick and synthesizes new DNA. This process is ubiquitous in paraffin-embedded tissues and precludes the direct incorporation of the labeled nucleotide for DNA targets *(3,15)*. It is of interest that one can eliminate the DNA repair pathway with overnight digestion in DNase, which is the cornerstone of reverse transcriptase (RT) *in situ* PCR *(3,5,8,11)*. The latter is actually simpler and quicker than PCR *in situ* hybridization for a DNA target, as the target-specific direct incorporation of the biotin- or digoxigenin-tagged nucleotide precludes the need for a hybridization step. Finally, one can use a labeled primer for methylation-specific PCR *in situ* hybridization and avoid the hybridization step. However, in my experience, they tend not to work as well compared with using a labeled probe after methylation-specific PCR *in situ* hybridization *(3)*. One exception may be the Sunrise fluorescence based system *(3–6)*.

3. There are two important technical tips regarding hot-start PCR *in situ* hybridization. First, it is very useful to use silane coated slides (PLUS slides) and for the technician to places two to three 4-μ sections per slide. This allows one to perform important negative controls (for example, omitting the polymerase) on the same slide in which the reaction is being done. Of course, three sections per slide also allows one to test methylation and no methylation on the same tissue sections on the same glass slide. Background signal is probably caused by the probe and *not* the PCR reaction; hence the most useful negative control is simply to omit the primers or polymerase. Second, there are several ways to keep the amplifying solution from drying out during the PCR process. One method is to use plastic covers and clips (Ampliclips, Applied Biosystems). Another is to cut polypropylene cover slips to size, anchor them to the slide with a small drop of superglue or nail polish, and place the slide in an aluminum boat, which is filled with mineral oil during cycling.

4. The correct probe concentration is best determined by trial and error using a sample known to have the target and another sample known not to contain the

target of interest. Start with an initial concentration of 100 n*M* and, with these two controls, determine what probe concentration yields a good signal with no to minimal background (*see* **Note 5**).

5. Background with *in situ* hybridization or methylation-specific PCR *in situ* hybridization is mostly likely caused by the probe *(3)*. When evident (either by positive nuclei in the tissue known not to have the target or in the sample in which either the polymerase or primer was excluded), first reduce the probe concentration to 1:10. If the background persists, then reduce the hybridization time by 50%. If it still persists, which is very unlikely, then increase the temperature of the stringent wash by 16°C. Another problem one may encounter is no signal. If this occurs, it is recommended that one use a consensus DNA probe (for example, against the repetitive *alu* sequence) to confirm that the fixative, protease, and detection arms of the assay are working properly. If a signal is generated with the *alu* probe, then redo the methylation-specific PCR *in situ* hybridization using a 10 times more concentrated probe with a doubling of the hybridization time.

6. There are many different chromogens to choose. The two most common in diagnostic pathology are diaminobenzidine and NBT/BCIP. Either will produce acceptable results; the former of course requires a peroxidase conjugate. The NBT/BCIP preparations commercially available from different companies behave very differently relative to signal and background. It is recommended to use the NBT/BCIP from Enzo Biochemicals at the manufacturer's recommended amounts.

Acknowledgments

The author would like to acknowledge the technical assistance of Ms. Maricella Suarez and the interesting and useful discussions regarding hypermethylation with Drs. Jim Herman, Steven Baylin, and Albert de la Chapelle. The financial support of the Lewis Foundation and MGN Labs is greatly appreciated.

References

1. Haase, A., Retzel, E., and Staskus, K. A. (1990) Amplification and detection of lentiviral DNA inside cells. *Proc. Natl. Acad. Sci. USA* **87,** 4971–4975.
2. Nuovo, G. J., Gorgone, G., MacConnell, P., and Goravic, P. (1992) *In situ* localization of human and viral cDNAs after PCR-amplification. *PCR Methods Applic.* **2,** 117–123.
3. Nuovo, G. J. (1996) *PCR* In Situ *Hybridization: Protocols and Applications*, 3rd ed. Raven, New York.
4. Nagai, N., Nuovo, G. J., Friedman, D., and Crum, C. P. (1987) Detection of papillomavirus nucleic acids in genital precancers with the *in situ* hybridization technique: a review. *Int. J. Gynecol. Pathol.* **6,** 366–379.

5. Bagasra, O. and Pomeranz, R. (1993) PCR in situ: intracellular amplification and detection of HIV-1 proviral DNA and other specific genes. *J. Immunol. Methods* **158,** 131–145.

6. Embretson, J., Ribas, J., Burke, A., and Haase, A. (1993). Analysis of HIV-1 infected tissues by amplification and in situ hybridization reveals latent and permissive infection at single cell resolution. *Proc. Natl. Acad. Sci. USA* **90,** 357–361.

7. Nuovo, G. J., Becker, J., Margiotta, M., Burke, M., Fuhrer, J., and Steigbigel, R. (1994) In situ detection of PCR-amplified HIV-1 nucleic acids in lymph nodes and peripheral blood in asymptomatic infection and advanced stage AIDS. *J. Acquired Immun. Def.* **7,** 916–923.

8. Issa, J., Ottaviano, Y., Celano, P., Hamilton, S., Davidson, N., and Baylin, S. (1994) Methylation of the estrogen receptor CpG islands links again and neoplasia in human colon. *Nature Genet.* **7,** 536–540.

9. Baylin, S., Herman, J., Graff, J., Vertino, P., and Issa, J. (1998) Alterations in DNA methylation: a fundamental aspect of neoplasia. *Adv. Cancer Res.* **72,** 141–196.

10. Nakagawa, H., Chadwick, R., Peltomaki, P., Plass, C., Nakamura, Y., and de la Chapelle, A. (2001) Loss of imprinting of the insulin-like growth factor II gene occurs by biallelic methylation in a core region of H19-associated CTCF-bidning sites in colorectal cancer. *Proc. Natl. Acad. Sci. USA* **98,** 591–596.

11. Nuovo, G. J., Baylin, S. B., Bolinsky, S., Herman, J. G., and Plaia, T. (1999) In situ detection of the hypermethylation-induced inactivation of the p16 gene as an early event in oncogenesis. *Proc. Natl. Acad. Sci. USA* **96,** 12754–12759.

12. Holst, C. R., Nuovo, G. J., Chew, K., Baylin, S., Herman, J. G., Cha, I., and Tlsty, T. (2003) Methylation of p16 (INK4a) promoters occurs in vivo in histologically normal human mammary epithelium. *Cancer Res.* **63,** 1596–1601.

13. Nakagawa, H., Nuovo, G. J., Zervos, E. E., Martin, E. W., Aaltonen, L. A., and delaChapelle, A. (2001) Age-related hypermethylation of MLH1 5' region in normal colonic mucosa is associated with microsatellite-unstable colorectal cancer development. *Cancer Res.* **61,** 6991–6995.

14. Chou, Q., Russell, M., Birch, D., and Bloch, W. (1992) Prevention of pre-PCR mispriming and primer dimerization improves low copy number amplification. *Nucleic Acid Res.* **20,** 1717–1723.

15. Nuovo, G. J., Gallery, F., Hom, R., MacConnell, P., and Bloch, W. (1993) Importance of different variables for optimizing in situ detection of PCR-amplified DNA. *PCR Method Applic.* **2,** 305–312.

16. Nuovo, G. J., Hohman, R. J., Nardone, G. A., and Nazarenko, I. A. (1993) In situ amplification using universal energy transfer labeled primers. *J. Histochem. Cytochem.* **47,** 273–279.

21

Relative Quantitation of DNA Methyltransferase mRNA by Real-Time RT-PCR Assay

John Attwood and Bruce Richardson

Summary

DNA methylation is one mechanism of epigenetic gene regulation and influences gene expression by recruiting methylcytosine-binding proteins and/or inducing changes in chromatin structure. In mammals, DNA methylation is mediated by at least four DNA methyltransferase (Dnmt) enzymes, including Dnmt1, Dnmt2, Dnmt3a, and Dnmt3b. To understand fully how DNA methylation is involved in gene regulation, knowledge of Dnmt mRNA transcript levels is required, both as a surrogate measure of Dnmt protein levels and also to facilitate an understanding of the regulation of expression of the corresponding genes. Measurement of transcript levels has traditionally been achieved by Northern blot analysis and more recently either by the ribonuclease protection assay or by reverse-transcription polymerase chain reaction (RT-PCR), followed by agarose gel electrophoresis. In the past few years, a form of PCR has been developed that measures the accumulation of PCR product in real time. In conjunction with RT, real-time RT-PCR has become a widely accepted tool for measuring mRNA transcript levels and is now probably the method of choice. This technique is both sensitive and specific and allows for the rapid assessment of Dnmt mRNA transcript levels as well transcripts for other genes that may be involved in DNA methylation.

Key Words: Epigenetic regulation; DNA methylation; CpG dinucleotide; DNA methyltransferase; Dnmt1; Dnmt2; Dnmt3a; Dnmt3b; real-time RT-PCR; mRNA transcript.

1. Introduction

In the past few years, there has been a remarkable expansion of interest in the epigenetic regulation of gene expression that includes changes in the methylation of genomic DNA. In higher eukaryotes, DNA methylation occurs at the 5' position of cytosine bases in the context of CpG dinucleotides and is catalyzed by DNA methyltransferases (Dnmts). To date, four Dnmts have been identified in humans and mice, namely, Dnmt1, Dnmt2, Dnmt3a, and Dnmt3b (1–3). DNA methylation influences gene expression during development and in somatic tissues. Aberrant DNA methylation in tumor cells may lead to

From: *Methods in Molecular Biology, vol. 287: Epigenetics Protocols*
Edited by: T. O. Tollefsbol © Humana Press Inc., Totowa, NJ

dysregulated gene expression. To understand the biology of these processes better, a knowledge of the activities of the various Dnmt's under these different circumstances is required. In addition, one needs to understand how the expression of Dnmts is regulated in various cells and tissues at the transcriptional or posttranscriptional level. This requires a reliable technique for analyzing the cellular levels of transcripts for each of the Dnmt genes.

Traditional techniques for measuring mRNA transcript levels include Northern blot analysis and the ribonuclease protection assay (RPA). Significant drawbacks with these techniques include the relatively large amount of RNA required, the use of radioactive probes, and the length of time taken to generate the probes and perform the assays. Following the development of the polymerase chain reaction (PCR), PCR has been applied to cDNA derived from RNA by reverse transcriptase (RT)-catalyzed reactions, a technique termed RT-PCR. RT-PCR can be performed either as a two-step procedure, with an initial RT step primed by random oligonucleotides followed by PCR using gene-specific primers, or as a one-step reaction with both the RT and polymerase together in the same tube in the presence of gene-specific primers.

Until recently, RT-PCR has relied on the analysis of products visualized following agarose gel electrophoresis. However, the ability to perform accurate quantitation (whether absolute or relative) by this method is poor, as the identification of the log linear phase of the PCR reaction, during which quantitative measurements of product can be made, requires multiple pilot experiments with differing numbers of PCR cycles. In fact, this may actually be impossible if there is a marked difference in the levels of the transcript of interest between the various samples, as the appropriate log linear phase may occur at quite different cycle numbers for different samples. More recently, real-time PCR techniques have been developed in which analysis of product at the end of each PCR cycle is achieved by the covalent or noncovalent incorporation of fluorescent markers or probes into the PCR product. In conjunction with software programs capable of analyzing the fluorescent data acquired in real time, this has permitted far more accurate absolute or relative quantitation of mRNA transcripts (**Fig. 1**).

A number of companies now supply real-time thermocyclers as well as appropriate one- and two-step real-time RT-PCR enzyme kits, allowing researchers to perform real-time RT-PCR experiments, often without the need for further optimization of the reaction conditions. However, because of the nature of the PCR reaction (a process of multiple rounds of amplification), any small differences in the quality or quantity of initial RNA or in the efficiency of the reaction may have quite significant effects on the measured outcome variable. One of the more important technical aspects of real-time RT-PCR experiments is therefore to reduce such potentially confounding issues.

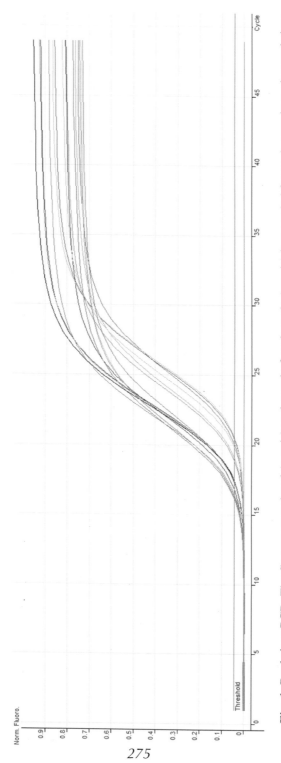

Fig. 1. Real-time PCR. The fluorescence level (y-axis) at the end of each cycle (x-axis) is recorded for each sample so that real-time changes in product concentration can be calculated. The upper horizontal "threshold" line is set by analytical software so as to determine the cycle number for each sample at which the sample fluorescence best reflects the initial transcript concentration. The lower horizontal line is the "no-RNA" negative control.

2. Materials

1. RNA isolation reagents: Trizol reagent (Invitrogen) or RNeasy Mini (also Midi and Maxi) Kit (Qiagen); RNase-free DNase (Qiagen).
2. RNA quantitation: Ultramicro quartz cuvettes (Fisher Scientific).
3. Primers: MacVector software (Accelrys) is used in our laboratory and has generated primer pair sequences used successfully by our group to measure human *(4)* and mouse *(5)* Dnmt1, -3a, and -3b. However, many primer design software programs are now available, including freely accessible on-line PCR design programs, freeware desktop programs, and commercial software. We have included examples of primer pair sequences for Dnmt1, -3a, and -3b, although these do not necessarily take into account the alternatively spliced isoforms that have been identified (**Table 1**).
4. Real-time thermocyclers: These are available from the following suppliers: Bio-Rad (iCycler iQ and MyiQ single-color Real-Time PCR Detection Systems); Cepheid (Smart Cycler II System); Corbett Research and Pyrosequencing (Rotor-Gene 3000); Idaho Technologies (R.A.P.I.D. System); MJ Research (DNA Engine Opticon and Opticon 2 Continuous Fluorescence Detection Systems); Applied Biosystems (ABI Prism 7000 and 7900HT and GeneAmp 5700 Sequence Detection Systems); Roche Applied Science (LightCycler and LightCycler 2.0 Instruments); and Stratagene (Mx3000P Real-Time and Mx4000 Multiplex Quantitative PCR Systems). We currently use the Rotor-Gene 3000 (*see* **Note 1**).
5. Kits for real-time PCR and/or RT-PCR: These are available from the following suppliers: Ambion, Applied Biosystems, Bio-Rad, EpiCentre, Eurogentec, Finnzymes, Genomics/Eurogentec, Invitrogen, Marligen Biosciences, MJ Research, Qiagen ,Roche Applied Science, Stratagene, and Takara.Mirus.Bio. Many of the real-time thermocycler vendors supply their own enzyme kits, as can be seen from this list. In addition, most of the kit suppliers identify the real-time thermocyclers with which their kits work for or which they have been optimized. We generally use the QuantiTect SYBR Green RT-PCR kit from Qiagen, which is designed for one-step RT-PCR and contains SYBR Green 1, a dye that fluoresces in the presence of double-stranded DNA. (For further information on PCR and RT-PCR kits, *see* **Note 2**.) The reverse transcriptase and polymerase enzymes should be maintained in a –20°C benchtop cooler when they are out of the freezer.

3. Methods

3.1. RNA Isolation

Both Trizol and the RNeasy kits are adequate for total RNA isolation (*see* **Note 3**). If removal of contaminating DNA is required, we isolate total RNA with the RNeasy kit that contains columns with RNA-binding silica gel-based membranes, and perform on-column DNA digestion using RNase-free DNase, also from Qiagen (*see* **Note 4**). Dissolve the purified RNA in nuclease-free water. In terms of positive controls, note that the Dnmts, especially Dnmt1, are

Table 1
Primer Pair Sequences (5' to 3') for Human and Mouse Dnmt1, Dnmt3a, and Dnmt3b

	Forward Primer	Reverse Primer
	Dnmt1:	
human	CGACTACATCAAAGGCAGCAACCTG	TGGAGTGGACTTGTGGGTGTTCTC
mouse	GGAAGGCTACCTGGCTAAAGTCAAG	ACTGAAAGGGTGTCACTGTCCGAC
	Dnmt3a:	
human	CGAGTCCAACCCTGTGATGATTG	GCTGGTCTTTGCCCTGCTTTATG
mouse	TGGAGAATGGCTGCTGTGTGAC	CACTCATCCCGTTTCCGTTTG
	Dnmt3b:	
human	TTGGAATAGGGGACCTCGTGTG	AGAGACCTCGGAGAACTTGCCATC
mouse	AGTGACCAGTCCTCAGACACGAAG	ATCAGAGCCATTCCCATCATCTAC

expressed ubiquitously in dividing cells but at significantly lower levels in most nondividing cells. For our work, we have found that Dnmt1, -3a, and -3b are detectable in both human and murine-activated T cells.

3.2. RNA Quantitation

Because small quantities of RNA may be isolated, using an ultramicro quartz cuvet with a chamber capacity of 50 µL ensures that as little as possible of the RNA is used for spectrophotometic quantitation. Adjust the final concentration of the RNA samples so that there is 100 ng (or whatever amount is used for each reaction) per 5 µL (*see* **Note 5**).

3.3. Primer Design

We use the commercial sequence analysis package MacVector (Accelrys) and have found this software adequate (*see* **Note 6**). Generally, for real-time RT-PCR, relatively short products of 75–200 bases work best. Primers can be synthesized in house or by commercial oligonucleotide synthesis vendors.

3.4. Real-Time RT-PCR

1. In the cold room, prepare a master mix that consists of a cocktail of all the necessary reaction components except for the RNA, and mix gently.
2. Transfer an appropriate volume of the master mix to each reaction tube or well.
3. Finally, add 100 ng (5 µL) of each RNA sample to the corresponding reaction tube or well (*see* **Note 7**).
4. Generate a standard curve by using known dilutions of a single RNA sample that has been identified in pilot experiments to have the highest concentration of the transcript of interest.

5. The fold of dilution will depend on the spread of concentrations of the transcript of interest in the various samples. For example, if there is approximately a 10-fold difference in RNA concentrations between the sample with the lowest amount of transcript and the one with the highest amount, then a standard curve generated from the sample found to contain the highest amount of transcript of interest and consisting of four twofold dilutions, i.e., 1X, 0.5X, 0.25X, 0.125X, and 0.0625X, will cover a 16-fold difference and therefore ensure that all samples lie within the standard curve. Note that *absolute* quantitation is rarely required and that *relative* quantitation suffices for most circumstances.

6. Run the RT-PCR in the appropriate real-time thermocycler following the protocol recommended by the RT-PCR kit vendor, including a final melting curve analysis step to confirm that a single product with identical melting curve characteristics is generated for each sample.

7. Samples should be saved and subjected to agarose gel electrophoresis to ensure that the anticipated product sizes are correct.

8. Additional confirmation of specificity may be obtained by the use of sequence-specific probes such as TaqMan or other dual-labeled probes.

3.5. Controls

To control for differences in RNA concentration, results may be normalized against levels of transcripts for housekeeping genes such as GAPDH, β-actin, and others. Because changes in levels of Dnmt transcripts occur with different stages of the cell cycle (**ref. 6** and our own unpublished observations), levels of histone H4 transcripts can be measured to determine whether there are differences in the cell cycle status between the different samples (*see* **Note 8**).

4. Notes

1. Choosing a real-time thermocycler. We have used the Light Cycler and more recently the Rotor-Gene 3000. Each thermocycler has its own advantages and disadvantages. For example, the design of the LightCycler and Rotor-Gene 3000 permits rapid temperature cycling, allowing multiple experiments to be performed on the same day. However, the LightCycler can only accept a maximum of 32 samples, whereas the Rotor-Gene 3000 is capable of up to 72 reactions, as well as incorporating a centrifugal design that provides temperature uniformity. Other thermocyclers such as the ABI Prism 7000, the iCycler, and the Mx3000P and Mx4000 systems are capable of performing up to 96 reactions simultaneously in a plate format. The ABI Prism 7900HT is designed for high throughput capable of processing 384 samples simultaneously. Finally, the ability to perform multiplex reactions using different fluoroprobes may vary between different thermocyclers depending on the nature and number of excitation sources and detection filters present in the thermocycler, as well as the versatility of the software.

2. PCR and RT-PCR kits. Options for real-time RT-PCR include a one-step kit, with both the RT and PCR components occurring in the same tube and with gene

specific primers in a real-time thermocycler, or a two-step kit, with an initial RT step usually with random primers, followed by real-time PCR with gene-specific primers. Although two-step RT-PCR tends to be more sensitive for detecting rare transcripts (*see* also **Note 5**), the sensitivity of one-step kits continues to improve. Because the reagents are available in commercial kit form, reaction conditions have usually been carefully optimized and are outlined in detail in the user manual that usually accompanies each of the kits. We have found this to be the case with a number of kits we have tried, and generally the user manuals are well written and helpful. In addition, many of the suppliers' websites contain reviews of real-time RT-PCR techniques as well as trouble-shooting tips. Therefore, we do not attempt to suggest any homemade approaches to determining experimental conditions for real-time RT-PCR, and we encourage researchers to read the accompanying user manual carefully and also to review the suppliers' websites for any additional useful information. Note, however, that each kit has not necessarily been optimized for all the real-time thermocyclers.

3. RNA isolation. For cells in culture, lysis is easily achievable by simply pipeting the loosened cell pellet up and down in whatever lysis buffer is used. For tissues, however, we usually homogenize in Trizol. We generally isolate total RNA and have found this to be suitable for real-time RT-PCR under most circumstances. However, when the RNA transcript of interest is present at low levels, isolation of mRNA rather than total RNA may improve sensitivity. Drawbacks with this approach include more expensive isolation kits, more difficult quantitation because of the much lower RNA concentrations, and the possibility that the relative levels of transcripts may change with mRNA isolation procedures because of differential recovery of different transcripts.

4. DNA contamination. In the absence of DNase treatment, most methods of isolating total RNA result in a small but significant amount of DNA contamination. DNA contamination is a potential problem primarily when the RNA transcript of interest is of low abundance, i.e., if the number of gene copies present in the contaminating DNA is approaching the magnitude of the number of cDNA copies of the relevant RNA transcript following reverse transcription. This may be the case with both Dnmt3a and Dnmt3b transcripts, as these are often present at relatively low copy numbers, whereas Dnmt1 is usually present at much higher copy numbers. The presence of DNA can be confirmed by performing RT-PCR and leaving out the RT enzyme. This is straightforward in the case of two-step RT-PCR, but for one-step RT-PCR this necessitates the RT being a separate component of the kit so as to be able to leave it out. Unfortunately, in some kits, both RT and polymerase are combined as an enzyme mix, which makes it impossible to leave out the RT selectively. There are two approaches for overcoming the problem of DNA contamination. First, the isolated RNA sample can be treated with RNase-free DNase. The most convenient way to perform this is by on-column treatment during isolation techniques that use columns containing silica gel-based membranes. Using Qiagen's RNase-free DNase for on-column treatment, we have found that although traces of DNA may

still be detectable by PCR, the level of contaminating DNA is usually sufficiently low so as not to interfere with the experimental results. An alternative, Ambion's DNA-free kit, contains a DNase Removal Reagent that itself can be removed from the RNA sample by a simple centrifugation step. This eliminates the need for heat treatment or phenol chloroform extraction to inactivate or remove the DNase, respectively. A second approach is to design primers that bind at either side of intron-exon boundaries and give rise to products of differing size, depending on whether they are generated from the gene or from the mature, processed mRNA transcript. However, this approach depends on knowing exactly where the intron-exon boundaries actually are. Furthermore, this can restrict the choice of primers and reduce the likelihood of primer design software generating suitable primer pair sequences.

5. RNA quantitation and concentration. Accurate quantitation of RNA is important, especially if normalization with housekeeping genes is not performed. This is usually straightforward provided the initial quality of the RNA sample is good, there is little contaminating DNA or protein, and the RNA concentration is not too low. One option for quantifying low-concentration RNA is to use the Agilent 2100 Bioanalyzer with the RNA 6000 Nano or Pico Lab Chip Kits (Agilent Technologies). An indication of comparable RNA concentrations in all the reaction tubes or wells during real-time RT-PCR can be obtained by comparing the fluorescence levels of the samples for the first few cycles of the PCR component of the experiment. This is because most of the fluorescence at that stage represents the weak binding of the SYBR green dye to the total RNA. We find that 100 ng of RNA per reaction generally works well, although lower concentrations may be possible provided the transcript of interest is present at sufficiently high levels. When transcript levels are very low, appropriate PCR product may be overwhelmed by unwanted primer dimer products, and increasing the amount of RNA per reaction or changing reaction conditions may not overcome the problem. Additional approaches to improving detection of low-level transcripts include performing a two-step RT-PCR rather than one-step RT-PCR in conjunction with RT kits designed for highly efficient reverse transcription such as the First-strand cDNA Synthesis System for Quantitative RT-PCR from Marlingen Biosciences. A second approach is to isolate mRNA rather than total RNA (*see* **Note 3**). Finally, it may also be necessary to redesign the primer pair sequences.

6. Primer design. Probably the most critical step in obtaining good-quality product is the initial design of suitable primer pair sequences. We believe that it is extremely difficult to design primers reliably without using one of the many primer design software tools now available. With the MacVector program, we have found that the primer pair sequences chosen by this software are usually suitable. Problems that may arise with poorly designed primers include early primer dimer-related product, as detected by melting curve analysis or by performing agarose gel electrophoresis on the real-time RT-PCR product. Although primer dimer product will eventually appear in the "no RNA" negative control with almost any primer

pair if a sufficient number of PCR cycles are performed, good primer design ensures that this will occur either not at all for whatever number of cycles are run, or else at a sufficiently high cycle number as to be unimportant. On the few occasions that a particular pair of primers does not seem to work well, we have found that a change in the reaction conditions such as altering the annealing temperature does little to improve the situation, and a new pair of primer sequences has to be redesigned. Occasionally, no primer pairs will be considered suitable by the primer design software, and in these instances, the best approach is to reduce gradually the stringency of the design parameter default settings determined by the software. We have found that it is best to avoid relaxing parameters that affect the likelihood of inappropriate primer interactions, but rather gradually to widen the acceptable percentage of C/G bases and/or the length of the predicted product until primer pairs are identified by the software. If all else fails, it is worth trying another primer design software suite. Another issue is that of splice variants, especially in the case of Dnmt3a and Dnmt3b *(7–10)*. The significance of these variants in different cell types and tissues remains largely unclear. However, when designing primers for the Dnmts, one needs at least to be familiar with the splice variants that have been reported in the literature and, unless specifically trying to determine levels of a particular splice variant, to try and design primers that are likely to detect most or all known variants.

7. Reproducibility. We usually prepare the experiment in the cold room. This ensures that pipets, pipet tips, kit reagents, and the RNA are all at about the same ambient temperature. Changes in temperature of the air within pipet tips during pipeting may lead to small but significant differences in the volumes pipeted. Ideally, RT-PCR should be performed at least in duplicate on each sample, and two or more further independent experiments should be performed under the conditions being examined. Occasionally, an aberrant result in one or more samples during a single experiment, especially owing to differences in PCR efficiency, as evidenced by differences in the slopes of the real-time curves, necessitates repeating the same experiment.

8. To normalize or not to normalize. Many researchers including ourselves control for RNA levels in their samples by normalizing with housekeeping genes such as GAPDH, β-actin, and others. The assumption is that levels of housekeeping genes do not change under the experimental conditions being examined. However, this is not always the case, and we and others have found, for example, that under the conditions of T-cell activation, levels of housekeeping genes may change. Accurate RNA quantitation may obviate the need for normalization, and in certain circumstances, we have dispensed with normalization of results using housekeeping transcript levels. However, because of the occasional very low levels of RNA in a sample, it may be difficult if not impossible to quantify the RNA accurately. Under these circumstances, normalization may be necessary, although newer techniques of quantifying RNA levels, using RNA-binding fluorescent dyes or the Agilent 2100 Bioanalyzer *(see* **Note 5**) may overcome this problem. In the case of Dnmt transcripts, an additional and important issue is how transcript lev-

els may change according to whether or not the cell has entered the cell cycle, and for cells in synchrony, at what stage of the cell cycle they are. This is especially important when comparing Dnmt levels in normal and cancer cell lines or tissues, as well as under conditions of signaling pathway inhibition, in which differences in cell cycle characteristics may be the primary explanation for any detectable differences in Dnmt levels. In addition to cell cycle analysis by flow cytometry, a simple method of determining whether cell or tissue samples differ in terms of their cell cycle characteristics is to assess histone H4 transcript levels, which are increased in cycling cells compared with cells in the G0 phase of the cell cycle *(6)*.

References

1. Bestor, T., Laudano, A., Mattaliano, R., and Ingram, V. (1988) Cloning and sequencing of a cDNA encoding DNA methyltransferase of mouse cells. The carboxyl-terminal domain of the mammalian enzymes is related to bacterial restriction methyltransferases. *J. Mol. Biol.* **203**, 971–983.
2. Xie, S., Wang, Z., Okano, M., Nogami, M., Li, Y., He, W. W., Okumura, K., and Li, E. (1999) Cloning, expression and chromosome locations of the human DNMT3 gene family. *Gene* **236**, 87–95.
3. Hermann, A., Schmitt, S., and Jeltsch, A. (2003) The human Dnmt2 has residual DNA-(cytosine-C5) methyltransferase activity. *J. Biol. Chem.* **278**, 31717–31721.
4. Zhang, Z., Deng, C., Lu, Q., and Richardson, B. (2002) Age-dependent DNA methylation changes in the ITGAL (CD11a) promoter. *Mech. Ageing Dev.* **123**, 1257–1268.
5. Yung, R., Ray, D., Eisenbraun, J. K., Deng, C., Attwood, J., Eisenbraun, M. D., Johnson, K., Miller, R. A., Hanash, S., and Richardson, B. (2001) Unexpected effects of a heterozygous dnmt1 null mutation on age-dependent DNA hypomethylation and autoimmunity. *J. Gerontol. A Biol. Sci. Med. Sci.* **56**, B268–276.
6. Lee, P. J., Washer, L. L., Law, D. J., Boland, C. R., Horon, I. L., and Feinberg, A. P. (1996) Limited up-regulation of DNA methyltransferase in human colon cancer reflecting increased cell proliferation. *Proc. Natl Acad. Sci. USA* **93**, 10366–10370.
7. Robertson, K. D., Uzvolgyi, E., Liang, G., Talmadge, C., Sumegi, J., Gonzales, F. A., and Jones, P. A. (1999) The human DNA methyltransferases (Dnmt's) 1, 3a and 3b: coordinate mRNA expression in normal tissues and overexpression in tumors. *Nucleic Acids Res.* **27**, 2291–2298.
8. Bonfils, C., Beaulieu, N., Chan, E., Cotton-Montpetit, J., and MacLeod, A. R. (2000) Characterization of the human DNA methyltransferase splice variant Dnmt1b. *J. Biol. Chem.* **275**, 10754–10760.
9. Weisenberger, D. J., Velicescu, M., Preciado-Lopez, M. A., Gonzales, F. A., Tsai, Y. C., Liang, G., and Jones, P. A. (2002) Identification and characterization of alternatively spliced variants of DNA methyltransferase 3a in mammalian cells. *Gene* **298**, 91–99.

10. Saito, Y., Kanai, Y., Sakamoto, M., Saito, H., Ishii, H., and Hirohashi, S. (2002) Overexpression of a splice variant of DNA methyltransferase 3b, DNMT3b4, associated with DNA hypomethylation on pericentromeric satellite regions during human hepatocarcinogenesis. *Proc. Natl Acad. Sci. USA* **99,** 10060–10065.

22

DMB (DNMT-Magnetic Beads) Assay

Measuring DNA Methyltransferase Activity In Vitro

Tomoki Yokochi and Keith D. Robertson

Summary

DNA methylation is an epigenetic modification of DNA that leads to heritable alterations in transcriptional regulation and conformational changes in chromatin structure of higher eukaryotes. Mammalian DNA methyltransferases, which are the enzymes responsible for DNA methylation, have attracted the attention of both basic and clinical researchers because they appear to participate in embryogenesis and carcinogenesis via chromatin modification. DNA methyltransferase catalyzes the transfer of a methyl group into DNA strands. Since traditional assays for DNA methyltransferase activity in vitro have insufficient reproducibility, there is a need in the art for more sensitive and quantitative methods for measuring enzymatic activity. We report a novel assay system, in which the activity of a DNA methyltransferase is measured as the incorporation of tritium into biotinylated DNA oligonucleotides. The DNA is immobilized onto magnetic beads with streptavidin covalently attached to the bead surface. The radioactive DNA can easily be separated from the unreacted radioactive substrate using a magnet. The radioactivity is counted by the liquid scintillation system. This DMB assay is simple and easy, has very low background, and, most importantly, is highly reproducible for the precise enzymatic analysis of any DNA methyltransferase *in vitro*.

Key Words: DNA methyltransferase; methylase; DNMT1; Dnmt3a; unmethylated DNA; hemimethylated DNA; magnetic beads; biotin; streptavidin; *S*-adenosyl-L-methionine; kinetics; enzymatic assay.

1. Introduction

The enzymatic activities of many DNA methyltransferases have been sufficiently robust to be detected by classical assays using a glass fiber or DEAE-cellulose filter sheet to trap the methylated substrate *(1,2)*. However, the main problem with these assays lies in the washing steps of the filters on which the radioactive DNA is captured for quantitation. Gentle washing of the filters yields a higher signal but also a higher background, whereas extensive wash-

From: *Methods in Molecular Biology, vol. 287: Epigenetics Protocols*
Edited by: T. O. Tollefsbol © Humana Press Inc., Totowa, NJ

ing may result in a lower background but also a lower signal. In any case, it is difficult to control the reproducibility of each enzymatic reaction; thus these assays could not be applied to the precise analysis of the enzymatic properties of a DNA methyltransferase having a slow reaction velocity, such as mammalian *de novo* DNA methyltransferase Dnmt3a *(3–6)*. Other techniques for the separation of radioactive substrates reported thus far utilize a solid matrix *(7)* or a biotin-coated microplate *(8)*; however, the preparation of materials for these assays is a time-consuming procedure.

To overcome these problems, we developed and optimized a novel assay system for the detection of methyltransferase activity, namely, the DMB (DNMT-magnetic beads) assay (**Fig. 1**). This assay is based on the affinity purification of biotinylated synthetic oligonucleotides of fixed length with a fixed amount of streptavidin-coated magnetic beads. The magnetic beads are pretreated with nonradiolabeled substrates to reduce the nonspecific binding, thereby yielding a very low background. Consequently, unreacted radioactive substrates can be washed out reproducibly from the DNA substrate after the methylation reaction. The protocol is very simple, easy, fast, and accurate. It also has low background in comparison with the traditional DNA methylase assays that use glass fiber filters. This assay was recently employed to analyze successfully the enzymatic kinetics of two mammalian DNA methyltransferases *(6)*.

In this report, we describe the step-by-step protocol of the DMB assay utilizing a mammalian maintenance DNA methyltransferase (DNMT1). A tritium-labeled methyl group is transferred from the methyl group donor, *S*-adenosyl-L-[^{3}H-*methyl*] methionine (AdoMet), to the position of 5-cytosine in CpG dinucleotides by DNMT1. Substrate specificity of DNMT1 is shown as the typical result of this assay (**Fig. 2**). DNMT1 showed a 20- to 25-fold preference for hemimethylated DNA substrates compared with unmethylated double-stranded DNA, whereas no methylation was detected using fully methylated double-stranded DNA controls.

2. Materials

2.1. Preparation of Recombinant DNA Methyltransferase

This is a brief protocol to purify recombinant mammalian DNA methyltransferases (DNMT1 and Dnmt3a) expressed in Sf9 cells utilizing a baculovirus system. If enzymes from other sources (e.g., bacterial methylases such as *Sss*I, M.*Eco*RI, *Hha*I, *dam*, and so on) are utilized, this section can be bypassed.

1. Pellet infected Sf9 cells and wash once with 1X phosphate-buffered saline (PBS). Sonicate the cell pellet in radioimmunoprecipitation (RIPA) buffer and centrifuge at 3000 rpm (~2000*g*) for 20 min. Save the supernatants as whole-cell extracts.

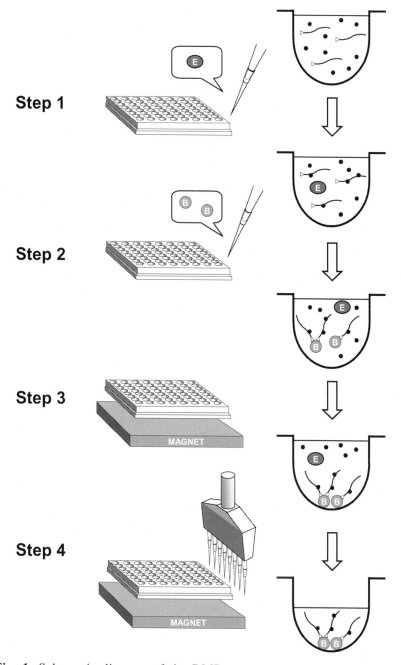

Fig. 1. Schematic diagram of the DMB assay protocol. Step 1, Add DNA methyltransferase (oval "E") to start enzymatic reactions. Step 2, After the reaction, add magnetic beads (gray circles "B") to immobilize biotinylated DNA fragments (curved lines). Step 3, Collect magnetic beads using a magnet. Step 4, Wash the magnetic beads to remove unreacted radioactive substrates (black circles).

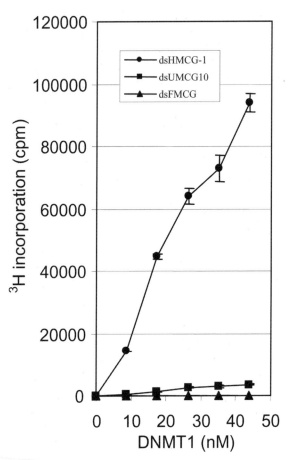

Fig. 2. Linearity of the methylation reaction as a function of enzyme concentration. Each reaction contains increasing amounts of DNMT1 (0, 8.8, 17.5, 26, 35, and 44 n*M*), 900 n*M* tritium-labeled AdoMet, and 125 n*M* double-stranded DNA. After incubation for 30 min at 37°C, tritium incorporation into DNA was assayed for DNA methyltransferase activity as described. DNA substrates utilized are as follows; hemimethylated DNA (dsHMCG-1, circles), unmethylated DNA (dsUMCG10, squares), and fully methylated DNA (dsFMCG, triangles). The mean values of independent duplicate experiments are plotted. The standard deviations are also shown as error bars.

2. Wash nickel-agarose resin once with 400 µL of Ni binding buffer, three times with 400 µL of Ni washing buffer 1, and then two times with 400 µL of Ni washing buffer 2. Elute His-tagged protein three times with 70 µL of Ni-elution buffer (total 210 µL) and pool. Snap-freeze aliquots in liquid nitrogen and store at –70°C until use. Protein solutions are allowed only one cycle of freeze-and-thaw to avoid a decrease in activity (*see* **Note 1**). The enzyme concentration is determined with the Protein Assay Kit (Bio-Rad).

2.2. Design and Preparation of the DNA Substrate

The DNA substrate for this assay must have a biotin molecule at one end. The DNA sequence should be designed to contain at least one recognition site for the DNA methyltransferase that will be employed (*see* **Note 2**). Double-stranded oligonucleotides are made by annealing two complementary single strands (*see* **Note 3**).

1. Mix equal volumes of two single-stranded DNA oligos that are adjusted to the same concentration.
2. Heat the mixture at 95°C for 5 min.
3. Cool down to room temperature gradually (1 h or more).

Typical synthetic DNA oligonucleotides we have utilized for mammalian CpG DNA methyltransferases are as follows:

1. dsUMCG10 (<u>d</u>ouble-<u>s</u>tranded, <u>u</u>n<u>m</u>ethylated DNA containing <u>10</u> <u>CpG</u> dinucleotides in each strand):

   ```
   5'-biotin-GAT CCG ACG ACG ACG CGC GCG CGA CGA CGA GAT C-3'
        3'-CTA GGC TGC TGC TGC GCG CGC GCT GCT GCT CTA G-5'
   ```
2. dsHMCG-1 (<u>d</u>ouble-<u>s</u>tranded, <u>h</u>emi<u>m</u>ethylated DNA containing 10 <u>CpG</u> dinucleotides in the top strand):

   ```
   5'-biotin-GAT CCG ACG ACG ACG CGC GCG CGA CGA CGA GAT C-3'
        3'-CTA GGM TGM TGM TGM GMG MGM GMT GMT GMT CTA G-5'
   ```
3. dsHMCG-2 (<u>d</u>ouble-<u>s</u>tranded, <u>h</u>emi<u>m</u>ethylated DNA containing 10 <u>CpG</u> dinucleotides in the bottom strand):

   ```
   5'-biotin-GAT CMG AMG AMG AMG MGM GMG MGA MGA MGA GAT C-3'
        3'-CTA GGC TGC TGC TGC GCG CGC GCT GCT GCT CTA G-5'
   ```
4. dsFMCG (<u>d</u>ouble-<u>s</u>tranded, <u>f</u>ully <u>m</u>ethylated DNA):

   ```
   5'-biotin-GAT CMG AMG AMG AMG MGM GMG MGA MGA MGA GAT C-3'
        3'-CTA GGM TGM TGM TGM GMG MGM GMT GMT GMT CTA G-5'
   ```

where M is 5-methylcytosine.

These double-stranded DNA oligonucleotides have 20 (dsUMCG10) or 10 (dsHMCG-1, dsHMCG-2) CpG dinucleotides that are acceptor sites for methylation. The dsFMCG has no unmethylated CpG dinucleotides and can be employed as a negative control. Both strands are carefully designed to anneal to each other correctly. They will have no self-annealing or irregular intermolecular annealing. For better reproducibility, a large amount of double-stranded DNA should be prepared at one time and stored in small aliquots until utilized.

2.3. Handling of Tritium-Labeled AdoMet

There are two points of caution when handling tritium-labeled AdoMet. First, it is a long-lived radioactive isotope. Second, in spite of the longevity of the radioactivity, the chemical structure of AdoMet is highly unstable and thus it will degrade easily. In some conditions, the half-life of the AdoMet is only 30 min in neutral pH, whereas the half-life of tritium is more than 12 yr.

S-adenosyl-L-[*methyl*-³H] methionine from Amersham Bioscience is supplied in dilute hydrochloric acid (pH 2.0–2.5). To minimize decomposition, AdoMet should be stored at –20°C. The manufacturer claims that storage at –70°C results in a higher rate of decomposition.

2.4. Preparation of Magnetic Beads

Magnetic beads should be washed before use to remove the preservative. TENT2M suspension of magnetic beads containing an excess of cold AdoMet is used not only for separation of biotinylated DNA oligos but also for terminating the reaction itself.

1. Put an appropriate amount (*see* **Note 4**) of Dynabeads M-280 (10 mg/mL) into a tube.
2. Place the tube in the Dynal MPC-S for a few seconds.
3. Remove the supernatant with a pipetman and then remove the tube from the magnet.
4. Add TENT2M to the same volume of the original suspension.
5. Shake vigorously and spin down with a microcentrifuge.
6. Place the tube in the magnet, remove the supernatant, and then remove the tube from the magnet.
7. Repeat **steps 4–6** (a total of three times).
8. Add an appropriate volume of TENT2M (*see* **Note 5**).
9. Add 1:10 vol of 100 mg/mL cold AdoMet (*see* **Note 6**) to the TENT2M-suspension.
10. Place on ice until ready to use (*see* **Note 7**).

2.5. Pretreatment of the Microtiterplate

To reduce the background, the microtiterplate should be pretreated with bovine serum albumin (BSA) (*see* **Note 8**).

1. Add 300 µL of BSA solution (10 mg/mL in water) to each well.
2. Incubate at room temperature for 15 min.
3. Discard the BSA solution just prior to adding the reaction solution.

2.6. Equipment

1. Scintillation counter: LS6000 Series Liquid Scintillation System (Beckman) or equivalent.
2. Magnetic beads and related products: 100 mg Dynabeads M-280 Streptavidin (Dynal, cat. no. 112.06), MPC-S magnetic particle concentrators (Dynal, cat. no. 120.20), MPC-96 magnet for 96-well plates (Dynal, cat. no. 120.05).
3. Microtiterplate: 96-well polypropylene plate, U-bottomed (VWR).
4. Multichannel pipetor: 8-channel, 30–300 µL (Eppendorf, cat. no. 2245120-1).

2.7. Reagents

For recombinant DNA methyltransferase preparation:

1. RIPA buffer: 1X PBS, 1% NP-40, 0.5% sodium deoxycholate, 0.1% sodium dodecyl sulfate (SDS), 10% glycerol, 0.5 mM phenylmethyl sulfonyl fluoride (PMSF), 5 µg/mL pepstatin A, 5 µg/mL antipain, 5 µg/mL chymostatin, 5 µg/mL leupeptin, 5 µg/mL aprotinin, 1 µg/mL E-64.
2. Ni binding buffer: 20 mM Tris-HCl, pH 8.0, 10% glycerol, 500 mM NaCl, 5 mM imidazole.
3. Ni washing buffer 1: 20 mM Tris-HCl, pH 8.0, 10% glycerol, 500 mM NaCl, 60 mM imidazole.
4. Ni washing buffer 2: 20 mM Tris-HCl, pH 8.0, 10% glycerol, 10 mM NaCl.
5. Ni elution buffer: 20 mM Tris-HCl, pH 8.0, 10% glycerol, 10 mM NaCl, 1 M imidazole.

For the methylation reaction:

6. DNA substrate: 5 µM dsHMCG-1, dissolved in 1X TE.
7. Tritium-labeled AdoMet: S-adenosyl-L-[*methyl*-^{3}H] methionine (Amersham Biosciences, cat. no. TRK581-1mCi) (*see* **Note 9**).
8. Enzyme: 1 µM DNMT1.
9. TENT2M: 20 mM Tris-HCl, pH 8.0, 2 mM EDTA, 0.01% Triton X-100, 2 M NaCl.
10. TENT1M: 10 mM Tris-HCl, pH 8.0, 1 mM EDTA, 0.005% Triton X-100, 1 M NaCl.
11. Cold (nonradioactive) AdoMet: 100 mg/mL (Sigma, cat. no. A7007), dissolved in water.
12. BSA: 10 mg/mL (Sigma, cat. no. A-2153), dissolved in water.
13. Liquid scintillation fluid: Ecoscint A (National Diagnostics, cat. no. LS-273).

3. Methods

3.1. The Methyl-Transfer Reaction

The methylation reaction protocol itself is straightforward. The reaction conditions are almost the same as traditional methylase assays using glass fiber filters. Biotinylated DNA oligonucleotides, however, are required as the substrate in the DMB assay. DNA, tritium-labeled AdoMet, and enzyme are incubated in the reaction buffer (*see* **Note 10**). The typical reaction condition (in final concentrations) is as follows:

1. Reaction buffer: 50 mM Tris-HCl, pH 8.0, 5 mM EDTA, 10% glycerol, 10 mM 2-mercaptoethanol, 0.5 mM PMSF.
2. DNA substrate: 125 nM dsHMCG-1.
3. Tritium-labeled AdoMet: 900 nM.
4. DNA methyltransferase: 30 nM DNMT1.

Reactions (in a total volume of 40 µL) are incubated for 30 min at 37°C (*see* **Note 11**) in a BSA-pretreated microtiterplate (*see* **Note 12**). The 2-mercaptoethanol and PMSF should be added just prior to use.

3.2. Separating and Washing the Magnetic Beads

Magnetic beads can be immobilized and washed on a magnet to remove the unreacted tritium donors.

1. After the reaction for 30 min, add 40 µL of magnetic beads (TENT2M suspension) (*see* **Note 13**).
2. Incubate for 15 min at room temperature using gentle rotation on a Nutator mixer or equivalent (*see* **Note 14**).
3. Separate magnetic beads, now coated with the biotinylated DNA fragment, using a Dynal MPC 96-well magnet. Leave the microtiterplate on the magnet for 1 min.
4. Remove the reaction solution with an 8-channel multipipettor (*see* **Note 15**).
5. Remove the microtiterplate from the magnet.
6. Add TENT1M with a single-channel pipettor and suspend the magnetic beads thoroughly (*see* **Note 16**).
7. Place the microtiterplate on the magnet. Leave the microtiterplate on the magnet for 5 min.
8. Remove supernatants with a multichannel pipettor (*see* **Note 17**).
9. Remove the microtiterplate from the magnet.
10. Repeat **steps 6–9** three more times (for a total of four cycles of washing).
11. Add 25 µL of TENT1M and suspend well.
12. Transfer the magnetic beads suspension into 10 mL of Ecoscint A in a scintillation vial.
13. Perform scintillation counting.

4. Notes

1. We found that snap freezing in liquid nitrogen did not affect the enzymatic activity. Purified DNMT1 is relatively stable and can be stored at −70°C for at least 3 mo. However, the activity of Dnmt3a was gradually lost at −70°C during 4 wk of storage after purification, probably because of the low salt concentration in the storage (elution) buffer. Since Dnmt3a is significantly more sensitive to salt in the reaction buffer, this storage condition was essential to obtain the maximum activity of Dnmt3a.
2. The DNA strand used as the substrate must have only one biotin molecule on one DNA molecule. If two single-stranded DNA oligos, each having a biotin molecule on one end, are annealed, the resulting double-stranded DNA will have two biotin molecules at both termini. This substrate acts as a "bridge" between two magnetic beads and causes significant aggregation of the beads-DNA complex. The unreacted AdoMet is difficult to remove from such a complex.
3. In most cases, we had a company synthesize the biotinylated DNA oligos; however, biotinylation of any DNA substrate can be carried out by following the product manual provided with the Dynabeads. Typically, synthetic DNA oligonucleotides (single-stranded) are adjusted to 10 µ*M*. Equal volumes of two complementary single-stranded DNA solutions (10 µ*M*) produce one double-stranded DNA solution (5 µ*M*).

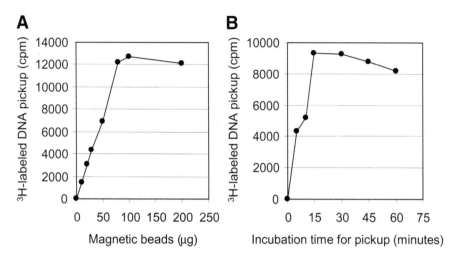

Fig. 3. Optimization of the conditions used to pick up the tritium-labeled DNA by magnetic beads. **(A)** Linearity of the pickup of radioactive DNA as a function of the dose of magnetic beads. Magnetic beads (0, 10, 20, 30, 50, 80, 100, and 200 µg) were incubated with a fixed amount (10 pmol) of radioactive DNA (dsUMCG10 methylated by DNMT1, 1200 cpm/pmol) for 15 min after the methyl-transfer reaction. **(B)** Time-course of the DNA binding to magnetic beads. Each reaction containing magnetic beads (100 µg) and radioactive DNA (10 pmol of dsUMCG10, 950 cpm/picomoles) was incubated at room temperature with gentle agitation. Incubations were terminated for analysis at 0, 5, 10, 15, 30, 45, and 60 min.

4. The manufacturer claims that 1 mg of Dynabeads will bind up to 200 pmol of biotinylated oligos (single-stranded DNA). However, the required amount of magnetic beads depends on the substrate (volume, structure, mole number, and length). In our experience, 1.6 mg of Dynabeads is required to pick up 200 pmol of our substrates (dsUMCG10 or dsHMCG-1) **(Fig. 3A)**. Thus, we decided to take 100 µg (10 µL of the original suspension) of Dynabeads for 10 pmol of our substrate as the standard (*see* **Note 18**). Further optimization, recommended by the manufacturer, may be required if longer oligos are utilized, since it lowers the binding capacity of the Dynabeads.

5. The manufacturer claims that 1 M NaCl (final concentration) is the optimal salt concentration for binding between biotin and streptavidin. TENT2M contains 2 M NaCl, so the volume of this magnetic bead suspension used will be the same as the volume of the reaction solution. That is, since the reaction volume is 40 µL (and contains no NaCl), the volume of the TENT2M-suspension will also be 40 µL (which contains 100 µg of magnetic beads) for each reaction, making the final NaCl concentration 1 M.

6. An excess amount of cold (nonradioactive) AdoMet is essential to reduce the background. This cold substrate is also expected to quench the reaction when it is

added to the reaction solution. To make a 100 mg/mL cold AdoMet stock solution, dissolve 100 mg of AdoMet in 1 mL of water. However, keep in mind that AdoMet is an extremely unstable compound. Do not make too much at one time. Make small aliquots and store them in a –20°C freezer.

7. Again, AdoMet is a highly unstable chemical. Keep it on ice.

8. The BSA solution must be freshly prepared, meaning that the BSA should be dissolved in water just before pretreatment of a microtiterplate. Use of an old BSA solution yields poor results, including low activity, lack of reproducibility, and inability to separate the magnetic beads. Bacteria or fungi can grow in BSA solutions and the microorganism's cell wall may have affinity for streptavidin or for DNA fragments.

9. The specific radioactivity of tritium-labeled AdoMet depends on each lot and manufacturer. When it is purchased from Amersham Bioscience (cat. no. TRK581-1mCi), the total radioactivity is 1 mCi/mL (37 MBq/mL). The specific radioactivity is usually 60–85 Ci/mmol, depending on the lot.

10. When this assay is attempted for the first time, the bacterial CpG methylase *SssI* (New England Biolabs, cat. no. M0226S) is a good choice as a positive control for the methylation reaction. Use of 0.5 μL of *SssI*, 125 nM dsUMCG10, and 900 nM AdoMet in a 40-μL reaction solution will yield 40,000–60,000 cpm. If necessary, negative controls can be done at the same time, such as "without enzyme," "without DNA," and "without AdoMet." They must be less than 100 cpm.

11. It is very important to set the temperature of the microtiterplate at 37°C as soon as possible. Here is a tip: always keep one metal heat block in a 37°C incubator. Place the microtiterplate on the preheated metal block to start the reaction. Without this "jump-start" on a heat block, enzymatic activity will be lower.

12. A 96-well microtiterplate is the best choice for this reaction scale. It should be noted that some microtiterplates are coated specifically to facilitate the adsorption of cells, antibodies, or proteins. They may or may not be compatible with this assay. A noncoated polypropylene microtiterplate is recommended. Do not forget the lid to prevent evaporation during incubation. A general lab adhesive tape, which is airtight and waterproof, can be utilized as a cover.

13. The manufacturer (Dynal) states, "The salt concentrations influence the efficiency of the binding of biotinylated DNA to Dynabeads-streptavidin. Extensive experience shows that for optimal binding, a salt concentration of 1 M is required in the binding buffer." Thus, the final salt concentration is adjusted to 1 M for binding. However, in our experience, the binding affinity of biotinylated DNA to magnetic beads did not change even when the final salt concentration was 2 M NaCl. Higher ionic strength may help to reduce the background.

14. An incubation time of 15 min is the manufacturer's recommendation. We tested several incubation times at this step and confirmed that 15 min is optimal (**Fig. 3B**). When incubated longer than 15 min, radioactive DNA oligos are gradually lost (*see* **Note 18**). The gentle rotation at this step is also essential. Without rotation, immobilizing ability is reduced. Tapping the microtiterplate for mixing is not recommended, since the reaction solution will splash on the underside of the lid and will be lost.

15. One should locate an adequate container in which to throw the radioactive liquid before starting this washing step. At this step, the researcher is handling a multi-channel pipetor containing a large amount of tritium liquid waste. These tips should not be discarded in a radioactive dry-waste box because the tritium liquid may splatter. The width of a multichannel pipetor may be wider than the standard opening of a radioactive liquid-waste tank. We recommend a large disposable weigh boat (14 × 14 × 2.5 cm) as a temporary liquid waste container.

16. The volume of TENT1M (washing solution) should be changed in each cycle of washing steps as follows:

    300 µL for the first washing.
    200 µL for the second washing.
    150 µL for the third washing.
    100 µL for the fourth washing.

    This washing procedure (four cycles with varied volumes of TENT1M) is necessary and sufficient to reduce the background. Although the manufacturer does not state this, 0.005% of Triton X-100 in all TENT solutions is essential. Without the detergent, the magnetic beads will repel water and make it difficult to remove the supernatant. On the other hand, 0.01% or above concentrations of Triton X-100 will make the reaction solution foam.

17. This is the most important step in the assay. Just 1 µL of the first reaction solution may contain over 100,000 counts (>100,000 cpm) of radioactivity. To reduce the background completely and ensure reproducibility, none of the high-count supernatant should be left over on the walls of the wells. Great attention has to be paid to avoid touching the wall of the well with tips of the multichannel pipetor. Less than 100 counts (<100 cpm) are considered background.

18. In addition to the optimization of the methyl-transfer reaction itself, the step of DNA binding to magnetic beads may require some preliminary experiments, mainly because of the use of different DNA substrates that depend on the sequence specificity of each methyltransferase. It should be noted that larger amounts of magnetic beads yield higher background by nonspecific binding of unreacted radioactive AdoMet, resulting in a significant decrease in reproducibility. Therefore, the linearity of the dose dependence and time-course of the DNA pickup efficiency by magnetic beads should be investigated for individual oligonucleotides. For 10 pmol of radioactive dsUMCG10, the pickup efficiency was maximized at 80–100 µg of magnetic beads and a 15-min incubation time (**Fig. 3**).

References

1. Reich, N. O. and Mashhoon, N. (1991) Kinetic mechanism of the *Eco*RI DNA methyltransferase. *Biochemistry* **30**, 2933–2939.
2. Pradhan, S., Bacolla, A., Wells, R. D., and Roberts, R. J. (1999) Recombinant human DNA (cytosine-5) methyltransferase. I. Expression, purification, and comparison of *de novo* and maintenance methylation. *J. Biol. Chem.* **274**, 33002–33010.

3. Okano, M., Bell, D. W., Haber, D. A., and Li, E. (1999) DNA methyltransferases Dnmt3a and Dnmt3b are essential for *de novo* methylation and mammalian development. *Cell* **99**, 247–257.

4. Lyko, F., Ramsahoye, B. H., Kashevsky, H., Tudor, M., Mastrangelo, M. A., Orr-Weaver, T. L., and Jaenisch, R. (1999) Mammalian (cytosine-5) methyltransferases cause genomic DNA methylation and lethality in *Drosophila*. *Nature Genet.* **23**, 363–366.

5. Gowher, H. and Jeltsch, A. (2001) Enzymatic properties of recombinant Dnmt3a DNA methyltransferase from mouse: the enzyme modifies DNA in a non-processive manner and also methylates non-CpG [correction of non-CpA] sites. *J. Mol. Biol.* **309**, 1201–1208.

6. Yokochi, T. and Robertson, K. D. (2002) Preferential methylation of unmethylated DNA by mammalian *de novo* DNA methyltransferase Dnmt3a. *J. Biol. Chem.* **277**, 11735–11745.

7. Hubscher, U., Pedrali-Noy, G., Knust-Kron, B., Doerfler, W., and Spadari, S. (1985) DNA methyltransferases: activity minigel analysis and determination with DNA covalently bound to a solid matrix. *Anal. Biochem.* **150**, 442–448.

8. Roth, M. and Jeltsch, A. (2000) Biotin-avidin microplate assay for the quantitative analysis of enzymatic methylation of DNA by DNA methyltransferases. *Biol. Chem.* **381**, 269–272.

Index

A

ADP–ribosylation, 137, 140–148
Aging, 2–8, 108, 121, 122, 129, 135, 176
Assay,
  chromatin, 2, 5, 9–11, 16, 45–53, 59–61, 75, 79, 83, 85, 99, 112, 113, 116, 120, 137, 140, 158, 273
  cross-linking, 249
  DNaseI hypersensitivity, 2, 5, 79–85
  DNA methyltransferase, 7, 260, 273, 287–296
  enzymatic, 137, 140–144, 287, 294, 296
  photocrosslinking oligonucleotide hybridization, 7, 233
  poly-ADP-ribosylation, 140–144
  methylation status, 193, 205, 234, 238, 249, 259
    quantitative determination of, 207
  RT-PCR, 94, 273–281

B

Biotin, 7, 123, 127, 140, 143, 144, 235–241, 263, 269, 287–296
Bisulfite,
  conversion, 171, 175, 176, 181, 197, 205–209, 220
  genomic sequencing, 169–179, 193, 204, 209
  modification, 67, 70–74, 170, 176, 181, 191, 207, 209, 219, 220, 226, 251, 252
  profiling, 169, 252
  sequencing, 6, 67, 70, 71, 169–179, 192, 193, 196, 204, 209
  single-strand conformation analysis, 6, 181

SNuPE, 6, 193–197, 200, 202, 205, 252
treatment, 6, 170–175, 181, 191, 193, 200, 207–209, 219, 225

C

Cancer,
  breast, 89, 95, 209, 260, 268
  cell lines, 89, 95, 254, 282
  clonal evolution, 208
  diagnostic, 233, 234, 251, 270
  human, 8, 89, 95, 96, 136, 169, 193, 234, 254, 260, 262, 270, 271, 282
  prostate, 89, 96
  tissues, 7, 181, 193, 262, 268, 271, 282
CDKN2A, 181, 193
ChIP,
  antibody, 13, 17, 27, 28, 32, 34, 41, 43, 48, 102–106, 111, 113, 117
  assay, 2, 4, 10, 11, 16, 112, 113, 205
  chromatin acetylation, 45
  elution buffer, 10, 14, 31, 32, 47, 49, 106, 112
  formaldehyde, 4, 9–12, 16, 18, 45–52, 101, 102
  histone acetylation, 2, 18, 43, 45, 51, 52, 99, 117, 158
  lysis buffer, 10–14, 28
  native, 2, 9, 18, 27, 31, 33, 39–43, 51, 99–104, 113
  nChIP, 2, 4, 9, 17, 18, 26–28, 31–34, 39–43
  Protein A, 10, 13, 14, 18, 27, 31, 32, 46, 106, 111, 112, 117
  Q-PCR, 4, 45–52
  technique, 2, 10, 18, 45–50, 258
  xChip, 4, 9, 10
ChIP-chip, 157, 158

Chromatin,
  acetylation, 1–5, 18, 27, 43–45, 51, 52,
    79, 86, 87, 93–96, 99–105, 116–
    119, 151, 158, 167
  active, 18, 19, 25–28, 34, 44, 80, 85, 86,
    139
    regions, 3, 42, 43, 53, 100, 103
  affinity purified antibody, 31
  deacetylation, 4, 5, 19, 87, 95, 96, 100,
    119, 167
  DNA analysis, 34
  DNaseI hypersensitivity analysis, 2
  histone methylation, 1–5, 99–102, 105,
    116, 118, 151, 167
  immunoprecipitation, 2, 8–13, 17–19,
    25–33, 39–48, 52, 99–102, 105,
    106, 111, 118, 119, 151, 158
  measuring changes, 65
  native, 2, 9, 15, 18, 25–33, 39–43, 51,
    99–105, 113, 118
  nucleosomal histones, 99
  open, 53, 57, 87
  remodeling, 2–5, 10, 60, 87, 95, 100,
    137, 151, 251
  structure, 2–5, 10–19, 44, 45, 53, 57–
    61, 65, 71, 79, 84–87, 95, 119,
    135–139, 148, 169, 195, 273
Chromosome,
  deletions, 159, 160, 249
  inversions, 159
  pericentric heterochromatin, 100, 119
  position effect, 121, 123, 127, 135
  telomere, 5, 121, 123, 127, 135, 163
  TPE (telomere position effect), 121
  X-chromosome,
    acetylation, 3, 100
    inactivation, 3, 100, 169
    methylation, 3, 100, 169
CpG,
  dinucleotide, 181, 207, 234, 251, 273
  doublets, 176
  island, 7, 86, 105, 219, 254, 260
  methylase, 192, 259, 294

  methylated, 6, 7, 65, 86, 175, 191, 193,
    196, 207, 209, 219, 231, 233, 237,
    253–260
  methylation,
    analyzing, 7, 181, 196, 252, 256
    detection, 52, 105, 192, 197, 205–
      208, 220, 225, 234, 271
    promoter regions, 234
    X-chromosome, 169
  unmethylated, 6, 7, 175, 176, 181, 191,
    192, 195–197, 207–209, 237,
    251–259, 289, 296
CpNpG, 65
Cross-linked, 18
Cytosine methylation, 4, 74, 75, 179, 195,
    196, 204, 207, 209, 224

D

Deletion, 132, 159, 162, 233, 234, 249
DHPLC, 195
DNA,
  coenzymic, 137, 139, 146
  Drosophila, 18, 61, 134, 148, 151, 162,
    163, 167, 168, 296
  domain, 4, 9, 26, 43, 118, 119, 145, 220,
    225–228
  heterochromatin, 3–5, 8, 26, 41, 42,
    100, 118, 119
  isolation, 16, 18, 25, 28, 43, 66, 67, 75,
    81–84, 172, 173, 207, 220, 228,
    231, 276, 279
  methylation,
    de novo, 3, 8, 295, 296
    detection, 52, 101, 117, 119, 151,
      179, 192, 197, 205–208, 220,
      224, 225, 234, 249, 262, 263, 267,
      270, 271
    hemimethylated, 3, 225, 288, 289
    hypermethylation, 3, 7, 169, 192,
      193, 251, 261, 262, 270, 271
    in situ hybridization, 7, 234, 249,
      261–263, 269–271

in vivo, 4, 5, 45, 52, 100, 119, 171, 271
sensitivity, 43, 118, 171, 178, 192, 193, 204, 234, 251, 261
transcriptional repression, 3, 52, 193, 207, 251
methyltransferase, 8, 167, 260, 273, 287–295
microarray, 2, 4, 7, 10, 157, 158, 167, 205, 251–260
quantitation, 56, 59, 61, 193, 205, 234, 273, 276, 279, 280
restriction, 2, 5, 53–61, 67, 70, 79–84, 107, 114, 121, 124, 129, 130, 170–173, 192, 196, 208, 224, 235, 237, 252
Southern blots, 34, 42, 56
unmethylated,
  cytosine, 176, 207–209, 296
  detection, 170, 192, 197, 207, 208, 263
  in vivo, 45, 171
  regions, 6, 45, 254, 257, 259
DNaseI, 80, 82
  hypersensitivity, 2, 5, 79–85
Drosophila, 18, 61, 134, 148, 151, 159–163, 166–168, 296

E

Epialleles, 151, 157–159, 168
Epigenetic,
  alteration, 75, 181
  consequences, 85
  expression, 1–7, 61, 65, 86, 87, 96–99, 158, 169, 195, 204, 233, 273
  inheritance, 1–3, 118, 151, 167
  imprinting, 3, 65, 167, 169, 204, 233
  microarray, 2, 4, 7, 157, 158, 167, 251, 259, 260
  modification, 2, 8, 137, 139, 159, 167, 181, 207, 209, 219, 233, 251
  phenomena, 53
  position effect, 61, 121

processes, 1–8, 53, 169, 259
quantitative, 2, 4, 45, 99, 151, 157–168, 193, 195, 207, 259, 260
regulation, 3, 61, 86, 87, 96, 99, 137, 139, 167, 169, 273
silencing, 5, 7, 65, 86, 119, 121, 167, 261

F

Formalin, 192, 261–263

G

Gene,
  deletion, 132, 233
  dosage, 7, 103, 115, 134, 233–245, 249
  duplication, 233
  expression, 1–7, 46, 61, 66, 74, 86–88, 93–96, 99, 100, 105, 115, 124, 132–135, 148, 158, 169, 195, 204, 233, 234, 273, 274, 282
  inactivation, 1, 3, 100, 119, 169, 193, 271
  promoter, 3–7, 39, 41, 53, 66, 80, 87, 88, 96, 123, 124, 128, 147, 148, 178, 193, 225, 226, 234, 259, 261, 282
  regulation, 3, 52, 61, 86–88, 94, 96, 99, 137, 139, 147, 148, 167, 169, 234, 273, 282
  silencing, 5, 7, 52, 86, 94, 119–123, 128, 133, 134, 167, 178, 196, 261
  transcription, 4, 8, 10, 43, 45, 52, 61, 80, 85–87, 134, 139, 140, 147, 169, 273, 279, 280
  unmethylated, 7, 45, 170, 171, 175, 176, 181, 195, 196, 204, 207, 209, 237, 251–254, 257, 259, 296
Globin,
  alpha, 28, 39–42, 118
  chicken, 26, 27, 39–44, 86, 118
  beta, 26, 27, 39–44, 118
  human, 44, 118

H

Healing, 121, 132
Heterochromatin,
  domains, 3, 100
  formation, 135
  methylation, 3–5, 8, 100, 118, 119
  pericentric, 100, 119
  regions, 3, 5, 42, 100, 118
High-throughput, 7, 193, 197, 207, 233,
    249, 251, 258, 260
Histone,
  acetylation, 1, 2, 5, 18, 27, 43, 51, 52,
    79, 86–88, 93–105, 116–119,
    151, 158, 161, 165, 167
  ADP–ribosylation, 137, 140–148
  antibodies, 17, 18, 28–32, 43, 47, 100,
    111, 116, 117
  core, 4, 18, 43, 51, 100, 118, 119
  deacetylase, 4, 84, 95, 96, 119, 128,
    136, 157
  H3, 4, 8, 17, 43, 47–51, 86, 94, 100,
    104, 105, 117–120, 140, 142,
    149, 167
  H4, 17, 18, 29, 30, 41, 43, 47–52, 93–
    97, 100, 104, 118, 119, 278, 282
  methylation, 1–5, 8, 43, 52, 79, 86, 96,
    99–105, 116–119, 151, 167, 195,
    282
  modification, 2, 4, 8, 17, 93, 102, 137,
    139, 142–146, 167
Hypersensitive, 5, 79–81, 84–86

I

Imprinting, 3, 65, 103, 105, 115, 167, 169,
    196, 204, 233, 234, 271
In situ hybridization, 7, 234, 249, 261–
    263, 269–271
Ion pair, 195, 205
ISH, 263, 267–271

K

Kinetic, 141, 295

M

Magnetic bead, 7, 123, 127, 234–237,
    241–243, 287, 290–294
Mammalian,
  cells, 7, 48, 74, 86, 100, 103, 121–123,
    129–135, 207, 240, 273, 282
  genes, 7, 8, 61, 74, 86, 100, 103, 119,
    123, 167, 168, 204, 207, 296
  model systems, 100, 134
  position effect, 61, 121, 123, 127–134
Mapping,
  analysis, 5, 6, 10, 27, 39, 151, 158, 170,
    178, 179, 193
  high–resolution, 10, 27
  DNaseI-hypersensitive sites, 79
  methylation sites, 170
  methylation, 5, 6, 52, 65, 70, 71, 75, 79,
    119, 151, 159, 178, 179, 193
Melting,
  map, 219, 225
  partial, 219, 228
  temperature, 34, 49, 219, 220, 225–228,
    259, 278
Methylation,
  conformation analysis, 6, 181, 193
  de novo, 3, 8, 295, 296
  histone, 1, 4, 5, 8, 43, 52, 79, 86, 96, 99–
    106, 116–119, 151, 159, 167,
    195, 282
  maintenance, 3, 169, 295
  microarray, 2, 4, 7, 167, 205, 251–260
  percentage, 6, 117, 201, 262
  promoter, 3–7, 66, 96, 178, 193, 225,
    226, 234, 259–262, 267, 268, 282
  X-chromosome, 3, 100, 169
Methylcytosine, 2, 65, 75, 169–171, 178,
    179, 204, 207, 208, 220, 251,
    252, 260, 273, 289
m5C, 65, 66, 70–73
Methyltransferase,
  adenine, 159, 167
  CpG, 7, 260, 273, 289, 296

Dnmt1, 3, 8, 273, 282, 288, 291, 293
Dnmt2, 3, 273, 282
Dnmt3a, 3, 8, 273, 296
Dnmt3b, 3, 8, 273, 296
  magnetic beads, 7, 290, 293, 295
  recombinant, 290, 295, 296
Microarray,
  ChIP-chip, 157, 158
  DamID, 157
  methylation-specific, 7, 205, 251–260
  oligonucleotide, 2, 7, 249–255, 258–260
Micrococcal nuclease,
  chromatin, 9, 17, 25, 44, 66
    changes, 2, 5, 65–75
    fractionated, 101
  digestion, 9, 25, 26, 44, 65–69, 74
  nChIP, 2, 9, 17, 26
  prepare nucleosomes using, 17
MS–SSCA, 6, 181, 191, 193
mRNA transcript, 273, 274, 280

N

NAD, 94, 137–146
Native chromatin immunoprecipitation, 25–33, 39–43
Nuclear enzyme, 137
Nucleosome,
  core region, 65, 69, 73
  destabilization, 87
  DNaseI hypersensitivity analysis, 2
  fragments, 28, 65, 72, 73, 79, 85, 101, 110, 118
  isolation, 28, 43, 66, 67, 75
  linker regions, 66, 70, 73
  methylation mapping, 65, 70, 71

O

Oligonucleotide,
  biotinylated, 7, 123, 127, 237, 239, 291, 292
  fluorescently labeled, 197

hybridization, 2, 7, 59, 197, 233, 234, 249–254, 257, 260
microarray, 2, 7, 251–260

P

PARP-1, 5, 137–149
PCR,
  allele-specific, 99, 105, 107, 114, 118, 120
  amplicon, 41, 42, 46, 49, 51
  bisulfite sequencing, 179
  ChIP assay, 4, 16, 45–51, 112
  efficiency, 16, 18, 49–51, 56, 59, 60, 72, 74, 112, 117, 171, 172, 175, 176, 208, 274, 281
  ligation-mediated, 53
  LM–PCR, 53–61
  lysis buffer, 12, 54, 58, 90, 279
  methylation-specific, 7, 193, 196, 205–208, 252, 255–263, 267–271
  MSP (methylation-specific PCR), 196, 197, 252
  MS–SSCA, 6, 191, 193
  purification kit, 172, 200, 254
  Q-PCR, 4, 45–52
  quantitative, 4, 6, 27, 34, 41, 45–52, 99–103, 107, 113, 179, 193, 197, 202, 205–208, 252, 259, 274, 276, 280
  real-time, 6, 7, 15, 32, 39–42, 52, 60, 61, 94, 103, 113, 197, 207–209, 273–281
  semiquantitative, 9, 12, 15, 17, 46, 67, 192
  SSCP–PCR, 108
  SSCP polymorphisms, 115
Photocrosslinking, 7, 233–235, 240–242
Poly-ADP-ribose, 144
Polypeptide posttranslational modification, 137
Position effect, 1, 6, 61, 121, 123, 127–134
Posttranslational modification, 2, 100, 137

Protease, 12, 14, 47–49, 270
  digestion, 25, 261–263, 269
  xChIP, 10

Q

Q-PCR, 4, 45–52
Quantitative,
  assessment, 46
    of methylation, 6, 208, 234, 237, 260
  methylation levels, 208, 252
    changes in, 207
  ChIP, 2, 4, 9, 12, 17, 27, 34, 41, 45–52,
    99, 101, 113, 157, 158, 197, 205,
    280
  DNA methylation analysis, 6, 193–197,
    205, 260
  epigenetics, 2, 6, 9, 45, 65, 99, 151,
    157–168, 181, 193, 195, 207
  inheritance, 2, 6, 151, 167
  manual quantitative PCR, 41
  PCR analysis, 41, 107, 113
  PCR–based SNuPE, 197
  Q-PCR, 4, 45–52
  RT-PCR, 274, 276, 280
  SNuPE, 6, 193–197, 202, 205, 252
  trait loci, 6, 151
  trait locus mapping, 158

R

Repression,
  inhibitor–induced gene repression, 94
  genes and chromosomal domains, 3,
    19, 52, 61, 75, 86, 94, 100, 121,
    133, 207, 251
  transcriptional, 3, 52, 66, 95, 100, 134,
    193, 207, 251
Restriction endonuclease, 54, 67, 79, 80,
    83, 107, 208, 221, 224
  accessibility, 2, 5, 53–60
Reverse-phase HPLC, 195, 197

S

Seeding, 121
Segregation of partly melted molecules,
    219, 220, 231

Sequencing
  bisulfite genomic, 169–179, 193
  bisulfite–converted DNA, 192, 196
  full-length cDNA clones, 162
  recessive lethality, testing for, 164
Silencing, 5, 7, 52, 65, 86, 94, 119–123,
    128, 133, 134, 167, 178, 196,
    261, 262
Single-strand conformation analysis, 6,
    181
SIRPH (SNuPe ion–pair reverse–phase
    high–performance   liquid
    chromatography), 195–205
SNuPE, 6, 193–197, 200–205, 252
SSCA, 6, 181, 191–193
Streptavidin, 7, 123, 127, 141, 144, 237,
    241, 243, 290, 293, 294
Subtelomeric, 121

T

Telomerase, 5, 87, 88, 95–97, 121, 128–
    133, 136
Telomere, 1, 5, 121, 123, 127, 128, 131–
    136, 163, 167
TIMP-3, 181, 191
Translocation, 5
Transcription,
  activation, 5, 52, 87, 94, 96, 147, 207
  local chromatin structure, 45
  control regions, 3
  factors, 3, 5, 8–10, 19, 87, 139
  inhibition, 86, 87, 93–96
  interference, 169
  repression, 3, 19, 52, 61, 66, 86, 94, 95,
    100, 134, 193, 207, 251
  start site, 80, 81
Transgene, 5, 121, 122, 133, 135, 167
Trans-modification, 139, 144, 145
Trichostatin A (TSA), 5, 87, 122
Truncation, 121–124, 128, 132, 133
Tumorigenesis, 2–5

V

Variegation, 61, 86, 121, 135, 167